THE PEGAN DIET COO

500+ TASTY AND WHOLESOME RECIPES THAT COMBINE PALEO AND VEGAN DIET TO EATING WELL, LOSE WEIGHT, AND FEELING VIBRANT.

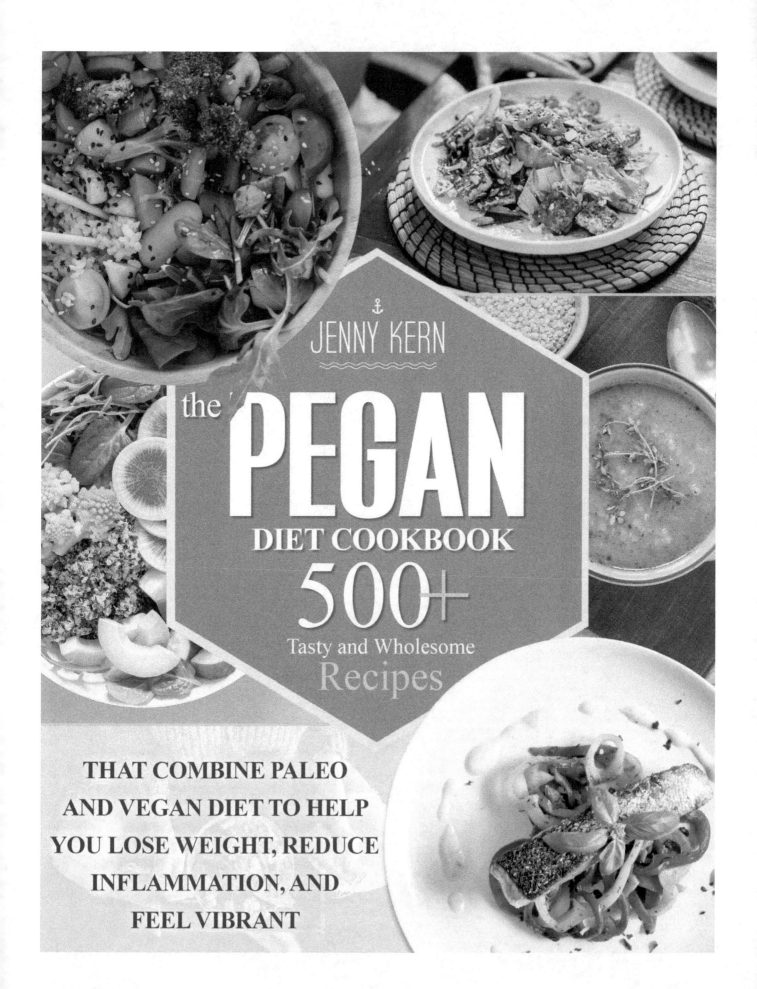

JENNY KERN

the PEGAN
DIET COOKBOOK
500+
Tasty and Wholesome
Recipes

THAT COMBINE PALEO
AND VEGAN DIET TO HELP
YOU LOSE WEIGHT, REDUCE
INFLAMMATION, AND
FEEL VIBRANT

Table of Contents

CHAPTER 10: DESSERT RECIPES 236

Introduction

Pegan Diet is a diet that's been proven to improve heart health, and also help combat diabetes. It's a diet that's been shown to be more effective than the Paleo Diet, and the Ketogenic Diet. The Pegan Diet is made up of 60% good carbs, 30% unrefined fat, and 10% lean protein for every meal.

The main ingredients are beans, potatoes, tomatoes, zucchini squash and spinach. You may also include cucumbers on occasion but no more than 5 times per week because it's high in sugar content. More importantly is the inclusion of lentils which are extremely high in fiber at 15 grams per cup cooked which has been shown to lower cholesterol levels by as much as 25%.

The Pegan Diet was created by Jimmy Moore and Tom Naughton who are both also part of the popular podcast "The Livin' La Vida Low-Carb Show". This diet was created from their experiences after being on the Paleo Diet and Ketogenic Diet.

Both Jimmy Moore and Tom Naughton had been on the Ketogenic Diet for over 5 years when they started to notice their own health deteriorating. They suffered from a feeling of being tired all the time, even when not doing any kind of physical work. They got aches and pains all over their joints, even while sitting in front of a computer screen all day long. Their hair started to fall out and they had a layer of fat that was starting to develop on their bellies.

Jimmy Moore was also diagnosed with a heart arrhythmia, which is known as atrial fibrillation. Jimmy Moore and Tom Naughton decided to ditch the Ketogenic Diet for good after this last event, along with the idea that it may be causing these conditions.

During this time, Jimmy Moore was already blogging about the Ketogenic Diet on his website called "Livin' La Vida Low-Carb". He has received a decent amount of popularity from this blog, especially when he wrote a book in 2010 called "Cholesterol Clarity".

He was due to write another book but the idea was to try something different. He created a stress-free and more balanced diet that would not leave them feeling like they were on a diet all the time. Jimmy Moore and Tom Naughton wanted to include carbs in their diet again so they could feel more energized throughout the day, as well as being able to have normal bowel movements without feeling like they have constipation all the time.

They also wanted to have a diet that would give them more energy in general throughout the day. Jimmy Moore and Tom Naughton wanted a diet that would address the issues of heart health, as well as diabetes, which they had both been diagnosed with. They also wanted a diet that wasn't so extreme on either end of the spectrum. They didn't want to do strict Paleo or Ketogenic Diet again because they had stopped feeling healthy after doing them for so long.

Some ideas for this new diet involved eating beans for protein but that was always met with resistance by Jimmy Moore's wife who said it would end up being just another fad diet. This was because in the past Jimmy Moore had tried to get her on the Ketogenic Diet, but she ended up not being able to handle it. She didn't like the feeling of not having any carbs in her body, although Jimmy was confident that the Pegan Diet would be different.

The Pegan Diet was created where 60% of your food is made up of carbs and they allow for more green vegetables than some other diets. The Pegan Diet also allows you to consume beans that have a variety of different nutrients including fiber and protein. The Pegan Diet is based on unrefined healthy fat as well as lean protein which are both important factors when it comes to heart health.

The Pegan Diet is similar to the Paleo Diet in that it does not allow refined carbs, processed foods or dairy products. It is also similar to the Ketogenic Diet in that it does not allow gluten or added sugars. The Pegan Diet is different from both of these diets because it allows for higher carbohydrate intake than either.

This is a recipe book that contains recipes which are all made from all-natural ingredients. Some of the recipes include a full day's worth of food while others only include one meal. There are 500 recipes in this Pegan Diet recipe book.

Other than the recipes, this book contains basic information about the Pegan Diet that every reader should know before starting the diet. This book also has information about the most common nutrients that are found in every single recipe and why they are important.

In this book, you'll find basic cooking instructions for every meal that includes a list of ingredients in each meal that will be needed to cook that particular meal.

This book is mainly focused on recipes while also providing some basic information about the Pegan Diet.

Chapter 1: What Pegan Diet is All About

What is Pegan Diet?

The Pegan Diet (a portmanteau of the words "paleo" and "vegan") is an eating regimen that combines the principles of a plant-based vegan diet with those of the Paleolithic diet.

Benefits of Paleo Diet

Here are some basic benefits of the Paleo Diet:

1. It is one of the clinically tested diets.
2. It gives a natural hunger suppressant action that controls your appetite.
3. The diet has been found to be very helpful in weight control and in keeping the weight from coming back after dieting is over. It also helps in preventing weight regain when calorie intake goes beyond the body's needs.
4. It makes your muscles more sensitive to insulin which reduces blood sugar level and keeps them from becoming resistant to this hormone, a major cause of diabetes mellitus type 2 cases in people who are overweight or obese.
5. The diet is rich in long-chain omega-3 acids which are major heart and neurologic system protectors that help in reducing the risk of cardiovascular disease, stroke, depression and Alzheimer's disease.
6. It helps maintain a healthy cholesterol level that reduces the chance of heart attack and stroke.
7. It contains an adequate amount of selenium and zinc which are vital for reproductive health, maintaining good immune function, and fighting cancer cells.

8. It has been found to control inflammation in the body which is one of the causes of chronic diseases like rheumatoid arthritis, asthma, inflammatory bowel disease, irritable bowel syndrome (IBS) and Crohn's disease.

Benefits of Vegan Diet:

Here are some of the basic benefits of the Vegan Diet:

1. It is rich in fiber which is necessary for digestive system health.
2. It has high amounts of phytonutrients that protect you from heart disease, cancer, and type 2 diabetes.
3. It is helpful in controlling blood pressure, cholesterol and other risk factors for heart disease and stroke.
4. It lowers your risk of developing some cancers and also helps in preventing overweight and obesity which are risk factors for cancer development and other diseases in the body.
5. It helps reduce the incidence of gallstones in women who are older than 40 years old. It also helps in reducing cholesterol and triglyceride levels in the body.
6. Vegan diets help regulate the blood sugar level and improve insulin sensitivity which reduces the risk of developing type 2 diabetes.
7. Vegan diets have high amounts of potassium, calcium, and magnesium which are essential for controlling high blood pressure or hypertension, a major risk factor for stroke, peripheral vascular disease (PVD), heart attack and kidney failure.
8. Vegan diets are rich in fiber, phytosterols, and phytoestrogens which all help reduce cholesterol levels in the body; thus, reducing risk factors for heart attack and stroke.

Foods to Eat on the Pegan Diet

The following are foods that are recommended on the Pegan Diet:

1. Cooked vegetables (any non-starchy variety)
2. Nuts and nut butters
3. Oily fish and other seafood (as a treat, not to be eaten too frequently)
4. Whole grains, legumes and beans in moderation (as a treat, not to be eaten too frequently)
5. Fruit in moderation
6. Olive oil as the main cooking oil
7. Turmeric
8. Raw foods (fruits, vegetables, nuts and seeds)
9. Spices, herbs and seasonings used sparingly
10. Water to drink in moderation (not to be drunk with meals)
11. Green tea to drink in moderation or not at all (not to be drunk with meals)
12. Wine and whiskey (optional, not to be drunk with meals)

Foods Not to Eat on the Pegan Diet:

1. Added sugars or sugary foods of any kind
2. Dairy products of any kind
3. Packaged processed foods of any kind
4. Oil used for cooking

5. Refined carbohydrates (white flour products, white rice, pasta)
6. Potatoes (unless they are home grown organic vegetables)
7. Processed salt and salty foods of any kind
8. Coffee of any kind
9. Any food or drink that contains artificial ingredients or preservatives of any kind
10. Any food that is fried in oil
11. Night shades (eggplant, tomato, potato, peppers)
12. Grains (wheat, corn, oats, rye)
13. Proteins (meat from animals: beef pork chicken goat lamb etc.) * *For vegans only

Chapter 2: Benefits of Pegan Diet

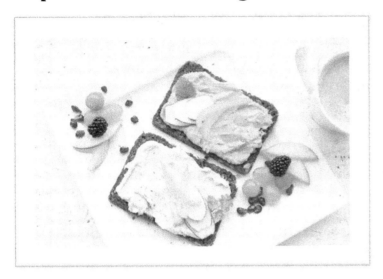

The benefits of Pegan Diet can be divided into three major groups: Disease Prevention, Weight Loss, and Brain and Gut Health. Let us talk in detail about each three major benefits of Pegan Diet:

Disease Prevention

Pegan Diet can prevent the following 12 diseases: high blood pressure, type 2 diabetes mellitus, stroke, heart attacks and other cardiovascular diseases, cancer, Alzheimer's disease, depression, Parkinson's disease, gallstones and gallbladder disease. How? Pegan Diet contains: plenty of fruits and vegetables, which are rich in fiber and antioxidants. Fiber can reduce the absorption of fat in the intestine, while antioxidants can prevent various diseases such as cancer.

Weight Loss

Pegan Diet includes about 50% of plant foods (fruits, vegetables and whole grains) that are low in calories but high in nutrition. The other 50% is rich proteins from plants, healthy fats from nuts, seeds, fish and seafoods and low-fat dairy products. In a word, Pegan Diet contains more nutrients rather than calories. Therefore, it will never make you obese or overweight because it has low calorie density (grams of calories per 100 grams).

Adopting Pegan Diet can help you to achieve an ideal weight without going through any kind of strict and hard dieting. This is because 1) Pegan Diet contains more fiber than any other diets. Fiber makes you feel full and satisfied so that you don't need to take a large portion of food. 2) Pegan Diet contains various plant foods from which you can select the ones that will be favorable to you. For example, if you like apples and oranges but dislike broccoli, you can easily make a choice. 3) Pegan Diet is designed to help you burn more calories than any other diets. This is because it contains both kinds of nutrients: fats and carbohydrates. When your body burns the nutrients for energy, it will produce heat. The larger the amount of nutrients, the more heat will be produced and in turn more calories will be burned.

Brain and Gut Health

Pegan Diet can provide your body with adequate nutrition for both brain and gut health.

The brains are made with 60% fats. Pegan Diet can improve your brain health in two ways: (1) it contains sufficient amount of omega 3 fatty acids, which are essential for the healthy function of the brain; (2) it includes nuts, seeds, legumes and whole grains which are excellent sources of vegetable protein and healthy fats.

Pegan Diet can improve your memory power and brain function generally; enhance gut health to promote healthy digestion and break down of undigested food in the intestines; reduce skin inflammation in acne patients; protect against eczema by stopping the chain of inflammatory reactions in skin cells. How does it improve your gut health? Pegan Diet contains two kinds of fiber: soluble fiber (found in fruits, vegetables, nuts and legumes, especially oats) and insoluble fiber (found in whole grains). Soluble fiber helps reduce the risk of diverticulosis and diverticulitis. Insoluble fiber reduces constipation.

Pegan Diet can reduce the risk of inflammatory bowel disease by reducing intestinal permeability; improve bowel movements and treat diarrhea; help to prevent colon cancer.

Pegan Diet can promote gastric ulcer healing; decrease the incidence of gallstones; cure itchy skin conditions like atopic dermatitis (eczema), urticaria (hives) and psoriasis.

Chapter 3: The 75 Percent Rule and How to Approach the Sugar

What is the 75% Rule?

The 75% Rule is a guideline used for the Pegan Diet that states that 75% of your meals should be made up of vegetables. Benefits: A diet high in vegetables has been shown to provide several health benefits including weight loss and lower blood pressure.

When Should You Apply the Rule?

The 75% Rule should be used for three weeks, then you may be able to gradually reduce the number of vegetables at a meal or eventually remove them altogether.

Prep Suggestions: Plan out your meals for the week and make sure each meal is aligned with the Pegan Diet, where you eat meat with vegetables.

Why Use the 75% Rule?

This guideline is set in place to help you feel satisfied, get all of your nutrients and vitamins, and have enough energy throughout the day to stay active. By eating mostly plant-based foods and limiting animal products, you will also find lasting weight loss results easier than if you were to try lowering calories alone.

How to Approach Sugar when in Pegan Diet?

Sugar is not necessarily unhealthy. The problem is that most people eat too much of it. Luckily, there are natural sugars in vegetables and fruits that you can enjoy on the Pegan Diet, along with other nutrients to keep your body feeling satisfied for hours.

In fact, those suffering from high blood sugar levels should enjoy more foods like sweet potatoes, carrots, and leafy greens (the green tops of broccoli and cauliflower). These have been shown to naturally balance blood sugar levels without the negative side effects of medication such as diabetes or increased risk for heart disease.

Sugar is a Recreational Drug

Think about how you feel when you indulge in sugar. Do you often find yourself overcome by a sudden burst of energy that quickly fades? Do your thoughts and behaviors change because of sugar? If so, sugar may be acting as a recreational drug for you. You may even become addicted to it! The chemical reactions and reward centers of our brains become accustomed to the effects of sugar on our bodies, so we seek it out again and again, even if we are already overweight or obese. The recommended limit for women is 100 calories per day (two small slices of cake) and 150 calories per day (one can of soda) from added sugars. The recommended limit for men is 150 calories per day (one can of soda) from added sugars.

How do you Use the Principle of Least Harm?

First, understand that the Pegan Diet is not exclusively vegan or vegetarian, but rather a fusion of the two. By following this approach, you will find that it is healthier than a regular meat-only diet and more sustainable than an all-vegan one.

The second step is to reduce your carbon footprint by cutting out processed foods and using organic meats, eggs, and produce whenever possible.

Peganism is the fusion of the Paleo and vegan diets. It's designed to provide maximum nutrition with minimum sacrifices. For example, a vegan may not eat fish or chicken because of their animal origin, while a Paleo dieter might not eat potatoes or winter squash. Peganism offers a solution for those like vegans who want to continue their current diet but still achieve similar health benefits as those on the Paleo diet.

Chapter 4: How to Get Started

If you are planning to start the Pegan Diet, here are the things that you should do and consider:

- Make sure to consult your doctor before starting any diet.
- Plan for this diet to be a permanent change in your lifestyle (even if you're looking for something that will help you lose weight).
- Try to keep your meals as varied as possible by choosing from the different Pegan food groups.
- Stay away from processed foods and fast food, and limit sugar as much as possible.
- If you need to lose some weight, make sure to eat the proper number of calories for your specific needs.
- Remember that this diet is meant for long-term consumption.
- Plan your meals properly, and take note of the amounts of food that you're eating by writing it down.

The Pegan Diet is a combination of two different diets - the Paleo diet and the Ketogenic diet - and it will require careful planning to ensure that it's balanced and healthy for your body. Here are some suggestions on how to get started:

- Eat plenty of lean proteins, vegetables, and fruits (at least 50% from each category). You should be consuming lean sources of protein that are low in fat. The meats that you should be getting should be lean cuts of beef, chicken, turkey, and pork. Seafood is also a great option for protein sources. Some examples of these are salmon, shrimp, tuna, and anchovies.
- Eat plenty of vegetables and fruits (50% each). Vegetables and fruits are important for getting the nutrients that your body needs to stay healthy. The vegetables that you should try to get are green leafy vegetables such as spinach or kale. Other great options include broccoli, bell pepper, tomatoes, onions, squash and cabbage. In terms of fruits: apples, cranberries, mangoes and strawberries are some good choices.
- Eat healthy fats (25%). Healthy fats are important for promoting body fat loss and keeping your body healthy. Healthy fats include: olive oil, avocado, nuts, fatty fish and seeds.
- Eat enough carbs (25%). Carbs are not the enemy in this diet - you just have to eat them in moderation to avoid gaining weight. Some good sources of carbs include beans, legumes, quinoa, oats, and whole grains like brown rice or whole wheat. You can also try using sweet potatoes as your source for carbs since they are full of vitamins and minerals.
- Take some time out to work out. This doesn't have to be a strenuous workout, but something simple like walking every day will do the trick. You should also consider taking up yoga or Pilates for added benefits in flexibility and strength.
- Don't forget to drink plenty of water. It's important that you keep yourself hydrated throughout the day with lots of water. This will ensure that you're getting enough nutrients, and it can help you stay full as well.
- Don't put your body under too much stress or pressure (no long workouts or too many heavy lifts).
- Avoid processed foods as much as possible - avoid anything that has more than five ingredients listed on its label.

Chapter 5: Breakfast Recipes

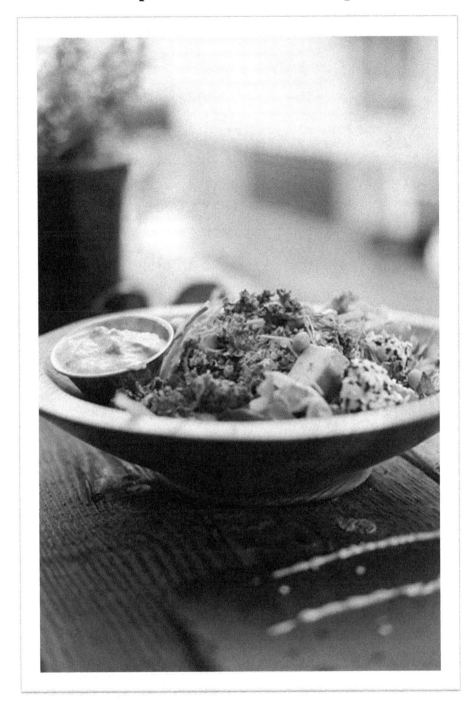

Green Breakfast Smoothie

Preparation Time: 10 minutes

Cooking time: 0 minutes

Servings: 2

Ingredients:

- 1/2 Banana, sliced
- 2 cups spinach
- 1 cup sliced berries of your choosing, fresh or frozen
- 1 orange, peeled and cut into segments
- 1 cup unsweetened nondairy milk
- 1 cup ice

Directions:

1. In a blender, combine all the ingredients.
2. Starting with the blender on low speed, begin blending the smoothie, gradually increasing blender speed until smooth. Serve immediately.

Nutrition:

Calories: 208;

Fat: 8g;

Protein: 14g;

Carbohydrates: 22g;

Fiber: 7g;

Sugar: 1g;

Sodium: 596mg

Warm Maple and Cinnamon Quinoa

Preparation Time: 5 minutes

Cooking time: 15 minutes

Servings: 4

Ingredients:

- 1 cup unsweetened nondairy milk
- 1 cup water
- 1 cup quinoa, rinsed
- 1 teaspoon cinnamon
- 1/4 cup chopped pecans
- 2 tablespoons pure maple syrup or agave

Directions:

1. Bring the almond milk, water, and quinoa to a boil. Lower the heat to medium-low and cover. Cook gently until the quinoa softens, about 15 minutes.
2. Turn off the heat and allow sitting, covered, for 5 minutes. Stir in the cinnamon, pecans, and syrup. Serve hot.

Nutrition:

Calories: 110;

Fat: 9g;

Protein: 15g;

Carbohydrates: 25g;

Fiber: 7g;

Sugar: 4g;

Sodium: 210mg

Blueberry and Chia Smoothie

Preparation Time: 10 minutes

Cooking time: 0 minutes

Servings: 2

Ingredients:

- 2 tablespoons chia seeds
- 2 cups unsweetened nondairy milk
- 2 cups blueberries, fresh or frozen
- 2 tablespoons pure maple syrup or agave
- 2 tablespoons cocoa powder

Directions:

1. Blend together the soaked chia seeds, almond milk, blueberries, maple syrup, and cocoa powder and blend until smooth. Serve immediately

Nutrition:

Calories: 100;

Fat: 18g;

Protein: 19g;

Carbohydrates: 20g;

Fiber: 9g;

Sugar: 4g;

Sodium: 500mg

Apple and Cinnamon Oatmeal

Preparation Time: 5 minutes

Cooking time: 15 minutes

Servings: 4

Ingredients:

- 1/4 cups apple cider
- 1 apple, peeled, cored, and chopped
- 2/3 cup rolled oats
- 1 teaspoon ground cinnamon

- 1 tablespoon pure maple syrup

Directions:

1. Take the apple cider to a boil over medium-high heat. Stir in the apple, oats, and cinnamon.

2. Bring the cereal to a boil and turn down heat to low. Simmer until the oatmeal thickens, 3 to 4 minutes. Spoon into two bowls and sweeten with maple syrup, if using. Serve hot.

Nutrition:

Calories: 110;

Fat: 9g;

Protein: 15g;

Carbohydrates: 25g;

Fiber: 7g;

Sugar: 4g;

Sodium: 210mg

Spiced Orange Breakfast Couscous

Preparation Time: 5 minutes

Cooking time: 15 minutes

Servings: 4

Ingredients:

- 3 cups orange juice
- 1.1/2 cups couscous
- 1 teaspoon ground cinnamon
- 1/4 teaspoon ground cloves
- 1/2 cup dried fruit
- 1/2 cup chopped almonds

Directions:

1. Take the orange juice to a boil. Add the couscous, cinnamon, and cloves and remove from heat. Shield the pan and allow sitting until the -couscous softens.

2. Fluff the couscous and stir in the dried fruit and nuts. Serve -immediately. Pecans and syrup. Serve hot.

Nutrition:

Calories: 110;

Fat: 9g;

Protein: 15g;

Carbohydrates: 25g;

Fiber: 7g;

Sugar: 4g;

Sodium: 210mg

Broiled Grapefruit with Cinnamon Pitas

Preparation Time: 5 minutes

Cooking time: 15 minutes

Servings: 4

Ingredients:

- 2 whole-wheat pitas cut into wedges
- 2 tablespoons coconut oil, melted
- 1 tablespoon ground cinnamon
- 2 tablespoons brown sugar
- 1 grapefruit, halved
- 2 tablespoons pure maple syrup or agave

Directions:

1. Preheat the oven to 375°F. Line a baking sheet with parchment paper.

2. Spread pita wedges in a single layer on a baking sheet and brush with melted coconut oil.

3. In a small bowl, combine the cinnamon and brown sugar and sprinkle over the pita wedges.

4. Bake in preheated oven until the wedges are crisp, about 8 minutes. Transfer the pita wedges to a plate and set aside.

5. Turn the oven to broil. Drip the maple syrup over the top of the grapefruit, if using. Broil until the syrup bubbles and begins to crystallize, 3 to 5 minutes. Serve immediately.

Nutrition:

Calories: 115;

Fat: 19g;

Protein: 25g;

Carbohydrates: 35g;

Fiber: 17g;

Sugar: 14g;

Sodium: 210mg

Breakfast Parfaits

Preparation Time: 5 minutes

Cooking time: 15 minutes

Servings: 4

Ingredients:

- One 14-ounce cans coconut milk, refrigerated overnight
- 1 cup granola
- 1/2 cup walnuts

- 1 cup sliced strawberries or other seasonal berries

Directions:

1. Pour off the canned coconut-milk liquid and retain the solids.

2. In two parfait glasses, layer the coconut-milk solids, granola, walnuts, and -strawberries. Serve immediately.

Nutrition:

Calories: 125;

Fat: 9g;

Protein: 15g;

Carbohydrates: 35g;

Fiber: 17g;

Sugar: 18g;

Sodium: 310mg

Orange French toast

Preparation Time: 5 minutes

Cooking time: 15 minutes

Servings: 4

Ingredients:

- 3 very ripe bananas
- 1 cup unsweetened nondairy milk
- Zest and juice of 1 orange
- 1 teaspoon ground cinnamon
- 1/4 teaspoon grated nutmeg
- 4 slices French bread
- 1 tablespoon coconut oil

Directions:

1. Blend the bananas, almond milk, orange juice and zest, cinnamon, and nutmeg and blend until smooth. Dip the bread in the mixture for 5 minutes on each side.

2. While the bread soaks, heat a griddle or sauté pan over medium-high heat. Melt the coconut oil in the pan and swirl to coat. Cook the bread slices until golden brown on both sides, about 5 minutes each. Serve immediately.

Nutrition:

Calories: 113;

Fat: 19g;

Protein: 25g;

Carbohydrates: 85g;

Fiber: 19g;

Sugar: 18g;

Sodium: 320mg

Pumpkin Pancakes

Preparation Time: 5 minutes

Cooking time: 15 minutes

Servings: 4

Ingredients:

- 2 cups unsweetened almond milk
- 1 teaspoon apple cider vinegar
- 2.1/2 cups whole-wheat flour
- 2 tablespoons baking powder
- 1/2 teaspoon baking soda
- 1 teaspoon sea salt
- 1 teaspoon pumpkin pie
- 1/2 cup canned pumpkin purée

- 1 cup water
- 1 tablespoon coconut oil

Directions:

1. Dip together the flour, baking powder, baking soda, salt and pumpkin pie spice.

2. In another large bowl, combine the almond milk mixture, pumpkin purée, and water, whisking to mix well.

3. Add the wet ingredients to the dry ingredients and fold together until the dry -ingredients are just moistened. You will still have a few streaks of flour in the bowl.

4. In a nonstick pan or griddle over medium-high heat, melt the coconut oil and swirl to coat. Pour the batter into the pan 1/4 cup at a time and cook until the pancakes are browned, about 5 minutes per side. Serve immediately.

Nutrition:

Calories: 113;

Fat: 19g;

Protein: 25g;

Carbohydrates: 85g;

Fiber: 19g;

Sugar: 18g;

Sodium: 320mg

Sweet Potato and Kale Hash

Preparation Time: 10 minutes

Cooking time: 15 minutes

Servings: 2

Ingredients:

- 1 sweet potato
- 2 tablespoons olive oil
- 1/2 onion, chopped
- 1 carrot, peeled and chopped
- 2 garlic cloves, minced
- 1/2 teaspoon dried thyme
- 1 cup chopped kale
- Sea salt
- Freshly ground black pepper

Directions:

1. Pierce the sweet potato and microwave on high until soft, about 5 minutes. Remove from the microwave and cut into 1/4-inch cubes.

2. In a large nonstick sauté pan, heat the olive oil over medium-high heat. Add the onion and carrot and cook until softened, about 5 minutes. Attach the garlic and thyme until the garlic is fragrant, about 30 seconds.

3. Add the sweet potatoes and cook until the potatoes begin to brown, about 7 -minutes. Add the kale and cook just until it wilts, 1 to 2 minutes. Season with salt and pepper. Serve immediately.

Nutrition:

Calories: 125;

Fat: 9g;

Protein: 15g;

Carbohydrates: 35g;

Fiber: 17g;

Sugar: 18g;

Sodium: 310mg

Savory Oatmeal Porridge

Preparation Time: 5 minutes

Cooking time: 20 minutes

Servings: 4

Ingredients:

- 2 1/2 cups vegetable broth
- 2 1/2 cups milk
- 1/2 cup steel-cut oats
- 1 tablespoon faro
- 1/2   cup slivered almonds
- 1/4 cup nutritional yeast
- 2 cups old-fashioned rolled oats
- 1/2 teaspoon salt (optional)

Directions:

1. Take the broth and almond milk to a boil. Add the oats, faro, almond slivers, and nutritional yeast. Cook over medium-high heat for 20 minutes, stirring occasionally.

2. Add the rolled oats and cook for another 5 minutes, until creamy. Stir in the salt (if using).

3. Divide into 4 single-serving containers. Let cool before sealing the lids.

Nutrition:

Calories: 152;

Fat: 16g;

Protein: 35g;

Carbohydrates: 55g;

Fiber: 25g;

Sugar: 18g;

Sodium: 245mg

Pumpkin Steel-Cut Oats

Preparation Time: 15 minutes

Cooking time: 25 minutes

Servings: 4

Ingredients:

- 3 cups water
- 1 cup steel-cut oats
- 1/2 cup canned pumpkin purée
- 1/4 cup pumpkin seeds (pipits)
- 2 tablespoons maple syrup
- Pinch salt

Directions:

1. Whip and reduce the heat to low. Simmer until the oats are soft, 20 to 30 minutes, continuing to stir occasionally.

2. Stir in the pumpkin purée and continue cooking on low for 3 to 5 minutes longer. Stir in the pumpkin seeds and maple syrup, and season with the salt.

3. Divide the oatmeal into 4 single-serving containers. Let cool before sealing the lids.

Nutrition:

Calories: 132;

Fat: 19;

Protein: 4535g;

Carbohydrates: 75g;

Fiber: 73; g

Sugar: 15; g

Sodium: 345mg

Cinnamon and Spice Overnight Oats

Preparation Time: 15 minutes

Cooking time: 20 minutes

Servings: 3

Ingredients:

- 2.1/2 cups old-fashioned rolled oats
- 5 tablespoons pumpkin seeds (pipits)
- 5 tablespoons chopped pecans
- 5 cups unsweetened plant-based milk
- 21/2 teaspoons maple syrup or agave syrup
- 1/2 to 1 teaspoon salt
- 1/2 to 1 teaspoon ground cinnamon
- 1/2 to 1 teaspoon ground ginger

Directions:

1. Line up 5 wide-mouth pint jars. In each jar, combine 1/2 cup of oats, 1 tablespoon of pumpkin seeds, 1 tablespoon of pecans, 1 cup of plant-based milk, 1/2 teaspoon of maple syrup, 1 pinch of salt, 1 pinch of cinnamon, and 1 pinch of ginger.
2. Stir the ingredients in each jar. Close the jars tightly with lids. To serve, top with fresh fruit (if using).

Nutrition:

Calories: 124;

Fat: 1927

Protein: 35g;

Carbohydrates: 80;

Fiber: 65 g

Sugar: 18 g

Sodium: 276

Barley Breakfast Bowl

Preparation Time: 5 minutes

Cooking time: 15minutes

Servings: 4

Ingredients:

- 1.1/2 cups pearl barley
- 3.3/4 cups water
- Large pinch salt
- 1.1/2 cups dried cranberries
- 3 cups sweetened vanilla plant-based milk
- 2 tablespoons slivered almonds (optional)

Directions:

1. Put the barley, water, and salt. Bring to a boil.
2. Divide the barley into 6 jars or single-serving storage containers. Attached the 1/4 cup of dried cranberries to each. Pour 1/2 cup of plant-based milk into each. Attached the 1 teaspoon of slivered almonds (if using) to each. Close the jars tightly with lids.

Nutrition:

Calories: 109;

Fat: 15g;

Protein: 24g;

Carbohydrates: 32g;

Fiber: 8g;

Sugar: 1g;

Sodium: 466mg

Sweet Potato and Black Bean Hash

Preparation Time: 10 minutes

Cooking time: 20minutes

Servings: 6

Ingredients:

- 1 teaspoon extra-virgin olive oil or 3 teaspoons vegetable broth
- 1 large sweet yellow onion, diced
- 2 teaspoons minced garlic (about 2 cloves)
- 1 large sweet potato, unpeeled, diced into ¾-inch pieces
- 2 teaspoons ground cumin
- 1 teaspoon dried oregano
- 1 (14.5-ounce) can black beans, rinsed and drained
- 1/4 teaspoon salt
- 1/4 teaspoon freshly ground black pepper

Directions:

1. In large skillet over medium-high heat, heat the olive oil. Attach the onion and garlic and cook for 5 minutes, stirring frequently.

2. Add the sweet potatoes, cumin, and oregano. Stir and cook for another 5 minutes. Cover the skillet, reduce the heat to low, and cook for 15 minutes.

3. After 15 minutes, increase the heat to medium-high and stir in the black beans, salt (if using), and pepper. Cook for another 5 minutes.

4. Divide evenly among 6 single-serving containers. Let cool before sealing the lids.

Nutrition:

Calories: 209;

Fat: 12g;

Protein: 34g;

Carbohydrates: 22g;

Fiber: 8g;

Sugar: 1g;

Sodium: 466mg

Smoothie Breakfast Bowl

Preparation Time: 10 minutes

Cooking time: 20minutes

Servings: 4

Ingredients:

- 4 bananas, peeled
- 1 cup dragon fruit or fruit of choice
- 1 cup Baked Granola
- 2 cups fresh berries
- 1/2 cup slivered almonds
- 4 cups plant-based milk

Directions:

1. Open 4 quart-size, freezer-safe bags, and layer in the following order: 1 banana (halved or sliced) and 1/4 cup dragon fruit.

2. Into 4 small jelly jars, layer in the following order: 1/4 cup granola, 1/2 cup berries, and 2 tablespoons slivered almonds.

3. To serve, take a frozen bag of bananas and dragon fruit and transfer to a blender. Add 1 cup of plant-based milk, and blend until smooth. Pour into a bowl. Add the contents of 1 jar of granola, berries, and almonds over the top of the smoothie, and serve with a spoon.

Nutrition:

Calories: 109;

Fat: 12g;

Protein: 24g;

Carbohydrates: 24g;

Fiber: 8g;

Sugar: 5g;

Sodium: 366mg

Tortilla Breakfast Casserole

Preparation Time: 20 minutes

Cooking time: 20minutes

Servings: 4

Ingredients:

- 1 recipe Tofu-Spinach Scramble
- 1 (14-ounce) can black beans
- 1/4 cup nutritional yeast
- 2 teaspoons hot sauce
- 10 small corn tortillas
- 1/2 cup shredded vegan Cheddar or pepper Jack cheese, divided

Directions:

1. Preheat the oven to 350ºF. Coat a 9-by-9-inch baking pan with cooking spray.

2. In a large bowl, combine the tofu scramble with the black beans, nutritional yeast, and hot sauce. Set aside.

3. In the bottom of the baking pan, place 5 corn tortillas. Spread half of the tofu and bean mixture over the tortillas. Spread 1/4 cup of cheese over the top. Layer the remaining 5 tortillas over the top of the cheese. Spread the reminder of the tofu and bean mixture over the tortillas. Spread the remaining 1/4 cup of cheese over the top.

4. Bake for 20 minutes.

5. Divide evenly among 6 single-serving containers. Let cool before sealing the lids.

Nutrition:

Calories: 132;

Fat: 10g;

Protein: 34g;

Carbohydrates: 54g;

Fiber: 9g;

Sugar: 4g;

Sodium: 254mg

Tofu-Spinach Scramble

Preparation Time: 15 minutes

Cooking time: 20minutes

Servings: 5

Ingredients:

- 1 (14-ounce) package water-packed extra-firm tofu
- 1 teaspoon extra-virgin olive oil or 1/4 cup vegetable broth
- 1 small yellow onion, diced
- 3 teaspoons minced garlic (about 3 cloves)
- 3 large celery stalks, chopped
- 2 large carrots, peeled (optional) and chopped
- 1 teaspoon chili powder
- 1/2 teaspoon ground cumin
- 1/2 teaspoon ground turmeric
- 1/2 teaspoon salt (optional)
- 1/4 teaspoon freshly ground black pepper
- 5 cups loosely packed spinach

Directions:

1. Drain the tofu by placing it, wrapped in a paper towel, on a plate in the sink. Place a cutting board over the tofu, then set a heavy pot, can, or cookbook on the cutting board. Remove after 10 minutes. (Alternatively, use a tofu press.)

2. In a medium bowl, crumble the tofu with your hands or a potato masher.

3. Heat the olive oil. Add the onion, garlic, celery, and carrots, and sauté for 5 minutes, until the onion is softened.

4. Add the crumbled tofu, chili powder, cumin, turmeric, salt (if using), and pepper, and continue cooking for 7 to 8 more minutes, stirring frequently, until the tofu begins to brown.

5. Add the spinach and mix well. Cover and reduce the heat to medium. Steam the spinach for 3 minutes.

6. Divide evenly among 5 single-serving containers. Let cool before sealing the lids.

Nutrition:

Calories: 122;

Fat: 15g;

Protein: 14g;

Carbohydrates: 54g;

Fiber: 8g;

Sugar: 1g;

Sodium: 354mg

Savory Pancakes

Preparation Time: 10 minutes

Cooking time: 15minutes

Servings: 4

Ingredients:

- 1 cup whole-wheat flour
- 1 teaspoon garlic salt
- 1 teaspoon onion powder
- 1/2 teaspoon baking soda
- 1/4 teaspoon salt
- 1 cup lightly pressed, crumbled soft or firm tofu
- 1/2 cup unsweetened plant-based milk
- 1/4 cup lemon juice
- 2 tablespoons extra-virgin olive oil
- 1/2 cup finely chopped mushrooms

- 1/2 cup finely chopped onion
- 2 cups tightly packed greens (arugula, spinach, or baby kale work great)

Directions:

1. Attach the flour, garlic salt, onion powder, baking soda, and salt. Mix well. In a blender, combine the tofu, plant-based milk, lemon juice, and olive oil. Purée on high speed for 30 seconds.

2. Pour the contents of the blender into the bowl of dry ingredients and whisk until combined well. Fold in the mushrooms, onion, and greens.

Nutrition:

Calories: 132;

Fat: 10g;

Protein: 12g;

Carbohydrates: 44g;

Fiber: 9g;

Sugar: 1g;

Sodium: 254mg

Quinoa Breakfast Porridge

Preparation Time: 10 minutes

Cooking time: 5 minutes

Servings: 3

Ingredients:

- 1 cup dry quinoa
- 2 cups almond milk
- 1 tbsp. agave or maple syrup
- 1/2 tsp. vanilla
- 1/2 tsp. cinnamon

- 1 tablespoon ground flax meal

Directions:

1. Combine quinoa, almond milk, sugar, vanilla, and cinnamon in a little pot. Heat to the point of boiling and lessen to a stew.

2. Allow the quinoa to cook until the majority of the fluid is retained, and quinoa is fleecy (15-20 minutes). Blend in the flax meal. Blend in any extra toppers or include INS, and appreciate.

Nutrition:

Calories: 122;

Fat: 12g;

Protein: 12g;

Carbohydrates: 34g;

Fiber: 9g;

Sugar: 5g;

Sodium: 154mg

Grapes and Green Tea Smoothie

Preparation Time: 5 Minutes

Cooking Time: 0 Minutes

Servings: 2

Ingredients:

- ½ cup green tea
- ½ cup of green grapes
- 1 banana, peeled
- 1-inch piece of ginger
- ½ cup of ice cubes
- 2 cups baby spinach
- ½ of a medium apple, peeled, diced

Directions:

1. Place all the ingredients into the jar of a high-speed food processor or blender in the order stated in the ingredients list and then cover it with the lid.
2. Pulse for 1 minute until smooth, and then serve.

Nutrition:

Calories: 150 Cal;

Fat: 2.5 g;

Protein: 1 g;

Carbs: 36.5 g;

Fiber: 9 g

Mango and Kale Smoothie

Preparation Time: 5 Minutes

Cooking Time: 0 Minutes

Servings: 2

Ingredients:

- 2 cups oats milk, unsweetened
- 2 bananas, peeled
- ½ cup kale leaves
- 2 teaspoons coconut sugar
- 1 cup mango pieces
- 1 teaspoon vanilla extract, unsweetened

Directions:

1. Place all the ingredients into the jar of a high-speed food processor or blender in the order stated in the ingredients list and then cover it with the lid.
2. Pulse for 1 minute until smooth, and then serve.

Nutrition:

Calories: 281 Cal;

Fat: 3 g;

Protein: 6 g;

Carbs: 63 g;

Fiber: 16 g

Pomegranate Smoothie

Preparation Time: 5 Minutes

Cooking Time: 0 Minutes

Servings: 2

Ingredients:

- 2 cups almond milk, unsweetened
- 2 medium apples, cored, sliced
- 2 bananas, peeled
- 2 cups frozen raspberries
- 1 cup pomegranate seeds
- 4 teaspoons agave syrup

Directions:

1. Place all the ingredients into the jar of a high-speed food processor or blender in the order stated in the ingredients list and then cover it with the lid.
2. Pulse for 1 minute until smooth, and then serve.

Nutrition:

Calories: 141.5 Cal;

Fat: 1.1 g;

Protein: 4.1 g;

Carbs: 30.8 g;

Fiber: 2.4 g

Coconut Water Smoothie

Preparation Time: 5 Minutes

Cooking Time: 0 Minutes

Servings: 2

Ingredients:

- 2 cups of coconut water
- 1 large apple, peeled, cored, diced
- 1 cup of frozen mango pieces
- 2 teaspoons peanut butter
- 4 teaspoons coconut flakes

Directions:

1. Place all the ingredients into the jar of a high-speed food processor or blender in the order stated in the ingredients list and then cover it with the lid.
2. Pulse for 1 minute until smooth, and then serve.

Nutrition:

Calories: 113.4 Cal;

Fat: 0.3 g;

Protein: 0.6 g;

Carbs: 29 g;

Fiber: 2 g

Apple, Banana, and Berry Smoothie

Preparation Time: 5 Minutes

Cooking Time: 0 Minutes

Servings: 2

Ingredients:

- 2 cups almond milk, unsweetened
- 2 cups frozen strawberries
- 2 bananas, peeled
- 1 large apple, peeled, cored, diced
- 2 tablespoons peanut butter

Directions:

1. Place all the ingredients into the jar of a high-speed food processor or blender in the order stated in the ingredients list and then cover it with the lid.

2. Pulse for 1 minute until smooth, and then serve.

Nutrition:

Calories: 156.1 Cal;

Fat: 3.2 g;

Protein: 3 g;

Carbs: 17 g;

Fiber: 5.8 g

Berry Ginger Zing Smoothie

Preparation Time: 5 Minutes

Cooking Time: 0 Minutes

Servings: 2

Ingredients:

- 2 cups almond milk, unsweetened
- 1 cup frozen raspberries
- 1 cup of frozen strawberries
- 1 cup cauliflower florets
- 1-inch pieces of ginger

Directions:

1. Place all the ingredients into the jar of a high-speed food processor or blender in the order stated in the ingredients list and then cover it with the lid.
2. Pulse for 1 minute until smooth, and then serve.

Nutrition:

Calories: 300 Cal;

Fat: 8 g;

Protein: 8 g;

Carbs: 30 g;

Fiber: 9 g

Dragon Fruit Smoothie Bowl

Preparation Time: 5 Minutes

Cooking Time: 0 Minutes

Servings: 2

Ingredients:

For the Bowl:
- ½ cup coconut milk, unsweetened
- 2 bananas, peeled
- ½ cup frozen raspberries
- 7 ounces frozen dragon fruit
- 3 tablespoons vanilla protein powder

  For the Toppings:
- 2 tablespoons coconut flakes
- 2 tablespoons hemp seeds

Directions:

1. Place all the ingredients for the bowl into the jar of a high-speed food processor or blender in the order stated in the ingredients list and then cover it with the lid.
2. Pulse for 1 minute until smooth, and then divide evenly between two bowls.
3. Sprinkle 1 tablespoon of coconut flakes and hemp seeds over the smoothie and then serve.

Nutrition:

Calories: 225 Cal;

Fat: 1.6 g;

Protein: 8.1 g;

Carbs: 48 g;

Fiber: 8.9 g

Chocolate Smoothie Bowl

Preparation Time: 5 Minutes

Cooking Time: 0 Minutes

Servings: 2

Ingredients:

For the Bowls:

- 2 cups almond milk, unsweetened
- 2 bananas, peeled
- 3 tablespoons cocoa powder
- 1 cup spinach leaves, fresh
- 2 tablespoons oat flour
- 4 Medjool dates, pitted
- 1/8 teaspoon salt
- 2 tablespoons vanilla protein powder
- 2 tablespoons peanut butter

For the Toppings:

- 2 tablespoons coconut flakes
- 2 tablespoons hemp seeds

Directions:

1. Place all the ingredients for the bowl into the jar of a high-speed food processor or blender in the order stated in the ingredients list and then cover it with the lid.
2. Pulse for 1 minute until smooth, and then divide evenly between two bowls.
3. Sprinkle 1 tablespoon of coconut flakes and hemp seeds over the smoothie and then serve.

Nutrition:

Calories: 382 Cal;

Fat: 14 g;

Protein: 22 g;

Carbs: 53 g;

Fiber: 9 g

Zucchini and Blueberry Smoothie

Preparation Time: 5 Minutes

Cooking Time: 0 Minutes

Servings: 2

Ingredients:

- 1 cup coconut milk, unsweetened
- 1 large celery stem
- 2 bananas, peeled
- ½ cup spinach leaves, fresh
- 1 cup frozen blueberries
- 2/3 cup sliced zucchini
- 1 tablespoon hemp seeds
- ½ teaspoon maca powder
- ¼ teaspoon ground cinnamon

Directions:

1. Place all the ingredients into the jar of a high-speed food processor or blender in the order stated in the ingredients list and then cover it with the lid.
2. Pulse for 1 minute until smooth, and then serve.

Nutrition:

Calories: 218 Cal;

Fat: 10.1 g;

Protein: 6.3 g;

Carbs: 31.8 g;

Fiber: 4.7 g

Hot Pink Beet Smoothie

Preparation Time: 5 Minutes

Cooking Time: 0 Minutes

Servings: 2

Ingredients:

- 2 cups almond milk, unsweetened
- 2 clementine, peeled
- 1 cup raspberries
- 1 banana, peeled
- 1 medium beet, peeled, chopped
- 2 tablespoons chia seeds
- 1/8 teaspoon sea salt
- ½ teaspoon vanilla extract, unsweetened
- 4 tablespoons almond butter

Directions:

1. Place all the ingredients into the jar of a high-speed food processor or blender in the order stated in the ingredients list and then cover it with the lid.
2. Pulse for 1 minute until smooth, and then serve.

Nutrition:

Calories: 260.8 Cal;

Fat: 1.3 g;

Protein: 13 g;

Carbs: 56 g;

Fiber: 9.3 g

Chickpea Flour Frittata

Preparation Time: 10 Minutes

Cooking Time: 50 Minutes

Servings: 6

Ingredients:

- 1 medium green bell pepper, cored, chopped
- 1 cup chopped greens
- 1 cup cauliflower florets, chopped
- ½ cup chopped broccoli florets
- ½ of a medium red onion, peeled, chopped
- ¼ teaspoon salt
- ½ cup chopped zucchini

For the Batter:

- ¼ cup cashew cream
- ½ cup chickpea flour
- ½ cup chopped cilantro
- ½ teaspoon salt
- ¼ teaspoon cayenne pepper
- ½ teaspoon dried dill
- ¼ teaspoon ground black pepper
- ¼ teaspoon dried thyme
- ½ teaspoon ground turmeric
- 1 tablespoon olive oil
- 1 ½ cup water

Directions:

1. Switch on the oven, then set it to 375 degrees F and let it preheat.
2. Take a 9-inch pie pan, grease it with oil, and then set aside until required.
3. Take a large bowl, place all the vegetables in it, sprinkle with salt and then toss until combined.
4. Prepare the batter and for this, add all of its ingredients in it except for thyme, dill, and cilantro and then pulse until combined and smooth.
5. Pour the batter over the vegetables, add dill, thyme, and cilantro, and then stir until combined.
6. Spoon the mixture into the prepared pan, spread evenly, and then bake for 45 to 50 minutes until done and inserted toothpick into frittata comes out clean.
7. When done, let the frittata rest for 10 minutes, cut it into slices, and then serve.

Nutrition:

Calories: 153 Cal;

Fat: 4 g;

Protein: 7 g;

Carbs: 20 g;

Fiber: 4 g

Potato Pancakes

Preparation Time: 10 Minutes

Cooking Time: 20 Minutes

Servings: 10

Ingredients:

- ½ cup white whole-wheat flour
- 3 large potatoes, grated
- ½ of a medium white onion, peeled, grated
- 1 jalapeno, minced
- 2 green onions, chopped
- 1 tablespoon minced garlic
- 1 teaspoon salt
- ¼ teaspoon baking powder
- ¼ teaspoon ground pepper
- 4 tablespoons olive oil

Directions:

1. Take a large bowl, place all the ingredients except for oil and then stir until well combined; stir in 1 to 2 tablespoons water if needed to mix the batter.
2. Take a large skillet pan, place it over medium-high heat, add 2 tablespoons of oil and then let it heat.
3. Scoop the pancake mixture in portions into the pan, shape each portion like a pancake and then cook for 5 to 7 minutes per side until pancakes turn golden brown and thoroughly cooked.
4. When done, transfer the pancakes to a plate, add more oil into the pan and then cook more pancakes in the same manner.
5. Serve straight away.

Nutrition:

Calories: 69 Cal;

Fat: 1 g;

Protein: 2 g;

Carbs: 12 g;

Fiber: 1 g

Chocolate Chip Pancakes

Preparation Time: 5 Minutes

Cooking Time: 10 Minutes

Servings: 6

Ingredients:

- 1 cup white whole-wheat flour
- ½ cup chocolate chips, vegan, unsweetened
- 1 tablespoon baking powder
- ¼ teaspoon salt
- 2 teaspoons coconut sugar
- ½ teaspoon vanilla extract, unsweetened
- 1 cup almond milk, unsweetened
- 2 tablespoons coconut butter, melted
- 2 tablespoons olive oil

Directions:

1. Take a large bowl, place all the ingredients except for oil and chocolate chips, and then stir until well combined.
2. Add chocolate chips, and then fold until just mixed.
3. Take a large skillet pan, place it over medium-high heat, add 1 tablespoon oil and then let it heat.
4. Scoop the pancake mixture in portions into the pan, shape each portion like a pancake and then cook for 5 to 7 minutes per side until pancakes turn golden brown and thoroughly cooked.
5. When done, transfer the pancakes to a plate, add more oil into the pan and then cook more pancakes in the same manner.
6. Serve straight away.

Nutrition:

Calories: 172 Cal;

Fat: 6 g;

Protein: 2.5 g;

Carbs: 28 g;

Fiber: 8 g

Turmeric Steel-Cut Oats

Preparation Time: 5 Minutes

Cooking Time: 10 Minutes

Servings: 2

Ingredients:

- ½ cup steel-cut oats
- 1/8 teaspoon salt
- 2 tablespoons maple syrup
- ½ teaspoon ground cinnamon
- 1/3 teaspoon turmeric powder
- ¼ teaspoon ground cardamom
- ¼ teaspoon olive oil
- ½ cups water
- 1 cup almond milk, unsweetened

For the Topping:

- 2 tablespoons pumpkin seeds
- 2 tablespoons chia seeds

Directions:

1. Take a medium saucepan, place it over medium heat, add oats, and then cook for 2 minutes until toasted.
2. Pour in the milk and water, stir until mixed, and then bring the oats to a boil.
3. Then switch heat to medium-low level, simmer the oats for 10 minutes, and add salt, maple syrup, and all spices.
4. Stir until combined, cook the oats for 7 minutes or more until cooked to the

desired level and when done, let the oats rest for 15 minutes.

5. When done, divide oats evenly between two bowls, top with pumpkin seeds and chia seeds and then serve.

Nutrition:

Calories: 234 Cal;

Fat: 4 g;

Protein: 7 g;

Carbs: 41 g;

Fiber: 5 g

Vegetable Pancakes

Preparation Time: 10 Minutes

Cooking Time: 20 Minutes

Servings: 10

Ingredients:

- 1/3 cup cooked and mashed sweet potato
- 2 cups grated carrots
- 1 cup chopped coriander
- 1 cup cooked spinach
- 2 ounces chickpea flour
- ½ teaspoon baking powder
- 1 ½ teaspoon salt
- 1 teaspoon ground turmeric
- 2 tablespoons olive oil
- ¾ cup of water

Directions:

1. Take a large bowl, place chickpea flour in it, add turmeric powder, baking powder, and salt, and then stir until combined.
2. Whisk in the water until combined, stir in sweet potatoes until well mixed and then add carrots, spinach, and coriander until well combined.

3. Take a large skillet pan, place it over medium-high heat, add 1 tablespoon oil and then let it heat.
4. Scoop the pancake mixture in portions into the pan, shape each portion like a pancake and then cook for 3 to 5 minutes per side until pancakes turn golden brown and thoroughly cooked.
5. When done, transfer the pancakes to a plate, add more oil into the pan and then cook more pancakes in the same manner.
6. Serve straight away.

Nutrition:

Calories: 74 Cal;

Fat: 0.3 g;

Protein: 3 g;

Carbs: 16 g;

Fiber: 2.7 g

Banana and Chia Pudding

Preparation Time: 25 Minutes

Cooking Time: 12 Minutes

Servings: 2

Ingredients:

For the Pudding:

- 2 bananas, peeled
- 4 tablespoons chia seeds
- 2 tablespoons coconut sugar
- ½ teaspoon pumpkin pie spice
- 1/8 teaspoon sea salt
- ½ cup almond milk, unsweetened

For the Bananas:

- 2 bananas, peeled, sliced
- 2 tablespoons coconut flakes
- 1/8 teaspoon ground cinnamon

- 2 tablespoons coconut sugar
- ¼ cup chopped walnuts
- 2 tablespoons almond milk, unsweetened

Directions:

1. Prepare the pudding and for this, place all of its ingredients in a blender except for chia seeds and then pulse until smooth.
2. Pour the mixture into a medium saucepan, place it over medium heat, bring the mixture to a boil and then remove the pan from heat.
3. Add chia seeds into the hot banana mixture, stir until mixed, and then let it sit for 5 minutes.
4. Whisk the pudding and then let it chill for 15 minutes in the refrigerator.
5. Meanwhile, prepare the caramelized bananas and for this, take a medium skillet pan, and place it over medium heat.
6. Add banana slices, sprinkle with salt, sugar, and nutmeg, drizzle with milk and then cook for 5 minutes until mixture has thickened.
7. Assemble the pudding and for this, divide the pudding evenly between two bowls, top with banana slices, sprinkle with walnuts, and then serve.

Nutrition:

Calories: 495 Cal;

Fat: 21 g;

Protein: 9 g;

Carbs: 76 g;

Fiber: 14 g

Tofu Scramble

Preparation Time: 5 Minutes

Cooking Time: 15 Minutes

Servings: 3

Ingredients:

- 12 ounces tofu, extra-firm, pressed, drained
- ½ of a medium red onion, peeled, sliced
- 1 cup baby greens mix
- 1 medium red bell pepper, cored, sliced
- ½ teaspoon garlic powder
- 1 teaspoon salt
- ½ teaspoon ground black pepper
- ¼ teaspoon turmeric powder
- ¼ teaspoon ground cumin
- 4 tablespoons olive oil, divided

Directions:

1. Take a large bowl, place tofu in it, and then break it into bite-size pieces.
2. Add salt, black pepper, turmeric, and 2 tablespoons of oil, and then stir until mixed.
3. Take a medium skillet pan, place it over medium heat, add garlic powder and cumin and then cook for 1 minute until fragrant.
4. Add tofu mixture, stir until mixed, switch heat to medium-high level, and then cook for 5 minutes until tofu turn golden brown.
5. When done, divide tofu evenly between three plates, keep it warm, and then set aside until required.
6. Return the skillet pan over medium-high heat, add remaining oil and let it heat until hot.
7. Add onion and bell peppers, cook for 5 to 7 minutes or until beginning to brown, and then season with a pinch of salt.
8. Add baby greens, toss until mixed, and then cook for 30 seconds until leaves begin to wilts.

9. Add vegetables evenly to the plates to scrambled tofu and then serve.

Nutrition:

Calories: 304 Cal;

Fat: 25.6 g;

Protein: 14.2 g;

Carbs: 6.6 g;

Fiber: 2.6 g

Pumpkin Spice Oatmeal

Preparation Time: 5 Minutes

Cooking Time: 8 Minutes

Servings: 2

Ingredients:

- ¼ cup Medjool dates, pitted, chopped
- 2/3 cup rolled oats
- 1 tablespoon maple syrup
- ½ teaspoon pumpkin pie spice
- ½ teaspoon vanilla extract, unsweetened
- 1/3 cup pumpkin puree
- 2 tablespoons chopped pecans
- 1 cup almond milk, unsweetened

Directions:

1. Take a medium pot, place it over medium heat, and then add all the ingredients except for pecans and maple syrup.
2. Stir all the ingredients until combined, and then cook for 5 minutes until the oatmeal has absorbed all the liquid and thickened to the desired level.
3. When done, divide oatmeal evenly between two bowls, top with pecans, drizzle with maple syrup and then serve.

Nutrition:

Calories: 175 Cal;

Fat: 3.2 g;

Protein: 5.8 g;

Carbs: 33 g;

Fiber: 6.1 g

Peanut Butter Bites

Preparation Time: 10 Minutes

Cooking Time: 0 Minutes

Servings: 5

Ingredients:

- 1 cup rolled oats
- 12 Medjool dates, pitted
- ½ cup peanut butter, sugar-free

Directions:

1. Plug in a blender or a food processor, add all the ingredients in its jar, and then cover with the lid.
2. Pulse for 5 minutes until well combined, and then tip the mixture into a shallow dish.
3. Shape the mixture into 20 balls, 1 tablespoon of mixture per ball, and then serve.

Nutrition:

Calories: 103.1 Cal;

Fat: 4.3 g;

Protein: 2.3 g;

Carbs: 15.4 g;

Fiber: 0.8 g

Maple and Cinnamon Overnight Oats

Preparation Time: 10 Minutes

Cooking Time: 0 Minutes

Servings: 4

Ingredients:

- 2 cups rolled oats
- ¼ cup chopped pecans
- ¾ teaspoon ground cinnamon
- 1 teaspoon vanilla extract, unsweetened
- 3 tablespoons coconut sugar
- 3 tablespoons maple syrup
- 2 cups almond milk, unsweetened

Directions:

1. Take four mason jars, and then add ½ cup oats, ¼ teaspoon vanilla, and ½ cup milk.
2. Take a small bowl, add maple syrup, cinnamon, and sugar, stir until mixed, add this mixture into the oats mixture and then stir until combined.
3. Cover the jars with the lid and then let them rest in the refrigerator for a minimum of 2 hours or more until thickened.
4. When ready to eat, top the oats with pecans, sprinkle with cinnamon, drizzle with maple syrup and then serve.

Nutrition:

Calories: 292 Cal;

Fat: 9 g;

Protein: 7 g;

Carbs: 48 g;

Fiber: 6 g

Breakfast Tomato and Eggs

Preparation Time: 5 Minutes

Cooking Time: 30 Minutes

Servings: 2

Ingredients:

- 2 eggs
- 2 tomatoes
- Salt and black pepper to taste
- 1 tsp. parsley, finely chopped

Directions:

1. Cut tomatoes tops, scoop flesh and arrange them on a lined baking sheet.
2. Crack an egg in each tomato.
3. Season with salt and pepper.
4. Introduce them in the oven at 150 degrees and bake for 30 minutes
5. Take tomatoes out of the oven, divide between plates, season with more salt and pepper, sprinkle parsley at the end and serve.
6. Enjoy!

Nutrition:

Calories: 186

Fat: 36g

Carbs: 2g

Protein: 14g

Fiber: 11.6g

Sugar: 0g

Breakfast Paleo Muffins

Preparation Time: 5 Minutes

Cooking Time: 30 Minutes

Servings: 4

Ingredients:

- 1 cup kale, chopped
- ¼ cup chives, finely chopped

- ½ cup almond milk
- 6 eggs
- Salt and black pepper to taste
- Some coconut oil for greasing the muffin cups

Directions:

1. In a bowl, mix eggs with chives and kale and whisk very well.
2. Add salt and black pepper to the taste and almond milk and stir well.
3. Divide this into eight muffin cups after you've greased it with some coconut oil.
4. Introduce this in preheated oven at 150 degrees and bake for 30 minutes
5. Take muffins out of the oven, leave them to cool down, transfer them to plates and serve warm.
6. Enjoy!

Nutrition:

Calories: 100

Fat: 5g

Carbs: 3g

Protein: 14g

Fiber: 10.6g

Sugar: 0g

Paleo Banana Pancakes

Preparation Time: 5 Minutes

Cooking Time: 5 Minutes

Servings: 2

Ingredients:

- 4 eggs
- A pinch of salt
- Two bananas, peeled and chopped
- ¼ tsp. baking powder
- Cooking spray

Directions:

1. In a bowl, mix eggs with chopped bananas, a pinch of salt and baking powder and whisk well.
2. Transfer this to your food processor and blend very well.
3. Heat up a pan over medium high heat after you've sprayed it with some cooking oil.
4. Add some of the pancakes batter, spread in the pan, cook for 1 minute, flip and cook for 30 seconds and transfer to a plate.
5. Serve and enjoy!

Nutrition:

Calories: 120

Fat: 2g

Carbs: 2g

Protein: 4g

Fiber: 6.6g

Sugar: 1g

Breakfast Eggs

Preparation Time: 5 Minutes

Cooking Time: 30 Minutes

Servings: 2

Ingredients:

- 2 eggs
- Salt and black pepper to taste
- 1 tsp. parsley, finely chopped

Directions:

1. Crack an egg in each tomato.
2. Season with salt and pepper.
3. Introduce them in the oven at 150 degrees and bake for 30 minutes

4. Divide between plates, season with more salt and pepper, sprinkle parsley at the end and serve.
5. Enjoy!

Nutrition:

Calories: 186

Fat: 10g

Carbs: 2g

Protein: 14g

Fiber: 6g

Sugar: 0g

Plantain Pancakes

Preparation Time: 5 Minutes

Cooking Time: 5 Minutes

Servings: 1

Ingredients:

- 3 eggs
- ¼ cup coconut flour
- ¼ cup coconut water
- 1 tsp. coconut oil
- ½ plantain, peeled and chopped
- ¼ tsp. cream of tartar
- ¼ tsp. baking soda
- A pinch of salt
- ¼ tsp. chai spice
- 1 tbsp. shaved coconut, toasted for serving
- 1 tbsp. coconut milk for serving

Directions:

1. In your food processor, mix eggs with a pinch of salt, coconut water and flour, plantain, cream of tartar, baking soda and chai spice and blend well.
2. Heat up a pan with the coconut oil over medium heat, add ¼ cup pancake batter, spread evenly, cook until it becomes golden, flip pancake and cook for one minute and transfer to a plate.
3. Serve pancakes with shaved coconut and coconut milk.

Nutrition:

Calories: 372

Fat: 17g

Carbs: 55g

Protein: 23g

Fiber: 5.6g

Sugar: 0g

Sweet Potato Waffles

Preparation Time: 5 Minutes

Cooking Time: 20 Minutes

Servings: 4

Ingredients:

- 2 sweet potatoes, peeled and finely grated
- 2 tbsp. melted coconut oil
- 3 eggs
- 1 tsp. cinnamon powder
- ½ tsp. nutmeg, ground
- Some apple sauce for serving

Directions:

1. In a bowl, mix eggs with sweet potatoes, coconut oil, cinnamon and nutmeg and whisk very well.
2. Cook waffles in your waffle iron, arrange them on plates and serve with apple sauce drizzled on top.
3. Enjoy!

Nutrition:

Calories: 227

Fat: 6g

Carbs: 37g

Protein: 6g

Fiber: 2g

Sugar: 2g

Eggplant French Toast

Preparation Time: 5 Minutes

Cooking Time: 5 Minutes

Servings: 2

Ingredients:

- 1 eggplant, peeled and sliced
- A pinch of sea salt
- 1 tsp. vanilla extract
- 2 eggs
- Stevia, to taste
- 1 tsp. coconut oil
- A pinch of cinnamon

Directions:

1. Arrange eggplant slices on a plate, sprinkle them with a pinch of salt, flip them and season with salt again and leave them aside for 2 minutes
2. In a bowl, mix eggs with vanilla, stevia, and cinnamon and whisk well.
3. Heat up a pan with the coconut oil over medium-high heat.
4. Dip eggplant slices in eggs mix, add to heated pan and cook until they become golden on each side.
5. Arrange them on plates and serve.
6. Enjoy!

Nutrition:

Calories: 125

Fat: 5g

Carbs: 13g

Protein: 7.8g

Fiber: 7.8g

Orange and Dates Granola

Preparation Time: 5 Minutes

Cooking Time: 25 Minutes

Servings: 6

Ingredients:

- 5 oz. dates, soaked in hot water
- Juice from 1 orange
- Grated rind of ½ orange
- 1 cup desiccated coconut
- ½ cup silvered almonds
- ½ cup pumpkin seeds
- ½ cup linseeds
- ½ cup sesame seeds
- Almond milk for serving

Directions:

1. In a bowl, mix almonds with orange rind, orange juice, linseeds, coconut, pumpkin and sesame seeds and stir well.
2. Drain dates, add them to your food processor and blend well.
3. Add this paste to almonds mix and stir well again.
4. Spread this on a lined baking sheet, introduce in the oven at 350 degrees and bake for 15 minutes, stirring every 4 minutes.
5. Take granola out of the oven, leave aside to cool down a bit and then serve with almond milk.
6. Enjoy!

Nutrition:

Calories: 208

Fat: 9g

Carbs: 3g

Protein: 6g

Fiber: 5g

Sugar: 0g

Breakfast Burrito

Preparation Time: 5 Minutes

Cooking Time: 5 Minutes

Servings: 2

Ingredients:

- 1 small yellow onion, finely chopped
- 4 eggs, egg yolks and whites separated
- ¼ cup canned green chilis, chopped
- 2 tomatoes, chopped
- 1 red bell pepper, cut into thin strips
- ¼ cup cilantro, finely chopped
- ½ cup chicken meat, already cooked and shredded
- Salt and black pepper to taste
- A drizzle of extra virgin olive oil
- 1 avocado, pitted, peeled and chopped
- Hot sauce for serving

Directions:

1. Put egg whites in a bowl, add a pinch of salt, whisk them well and leave them aside for now.
2. Heat up a pan with a drizzle of oil over medium-high heat, add half of the egg whites, spread evenly, cover the pan and cook for 30 seconds.
3. Repeat this with the rest of the egg whites and leave the two "tortillas" aside.
4. Heat up the same pan with another drizzle of oil over medium-high heat, add onions, stir and cook for 1 minute.

5. Add red bell pepper, green chilis, tomato, meat and cilantro and stir.
6. Add egg yolks to the pan and scramble the whole mix.
7. Add avocado, stir, take off heat and spread evenly on the two egg whites' "tortillas".
8. Roll them, arrange on plates and serve with some hot sauce.
9. Enjoy!

Nutrition:

Calories: 170

Fat: 5g

Carbs: 1g

Protein: 6g

Fiber: 0g

Sugar: 0.6g

Spinach Frittata

Preparation Time: 5 Minutes

Cooking Time: 25 Minutes

Servings: 4

Ingredients:

- ½ lb. sausage, ground
- 2 tbsp. ghee
- 1 cup mushrooms, thinly sliced
- 1 cup spinach leaves, chopped
- 10 eggs, whisked
- 1 small yellow onion, finely chopped
- Salt and black pepper to taste

Directions:

1. Heat up a pan with the ghee over medium-high heat, add onion, stir and cook until it browns.
2. Add sausage, stir and also cook until it browns.

3. Add spinach and mushrooms and cook for 4 minutes, stirring from time to time.
4. Take the pan off the heat, add eggs, spread evenly, introduce frittata in the oven at 150 degrees and bake for 20 minutes
5. Take frittata out of the oven, leave it aside for a few moments to cool down, cut, arrange on plates and serve.
6. Enjoy!

Nutrition:

Calories: 233

Fat: 13g

Carbs: 4g

Protein: 21g

Fiber: 1.2g

Sugar: 0g

Squash Blossom Frittata

Preparation Time: 5 Minutes

Cooking Time: 30 Minutes

Servings: 2

Ingredients:

- 10 eggs, whisked
- Salt and black pepper to taste
- ¼ cup heavy cream
- 1 yellow onion, finely chopped
- 1 leek, thinly sliced
- 2 scallions, thinly sliced
- 2 zucchinis, chopped
- 8 squash blossoms
- Butter

Directions:

1. In a bowl, mix eggs with heavy cream, salt and black pepper to the taste and stir well.

2. Heat up a pan with a lot of butter over medium high heat, add leek and onions, stir and cook for 5 minutes
3. Add zucchini, stir and cook for ten more minutes.
4. Add eggs, spread, reduce heat to low, cook for 5 minutes
5. Sprinkle scallions and arrange squash blossoms on frittata, press flowers into eggs, introduce everything in the oven at 150 degrees and bake for 20 minutes
6. Take frittata out of the oven, leave it to cool down, cut, arrange on plates and serve it.
7. Enjoy!

Nutrition:

Calories: 123

Fat: 8g

Carbs: 2g

Protein: 7g

Fiber: 4.6g

Sugar: 0g

Breakfast Burger

Preparation Time: 5 Minutes

Cooking Time: 30 Minutes

Servings: 4

Ingredients:

- 5 eggs
- 1 lb. ground beef meat
- ½ cup sausages, ground
- 8 slices bacon
- 3 sun-dried tomatoes, chopped
- 2 tbsp. almond meal
- 2 tsp. basil leaves, chopped
- 1 tsp. garlic, finely minced
- A drizzle of vegetable oil

- Salt and black pepper to taste

Directions:

1. In a bowl, mix beef meat with one egg, almond meal, tomatoes, basil, salt and pepper and garlic, stir well and form 4 burgers.
2. Heat up a pan over medium high heat, add burgers, cook them 5 minutes on each side, transfer them to plates and leave aside for now.
3. Heat up the same pan over medium-high heat, add sausages, stir, cook for 5 minutes and transfer them to a plate.
4. Heat up the pan again, add bacon, cook for 4 minutes, drain excess grease and also leave aside on a plate.
5. Fry the four eggs in a pan with a drizzle of oil over medium-high heat and place them on top of burgers.
6. Add sausage and bacon and serve.
7. Enjoy!

Nutrition:

Calories: 264

Fat: 12g

Carbs: 5g

Protein: 32g

Fiber: 0.3g

Sugar: 0.7g

Maple Nut Porridge

Preparation Time: 5 Minutes

Cooking Time: 10 Minutes

Servings: 2

Ingredients:

- 2 tbsp. coconut butter
- ½ cup pecans, soaked

- ¾ cup hot water
- 1 banana, peeled and chopped
- ½ tsp. cinnamon
- A pinch of salt
- 2 tsp. maple syrup

Directions:

1. In your food processor, mix pecans with water, coconut butter, banana, cinnamon, a pinch of salt and maple syrup and blend well.
2. Transfer this to a pan, heat up over medium heat until it thickens, pour into bowls and serve.
3. Enjoy!

Nutrition:

Calories: 170

Fat: 9g

Carbs: 20g

Protein: 6g

Fiber: 6g

Breakfast Sandwich

Preparation Time: 5 Minutes

Cooking Time: 5 Minutes

Servings: 2

Ingredients:

- 3.5 oz. pumpkin flesh, peeled
- 4 slices whole grain bread
- 1 small avocado, pitted and peeled
- 1 carrot, finely grated
- 1 lettuce leaf, torn into four pieces

Directions:

1. Put pumpkin in a tray, introduce in the oven at 350 degrees and bake for 10 minutes.

2. Take pumpkin out of the oven, leave aside for 2-3 minutes, transfer to a bowl and mash it a bit
3. Put avocado in another bowl and also mash it with a fork.
4. Spread avocado on two bread slices, add grated carrot, mashed pumpkin and two lettuce pieces on each and top them with the rest of the bread slices.
5. Enjoy!

Nutrition:

Calories: 340

Fat: 7g

Carbs: 13g

Protein: 4g

Fiber: 8g

Sugar: 1g

Turkey Breakfast Sandwich

Preparation Time: 5 Minutes

Cooking Time: 5 Minutes

Servings: 1

Ingredients:

- 2 oz. turkey meat, roasted and thinly sliced
- 2 tbsp. pecans, toasted and chopped
- 2 oz. Brie cheese, sliced
- 2 slices sourdough bread
- 2 tbsp. cranberry chutney
- ¼ cup arugula

Directions:

1. In a bowl, mix pecans with chutney and stir well.
2. Spread this on bread slice, add turkey slices, brie cheese and arugula and top with the other bread slice.

3. Serve right away.
4. Enjoy!

Nutrition:

Calories: 100

Fat: 11g

Carbs: 52g

Protein: 32g

Fiber: 4g

Sugar: 0g

Eggplant Breakfast Spread

Preparation Time: 5 Minutes

Cooking Time: 15 Minutes

Servings: 2

Ingredients:

- 4 tbsp. olive oil
- 2 lb. eggplants, peeled and roughly chopped
- 4 garlic cloves, minced
- A pinch of salt and black pepper
- 1 cup water
- ¼ cup lemon juice
- 1 tbsp. sesame seeds paste
- ¼ cup black olives, pitted
- A few sprigs thyme, chopped
- A drizzle of olive oil

Directions:

1. Set your instant pot on sauté mode, add oil, heat it up, add eggplant pieces, stir and sauté for 5 minutes
2. Add garlic, salt, pepper and the water, stir gently, cover and cook on High for 5 minutes.
3. Discard excess water, add sesame seeds paste, lemon juice and olives and blend using an immersion blender.

4. Transfer to a bowl, sprinkle chopped thyme, drizzle some oil and serve for a fancy breakfast.

Nutrition:

Calories: 163

Fat: 2g

Carbs: 5g

Protein: 7g

Fiber: 1g

Sugar: 0g

Chicken Liver Breakfast Spread

Preparation Time: 5 Minutes

Cooking Time: 15 Minutes

Servings: 2

Ingredients:

- 1 tsp. olive oil
- ¾ lb. chicken livers
- 1 yellow onion, chopped
- ¼ cup water
- 1 bay leaf
- 2 anchovies
- 1 tbsp. capers
- 1 tbsp. ghee
- A pinch of salt and black pepper

Directions:

1. Put the olive oil in your instant pot, add onion, salt, pepper, chicken livers, water and the bay leaf, stir, cover and cook on high for 10 minutes.
2. Discard bay leaf, add anchovies, capers and the ghee and pulse everything using your immersion blender.
3. Add salt and pepper, blend again, divide into bowls and serve for breakfast.

Nutrition:

Calories: 152

Fat: 4g

Carbs: 3g

Protein: 7g

Fiber: 2g

Sugar: 0g

Mushroom Spread

Preparation Time: 5 Minutes

Cooking Time: 25 Minutes

Servings: 2

Ingredients:

- 1 oz. porcini mushrooms, dried
- 1 lb. button mushrooms, sliced
- 1 cup hot water
- 1 tbsp. ghee
- 1 tbsp. olive oil
- 1 shallot, chopped
- ¼ cup cold water
- A pinch of salt and pepper
- 1 bay leaf

Directions:

1. Put porcini mushrooms in a bowl, add 1 cup hot water and leave aside for now.
2. Set your instant pot on sauté mode, add ghee and oil and heat it up.
3. Add shallot, stir and sauté for 2 minutes
4. Add porcini mushrooms and their liquid, fresh mushrooms, cold, salt, pepper and bay leaf, stir, cover and cook on high for 12 minutes,
5. Discard bay leaf and some of the liquid and blend mushrooms mix using an immersion blender.
6. Transfer to small bowls and serve as a breakfast spread.

Nutrition:

Calories: 120

Fat: 1g

Carbs: 1g

Protein: 10g

Fiber: 3g

Sugar: 0g

Breakfast Chia Pudding

Preparation Time: 5 Minutes

Cooking Time: 5 Minutes

Servings: 2

Ingredients:

- ½ cup chia seeds
- 2 cups almond milk
- ¼ cup almonds
- ¼ cup coconut, shredded
- 4 tsp. sugar

Directions:

1. Put chia seeds in your instant pot.
2. Add milk, almonds and coconut flakes, stir, cover and cook at high for 3 minutes
3. Release the pressure quick, divide the pudding between bowls, top each with a teaspoon of sugar and serve.

Nutrition:

Calories: 130

Fat: 1g

Carbs: 2g

Protein: 14g

Fiber: 5g

Sugar: 0g

Breakfast Sweet Potatoes

Preparation Time: 5 Minutes

Cooking Time: 15 Minutes

Servings: 2

Ingredients:

- 4 sweet potatoes
- 2 tsp. Italian seasoning
- 1 tbsp. bacon fat
- 1 cup chives, chopped for serving.
- Water
- Salt and pepper to taste

Directions:

1. Put potatoes in your instant pot, add water to cover them, cover the pot and cook at high for 10 minutes.
2. Release the pressure naturally, transfer potatoes to a working surface and leave them to cool down.
3. Peel potatoes, transfer them to a bowl and mash them a bit with a fork.
4. Set your instant pot on sauté mode, add bacon fat and heat up.
5. Add potatoes, seasoning, salt and pepper to the taste, stir, cover the pot and cook at high for 1 minute.
6. Release the pressure quickly, stir potatoes again, divide them between plates and serve with chives sprinkled on top.

Nutrition:

Calories: 90

Fat: 3g

Carbs: 6g

Protein: 7g

Fiber: 1g

Sugar: 0g

Eggs with Zucchini Noodles

Preparation Time: 10 Minutes

Cooking Time: 11 Minutes

Servings: 2

Ingredients:

- 2 tablespoons extra-virgin olive oil
- 3 zucchinis, cut with a spiralizer
- 4 eggs
- Salt and black pepper to the taste
- A pinch of red pepper flakes
- Cooking spray
- 1 tablespoon basil, chopped

Directions:

1. In a bowl, combine the zucchini noodles with salt, pepper, and the olive oil, and toss well.
2. Grease a baking sheet with cooking spray and divide the zucchini noodles into 4 nests on it.
3. Crack an egg on top of each nest, sprinkle salt, pepper, and the pepper flakes on top, and bake at 350 degrees F for 11 minutes.
4. Divide the mix between plates, sprinkle the basil on top, and serve.

Nutrition:

Calories: 296

Protein: 15 g

Fat: 24 g

Carbs: 11 g

Smoked Salmon and Poached Eggs on Toast

Preparation Time: 10 Minutes

Cooking Time: 4 Minutes

Servings: 4

Ingredients:

- 2 oz avocado smashed
- 2 slices of bread toasted
- Pinch of kosher salt and cracked black pepper
- 1/4 tsp freshly squeezed lemon juice
- 2 eggs see notes, poached
- 3.5 oz smoked salmon
- 1 TBSP. thinly sliced scallions
- Splash of Kikkoman soy sauce optional
- Microgreens are optional

Directions:

1. Take a small bowl and then smash the avocado into it. Then, add the lemon juice and also a pinch of salt into the mixture. Then, mix it well and set aside.
2. After that, poach the eggs and toast the bread for some time.
3. Once the bread is toasted, you will have to spread the avocado on both slices and after that, add the smoked salmon to each slice.
4. Thereafter, carefully transfer the poached eggs to the respective toasts.
5. Add a splash of Kikkoman soy sauce and some cracked pepper; then, just garnish with scallions and microgreens.

Nutrition:

Calories: 459

Protein: 31 g

Fat: 22 g

Carbs: 33 g

Mediterranean Breakfast Salad

Preparation Time: 10 Minutes

Cooking Time: 20 Minutes

Servings: 4

Ingredients:

- 4 whole eggs
- 2 cups of cherry tomatoes or heirloom tomatoes cut in half or wedges
- 10 cups of arugula
- A 1/2 chopped seedless cucumber
- 1 large avocado
- 1 cup cooked or cooled quinoa
- 1/2 cup of chopped mixed herbs like dill and mint
- 1 cup of chopped Almonds
- 1 lemon
- extra virgin olive oil
- sea salt
- freshly ground black pepper

Directions:

1. In this recipe, the eggs are the first thing that needs to be cooked. Start with soft boiling the eggs. To do that, you need to get water in a pan and let it sit to boil. Once it starts boiling, reduces the heat to simmer and lower the eggs into the water and let them cook for about 6 minutes. After they are boiled, wash the eggs with cold water and set aside. Peel them when they are cool and ready to use.
2. Combine quinoa, arugula, cucumbers, and tomatoes in a bowl and add a little bit of olive oil over the top. Toss it with salt and pepper to equally season all of it.
3. Once all that is done, serve the salad on four plates and garnish it with sliced avocados and the halved eggs. After that, season it with some more pepper and salt.
4. To top it all off, then use almonds and sprinkle some herbs along with some lemon zest and olive oil.

Nutrition:

calories: 85

protein: 3.4 g

fat: 3.46 g

carbs: 6.71 g

Honey Almond Ricotta Spread with Peaches

Preparation Time: 5 Minutes

Cooking Time: 8 Minutes

Servings: 4

Ingredients:

- 1/2 cup Fisher Sliced Almonds
- 1 cup whole milk ricotta
- 1/4 teaspoon almond extract
- zest from an orange, optional
- 1 teaspoon honey
- hearty whole-grain toast
- English muffin or bagel
- extra Fisher sliced almonds
- sliced peaches
- extra honey for drizzling

Directions:

1. Cut peaches into a proper shape and then brush them with olive oil. After that, set it aside.
2. Take a bowl; combine the ingredients for the filling. Set aside.
3. Then just pre-heat grill to medium.
4. Place peaches cut side down onto the greased grill.
5. Close lid cover and then just grill until the peaches have softened, approximately 6-10 minutes, depending on the size of the peaches.
6. Then you will have to place peach halves onto a serving plate.
7. Put a spoon of about 1 tablespoon of ricotta mixture into the cavity (you are also allowed to use a small scooper).

8. Sprinkle it with slivered almonds, crushed amaretti cookies, and honey.
9. Decorate with the mint leaves.

Nutrition:

Calories: 187

Protein: 7 g

Fat: 9 g

Carbs: 18 g

Mediterranean Eggs Cups

Preparation Time: 10 Minutes

Cooking Time: 20 Minutes

Servings: 8

Ingredients:

- 1 cup spinach, finely diced
- 1/2 yellow onion, finely diced
- 1/2 cup sliced sun-dried tomatoes
- 4 large basil leaves, finely diced
- Pepper and salt to taste
- 1/3 cup feta cheese crumbles
- 8 large eggs
- 1/4 cup milk (any kind)

Directions:

1. You have to heat the oven to 375°F.
2. Then, roll the dough sheet into a 12x8-inch rectangle
3. Then, cut in half lengthwise
4. After that, you will have to cut each half crosswise into 4 pieces, forming 8 (4x3-inch) pieces dough. Then, press each into the bottom and up sides of the ungreased muffin cup.
5. Trim dough to keep the dough from touching, if essential. Set aside.
6. Then, you will have to combine the eggs, salt, pepper in the bowl and beat it with a whisk until well mixed. Set aside.

7. Melt the butter in 12-inch skillet over medium heat until sizzling; add bell peppers.
8. You will have to cook it, stirring occasionally, 2-3 minutes or until crisply tender.
9. After that, add spinach leaves; continue cooking until spinach is wilted. Then just add egg mixture and prosciutto.
10. Divide the mixture evenly among prepared muffin cups.
11. Finally, bake it for 14-17 minutes or until the crust is golden brown.

Nutrition:

Calories: 240

Protein: 9 g

Fat: 16 g

Carbs: 13 g

Low-Carb Baked Eggs with Avocado and Feta

Preparation Time: 10 Minutes

Cooking Time: 15 Minutes

Servings: 2

Ingredients:

- 1 avocado
- 4 eggs
- 2-3 tbsp. crumbled feta cheese
- Nonstick cooking spray
- Pepper and salt to taste

Directions:

1. First, you will have to preheat the oven to 400 degrees F.
2. After that, when the oven is on the proper temperature, you will have to put the gratin dishes right on the baking sheet.

47

3. Then, leave the dishes to heat in the oven for almost 10 minutes
4. After that process, you need to break the eggs into individual ramekins.
5. Then, let the avocado and eggs come to room temperature for at least 10 minutes
6. Then, peel the avocado properly and cut it each half into 6-8 slices
7. You will have to remove the dishes from the oven and spray them with the non-stick spray
8. Then, you will have to arrange all the sliced avocados in the dishes and tip two eggs into each dish
9. Sprinkle with feta, add pepper and salt to taste

Nutrition:

Calories: 280

Protein: 11 g

Fat: 23 g

Carbs: 10 g

Mediterranean Eggs White Breakfast Sandwich with Roasted Tomatoes

Preparation Time: 15 Minutes

Cooking Time: 10 Minutes

Servings: 2

Ingredients:

- Salt and pepper to taste
- ¼ cup egg whites
- 1 teaspoon chopped fresh herbs like rosemary, basil, parsley,
- 1 whole-grain seeded ciabatta roll
- 1 teaspoon butter
- 1-2 slices Muenster cheese
- 1 tablespoon pesto
- About ½ cup roasted tomatoes
- 10 ounces grape tomatoes
- 1 tablespoon extra-virgin olive oil
- Black pepper and salt to taste

Directions:

1. First, you will have to melt the butter over medium heat in the small nonstick skillet.
2. Then, mix the egg whites with pepper and salt.
3. Then, sprinkle it with the fresh herbs
4. After that cook it for almost 3-4 minutes or until the eggs are done, then flip it carefully
5. Meanwhile, toast ciabatta bread in the toaster
6. After that, you will have to place the egg on the bottom half of the sandwich rolls, then top with cheese
7. Add roasted tomatoes and the top half of roll.
8. To make a roasted tomato, preheat the oven to 400 degrees.
9. Then, slice the tomatoes in half lengthwise.
10. Place on the baking sheet and drizzle with olive oil.
11. Season it with pepper and salt and then roast in the oven for about 20 minutes. Skins will appear wrinkled when done.

Nutrition:

Calories: 458

Protein: 21 g

Fat: 24 g

Carbs: 51 g

Greek Yogurt Pancakes

Preparation Time: 10 Minutes

Cooking Time: 5 Minutes

Servings: 2

Ingredients:

- 1 cup all-purpose flour
- 1 cup whole-wheat flour
- 1/4 teaspoon salt
- 4 teaspoons baking powder
- 1 Tablespoon sugar
- 1 1/2 cups unsweetened almond milk
- 2 teaspoons vanilla extract
- 2 large eggs
- 1/2 cup plain 2% Greek yogurt
- Fruit, for serving
- Maple syrup, for serving

Directions:

1. First, you will have to pour the curds into the bowl and mix them well until creamy.
2. You will have to put egg whites then mix them well until combined.
3. Then take a distinct bowl, pour the wet mixture into the dry mixture. Stir to combine. The batter will be extremely thick.
4. Spoon the batter onto the sprayed pan heated to medium-high.
5. Then, you will have to flip the pancakes once when they begin to bubble a bit on the surface. Cook until golden brown on both sides.

Nutrition:

Calories: 166

Protein: 14 g

Fat: 5 g

Carbs: 52g

Mediterranean Feta and Quinoa Egg Muffins

Preparation Time: 15 Minutes

Cooking Time: 15 Minutes

Servings: 12

Ingredients:

- 2 cups baby spinach finely chopped
- 1 cup chopped or sliced cherry tomatoes
- 1/2 cup finely chopped onion
- 1 tablespoon chopped fresh oregano
- 1 cup crumbled feta cheese
- 1/2 cup chopped {pitted} kalamata olives
- 2 teaspoons high oleic sunflower oil
- 1 cup cooked quinoa
- 8 eggs
- 1/4 teaspoon salt

Directions:

1. Pre-heat oven to 350 degrees Fahrenheit
2. Make 12 silicone muffin holders on the baking sheet, or just grease a 12-cup muffin tin with oil and set aside.
3. Finely slice the vegetables
4. Heat the skillet to medium.
5. Add the vegetable oil and onions and sauté for 2 minutes.
6. Then, add tomatoes and sauté for another minute, then add spinach and sauté until wilted, about 1 minute.
7. Put the beaten egg into a bowl and then add lots of vegetables like feta cheese, quinoa, veggie mixture as well as salt, and then stir well until everything is properly combined.
8. Pour the ready mixture into greased muffin tins or silicone cups, dividing the mixture equally. Then, bake it in an oven for 30 minutes or so, or until the eggs set nicely, and the muffins turn a light golden brown in color.

Nutrition:

Calories: 113

Protein: 6 g

Fat: 7 g

Carbs: 5 g

Mediterranean Eggs

Preparation Time: 15 Minutes

Cooking Time: 20 Minutes

Servings: 2

Ingredients:

- 5 tbsp. of divided olive oil
- 2 diced medium-sized Spanish onions
- 2 diced red bell peppers
- 2 minced cloves garlic
- 1 teaspoon cumin seeds
- 4 diced large ripe tomatoes
- 1 tablespoon of honey
- Salt
- Freshly ground black pepper
- 1/3 cup crumbled feta
- 4 eggs
- 1 teaspoon zaatar spice
- Grilled pita during serving

Directions:

1. To start with, you have to add 3 tablespoons of olive oil into a pan and heat it over medium heat. Along with the oil, sauté the cumin seeds, onions, garlic, and red pepper for a few minutes.
2. After that, add the diced tomatoes and salt and pepper to taste and cook them for about 10 minutes till they come together and form a light sauce.
3. With that, half the preparation is already done. Now you just have to break the eggs directly into the sauce and poach them. However, you must keep in mind to cook the egg whites but keep the yolks still runny. This takes about 8 to 10 minutes.
4. While plating adds some feta and olive oil with zaatar spice to further enhance the flavors. Once done, serve with grilled pita.

Nutrition:

Calories: 304

Protein: 12 g

Fat: 16 g

Carbs: 28 g

Pastry-Less Spanakopita

Preparation Time: 5 Minutes

Cooking Time: 20 Minutes

Servings: 4

Ingredients:

- 1/8 teaspoons black pepper, add as per taste
- 1/3 cup of virgin olive oil
- 4 lightly beaten eggs
- 7 cups of Lettuce, preferably a spring mix (mesclun)
- 1/2 cup of crumbled Feta cheese
- 1/8 teaspoon of Sea salt, add to taste
- 1 finely chopped medium Yellow onion

Directions:

1. For this delicious recipe, you need to first start by preheating the oven to 180C and grease the flan dish.
2. Once done, pour the extra virgin olive oil into a large saucepan and heat it over medium heat with the onions, until they are translucent. To that, add greens and keep stirring until all the ingredients are wilted.
3. After completing that, you should season it with salt and pepper and transfer the greens to the prepared dish and sprinkle on some feta cheese.
4. Pour the eggs and bake it for 20 minutes till it is cooked through and slightly brown.

Nutrition:

Calories: 325

Protein: 11.2 g

Fat: 27.9 g

Carbs: 7.3 g

Date and Walnut Overnight Oats

Preparation Time: 5 Minutes

Cooking Time: 20 Minutes

Servings: 2

Ingredients:

- ¼ Cup Greek Yogurt, Plain
- 1/3 cup of yogurt
- 2/3 cup of oats
- 1 cup of milk
- 2 tsp date syrup or you can also use maple syrup or honey
- 1 mashed banana
- ¼ tsp cinnamon
- ¼ cup walnuts
- pinch of salt (approx.1/8 tsp)

Directions:

1. Firstly, get a mason jar or a small bowl and add all the ingredients.
2. After that stir and mix all the ingredients well.
3. Cover it securely, and cool it in a refrigerator overnight.
4. After that, take it out the next morning, add more liquid or cinnamon if required, and serve cold. (However, you can also microwave it for people with a warmer palate.)

Nutrition:

Calories: 350

Protein: 14 g

Fat: 12 g

Carbs: 49 g

Greek Quinoa Breakfast Bowl

Preparation Time: 10 Minutes

Cooking Time: 20 Minutes

Servings: 2

Ingredients:

- 2 large eggs
- 3/4 cup Greek yogurt
- 2 cups of cooked quinoa
- 3/4 cup muhammara
- 3 ounces of baby spinach
- 4 ounces of marinated kalamata olives
- 6 ounces of sliced cherry tomatoes
- 1 halved lemon
- hot chili oil
- salt & pepper to taste
- fresh dill and sesame seeds to garnish

Directions:

1. Add all the ingredients, Greek yogurt, granulated garlic, onion powder, salt, and pepper, and whisk them all together and set aside.
2. In a different large saucepan, heat the olive oil on medium-high heat and add the spinach. You have to keep in mind to cook the spinach till it is slightly wilted. This takes about 3-4 minutes.
3. After that, cook the cherry tomatoes in the same skillet for 3-4 minutes till they are softened.
4. Stir in the egg mixture into this for about 7 to 9 minutes, until it has set and cooked them so that they get scrambled.
5. After the eggs have set, stir in the quinoa and feta and cook until it is heated all the way through and serve it hot with some fresh dill and sesame seeds to garnish.

Nutrition:

Calories: 357

Protein: 23 g

Fat: 20 g

Carbs: 20 g

Mediterranean Frittata

Preparation Time: 8 Minutes

Cooking Time: 6 Minutes

Servings: 4

Ingredients:

- Two teaspoons of olive oil
- 3/4 cup of baby spinach, packed
- Two green onions
- Four egg whites, large
- Six large eggs
- 1/3 cup of crumbled feta cheese, (1.3 ounces) along with sun-dried tomatoes and basil
- Two teaspoons of salt-free Greek seasoning
- 1/4 teaspoon of salt

Directions:

1. Take a boiler and preheat it
2. Take a ten-inch ovenproof skillet and pour the oil into it and keep the skillet on a medium flame.
3. While the oil gets heated, chop the spinach roughly and the onions.
4. Put the eggs, egg whites, Greek seasoning, cheese, as well as salt in a large mixing bowl and mix it thoroughly using a whisker.
5. Add the chopped spinach and onions into the mixing bowl and stir it well.
6. Pour the mixture into the pan and cook it for 2 minutes or more until the edges of the mixture set well. Lift the edges of the mixture gently and tilt the pan so that the uncooked portion can get underneath it. Cook for additional two minutes so that the whole mixture gets cooked properly.
7. Broil for two to three minutes till the center gets set.
8. Your Frittata is now ready. Serve it hot by cutting it into four wedges.

Nutrition:

Calories: 178

Protein: 16 g

Fat: 12 g

Carbs: 2.2 g

Honey-Caramelized Figs with Greek Yogurt

Preparation Time: 5 Minutes

Cooking Time: 5 Minutes

Servings: 4

Ingredients:

- Four fresh halved figs
- Two tablespoons of melted butter, 30ml
- Two tablespoons of brown sugar, 30ml
- Two cups of Greek yogurt 500ml
- 1/4 cup of honey, 60ml

Directions:

1. Take a non-stick skillet and preheat it over a medium flame
2. Put the butter on the pan and toss the figs into it and sprinkle in some brown sugar over it.
3. Put the figs on the pan and cut off the side of the figs.
4. Cook the figs on a medium flame for 2-3 minutes until they turn a golden brown.
5. Turn over the figs and cook them for 2-3 minutes again

6. Remove the figs from the pan and let it cool down a little.
7. Take a plate and put a scoop of Greek yogurt on it. Put the cooked figs over the yogurts and drizzle the honey over it

Nutrition:

Calories: 350

Protein: 6 g

Fat: 19 g

Carbs: 40 g

Savory Quinoa Egg Muffins with Spinach

Preparation Time: 15 Minutes

Cooking Time: 20 Minutes

Servings: 2

Ingredients:

- One cup of quinoa
- Two cups of water/ vegetable broth)
- Four ounces of spinach which is about one cup
- Half chopped onion
- Two whole eggs
- 1/4 cup of grated cheese
- Half teaspoon of oregano or thyme
- Half teaspoon of garlic powder
- Half teaspoon of salt

Directions:

1. Take a medium saucepan and put water in it. Add the quinoa in the water and bring the whole thing to a simmer. Cover the pan and cook it for 10 minutes till the water gets absorbed by the quinoa. Remove the saucepan from the heat and let it cool down.
2. Take a nonstick pan and heat the onions till they turn soft and then add spinach. Cook all of them together till the spinach

gets a little wilted and then remove it from the heat.
3. Preheat the oven to 176.667 C
4. Take a muffin pan and grease it lightly
5. Take a large bowl and add the cooked quinoa along with the cooked onions, spinach, and add cheese, eggs, thyme or oregano, salt, garlic powder, pepper and mix them together.
6. Put a spoonful of the mixture into a muffin tin. Make sure it is ¼ of a cup.
7. In the preheated pan, put it in the pan and bake it for around 20 minutes.

Nutrition:

Calories: 61

Protein: 4 g

Fat: 3 g

Carbs: 6 g

Avocado Tomato Gouda Socca Pizza

Preparation Time: 20 Minutes

Cooking Time: 20 Minutes

Servings: 2

Ingredients:

- One and 1/4 cups of chickpea or garbanzo bean flour
- One and 1/4 cups of cold water
- 1/4 teaspoon of pepper and sea salt each
- Two teaspoons of avocado or olive oil. Take one teaspoon extra for heating the pan
- One teaspoon of minced Garlic which will be around two cloves
- One teaspoon of Onion powder/other herb seasoning powder
- Ten to twelve-inch cast iron pan
- One sliced tomato
- Half avocado

- Two ounces of thinly sliced Gouda
- 1/4-1/3 cup of Tomato sauce
- Two or three teaspoons of chopped green scallion/onion
- Sprouted greens for green
- Extra pepper/salt for sprinkling on top of the pizza
- Red pepper flakes

Directions:

1. Mix the flour with two teaspoons of olive oil, herbs, water, and whisk it until a smooth mixture form. Keep it at room temperature for around 15-20 minutes to let the batter settle
2. In the meantime, preheat the oven and place the pan inside the oven and let it get heated for around 10 minutes
3. When the pan gets preheated, chop up the vegetables into fine slices
4. Remove the pan after ten minutes using oven mitts
5. Put one teaspoon of oil and swirl it all around to coat the pan
6. Pour the batter into the pan then slant the pan so that the batter spreads evenly throughout the pan.
7. Turn down the over to 425f and place back the pan for 5-8 minutes
8. Remove the pan from the oven and add the sliced avocado, tomato and on top of that, add the gouda slices and the onion slices
9. Put the pizza into the oven then wait till the cheese get melted or the sides of the bread gets crusty and brown
10. Remove the pizza from the pan and add the microgreens on top, along with the toppings.

Nutrition:

Calories: 416

Protein: 15 g

Fat: 10 g

Carbs: 37 g

Sunny-Side Up Baked Eggs with Swiss Chard, Feta, and Basil

Preparation Time: 15 Minutes

Cooking Time: 10 Minutes

Servings: 4

Ingredients:

- 4 bell peppers, any color
- 1 tablespoon extra-virgin olive oil
- 8 large eggs
- ¾ teaspoon kosher salt, divided
- ¼ teaspoon freshly ground black pepper, divided
- 1 avocado, peeled, pitted, and diced
- ¼ cup red onion, diced
- ¼ cup fresh basil, chopped
- Juice of ½ lime

Directions:

1. Stem and seed the bell peppers. Cut 2 (2-inch-thick) rings from each pepper. Chop the remaining bell pepper into small dice and set aside.
2. Heat the olive oil in a large skillet over medium heat. Add 4 bell pepper rings, then crack 1 egg in the middle of each ring. Season with ¼ teaspoon of the salt and 1/8 teaspoon of the black pepper. Cook until the egg whites are generally set, but the yolks are still runny 2 to 3 minutes. Gently flip and cook 1 additional minute for over easy. Move the egg–bell pepper rings to a platter or onto plates and repeats with the remaining 4 bell pepper rings.
3. In a medium bowl, blend the avocado, onion, basil, lime juice, reserved diced bell pepper, the remaining ¼ teaspoon kosher salt, and the remaining 1/8

teaspoon black pepper. Divide among the 4 plates.

Nutrition:

Calories: 270

Protein: 15 g

Fat: 19 g

Carbs: 12 g

Polenta with Sautéed Chard and Fried Eggs

Preparation Time: 5 Minutes

Cooking Time: 20 Minutes

Servings: 4

Ingredients:

- 2½ cups water
- ½ teaspoon kosher salt
- ¾ cups whole-grain cornmeal
- ¼ teaspoon freshly ground black pepper
- 2 tablespoons grated Parmesan cheese
- 1 tablespoon extra-virgin olive oil
- 1 bunch (about 6 ounces) Swiss chard, leaves and stems chopped and separated
- 2 garlic cloves, sliced
- ¼ teaspoon kosher salt
- 1/8 teaspoon freshly ground black pepper
- Lemon juice (optional)
- 1 tablespoon extra-virgin olive oil
- 4 large eggs

Directions:

TO MAKE THE POLENTA

1. Le the water and salt to boil in a medium saucepan over high heat.

Slowly add the cornmeal, whisking constantly.
2. Decrease the heat to low, cover, and cook for 10 to 15 minutes, stirring often to avoid lumps. Stir in the pepper and Parmesan and divide among 4 bowls.

TO MAKE THE CHARD

1. Heat the oil in a large frying pan on medium heat. Add the chard stems, garlic, salt, and pepper; sauté for 2 minutes. Add the chard leaves and cook until wilted, about 3 to 5 minutes.
2. Add a spritz of lemon juice (if desired), toss together, and divide evenly on top of the polenta.

TO MAKE THE EGGS

1. Heat the oil in the same large skillet over medium-high heat. Crack each egg into the skillet, taking care not to crowd the skillet and leaving space between the eggs. Cook until the whites are set and golden around the edges, about 2 to 3 minutes.
2. Serve sunny-side up or flip the eggs over carefully and cook 1 minute longer for over easy. Put one egg on top of the polenta and chard in each bowl.

Nutrition:

Calories: 310

Protein: 17 g

Fat: 18 g

Carbs: 21 g

Smoked Salmon Egg Scramble with Dill and Chives

Preparation Time: 5 Minutes

Cooking Time: 5 Minutes

Servings: 2

Ingredients:

- 4 large eggs
- 1 tablespoon milk
- 1 tablespoon fresh chives, minced
- 1 tablespoon fresh dill, minced
- ¼ teaspoon kosher salt
- 1/8 teaspoon freshly ground black pepper
- 2 teaspoons extra-virgin olive oil
- 2 ounces smoked salmon, thinly sliced

Directions:

1. In a large bowl, blend together the eggs, milk, chives, dill, salt, and pepper.
2. Heat the olive oil in a medium skillet or sauté pan over medium heat. Add the egg mixture and cook for about 3 minutes, stirring occasionally.
3. Add the salmon and cook until the eggs are set but moist about 1 minute.

Nutrition:

Calories: 325

Protein: 23 g

Fat: 26 g

Carbs: 1 g

Chapter 6: Soup and Salad Recipes

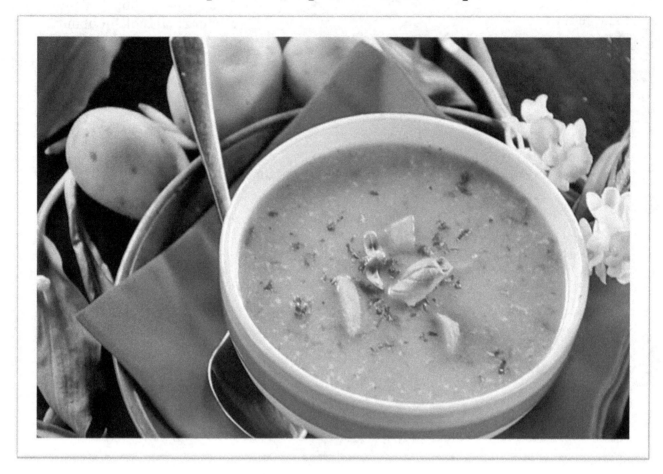

Classic Lentil Soup with Swiss Chard

Preparation time: 10 minutes

Cooking Time: 25 minutes

Servings: 5

Ingredients:

- 2 tablespoons olive oil
- 1 white onion, chopped
- 1 teaspoon garlic, minced
- 2 large carrots, chopped
- 1 parsnip, chopped
- 2 stalks celery, chopped
- 2 bay leaves
- 1/2 teaspoon dried thyme
- 1/4 teaspoon ground cumin
- 5 cups roasted vegetable broth
- 1 ¼ cups brown lentils, soaked overnight and rinsed
- 2 cups Swiss chard, torn into pieces

Directions:

1. In a heavy-bottomed pot, heat the olive oil over a moderate heat. Now, sauté the vegetables along with the spices for about 3 minutes until they are just tender.

2. Add in the vegetable broth and lentils, bringing it to a boil. Immediately turn the heat to a simmer and add in the bay leaves. Let it cook for about 15 minutes or until lentils are tender.

3. Add in the Swiss chard, cover and let it simmer for 5 minutes more or until the chard wilts.

4. Serve in individual bowls and enjoy!

Nutrition: Calories: 148; Fat: 7.2g; Carbs: 14.6g; Protein: 7.7g

Spicy Winter Farro Soup

Preparation time: 10 minutes

Cooking Time: 30 minutes

Servings: 4

Ingredients:

- 2 tablespoons olive oil
- 1 medium-sized leek, chopped
- 1 medium-sized turnip, sliced
- 2 Italian peppers, seeded and chopped
- 1 jalapeno pepper, minced
- 2 potatoes, peeled and diced
- 4 cups vegetable broth
- 1 cup farro, rinsed
- 1/2 teaspoon granulated garlic
- 1/2 teaspoon turmeric powder
- 1 bay laurel
- 2 cups spinach, turn into pieces

Directions:

1. In a heavy-bottomed pot, heat the olive oil over a moderate heat. Now, sauté the leek, turnip, peppers and potatoes for about 5 minutes until they are crisp-tender.

2. Add in the vegetable broth, farro, granulated garlic, turmeric and bay laurel; bring it to a boil.

3. Immediately turn the heat to a simmer. Let it cook for about 25 minutes or until farro and potatoes have softened.

4. Add in the spinach and remove the pot from the heat; let the spinach sit in the residual heat until it wilts. Bon appétit!

Nutrition: Calories: 298; Fat: 8.9g; Carbs: 44.6g; Protein: 11.7g

Rainbow Chickpea Salad

Preparation time: 10 minutes

Cooking Time: 30 minutes

Servings: 4

Ingredients:

- 16 ounces canned chickpeas, drained
- 1 medium avocado, sliced
- 1 bell pepper, seeded and sliced
- 1 large tomato, sliced
- 2 cucumber, diced
- 1 red onion, sliced
- 1/2 teaspoon garlic, minced
- 1/4 cup fresh parsley, chopped
- 1/4 cup olive oil
- 2 tablespoons apple cider vinegar
- 1/2 lime, freshly squeezed
- Sea salt and ground black pepper, to taste

Directions:

1. Toss all the Ingredients in a salad bowl.

2. Place the salad in your refrigerator for about 1 hour before serving.

3. Bon appétit!

Nutrition: Calories: 378; Fat: 24g; Carbs: 34.2g; Protein: 10.1g

Mediterranean-Style Lentil Salad

Preparation time: 10 minutes

Cooking Time: 20 minutes + chilling time

Servings: 5

Ingredients:

- 1 ½ cups red lentil, rinsed
- 1 teaspoon deli mustard
- 1/2 lemon, freshly squeezed
- 2 tablespoons tamari sauce
- 2 scallion stalks, chopped
- 1/4 cup extra-virgin olive oil
- 2 garlic cloves, minced
- 1 cup butterhead lettuce, torn into pieces
- 2 tablespoons fresh parsley, chopped
- 2 tablespoons fresh cilantro, chopped
- 1 teaspoon fresh basil
- 1 teaspoon fresh oregano
- 1 ½ cups cherry tomatoes, halved
- 3 ounces Kalamata olives, pitted and halved

Directions:

1. In a large-sized saucepan, bring 4 ½ cups of the water and the red lentils to a boil.

2. Immediately turn the heat to a simmer and continue to cook your lentils for about 15 minutes or until tender. Drain and let it cool completely.

3. Transfer the lentils to a salad bowl; toss the lentils with the remaining Ingredients until well combined.

4. Serve chilled or at room temperature. Bon appétit!

Nutrition: Calories: 348; Fat: 15g; Carbs: 41.6g; Protein: 15.8g

Roasted Asparagus and Avocado Salad

Preparation time: 10 minutes

Cooking Time: 20 minutes + chilling time

Servings: 4

Ingredients:

- 1 pound asparagus, trimmed, cut into bite-sized pieces
- 1 white onion, chopped
- 2 garlic cloves, minced
- 1 Roma tomato, sliced
- 1/4 cup olive oil
- 1/4 cup balsamic vinegar
- 1 tablespoon stone-ground mustard
- 2 tablespoons fresh parsley, chopped
- 1 tablespoon fresh cilantro, chopped
- 1 tablespoon fresh basil, chopped
- Sea salt and ground black pepper, to taste
- 1 small avocado, pitted and diced
- 1/2 cup pine nuts, roughly chopped

Directions:

1. Begin by preheating your oven to 420 degrees F.

2. Toss the asparagus with 1 tablespoon of the olive oil and arrange them on a parchment-lined roasting pan.

3. Bake for about 15 minutes, rotating the pan once or twice to promote even cooking. Let it cool completely and place in your salad bowl.

4. Toss the asparagus with the vegetables, olive oil, vinegar, mustard and herbs. Salt and pepper to taste.

5. Toss to combine and top with avocado and pine nuts. Bon appétit!

Nutrition: Calories: 378; Fat: 33.2g; Carbs: 18.6g; Protein: 7.8g

Creamed Green Bean Salad with Pine Nuts

Preparation time: 10 minutes

Cooking Time: 10 minutes + chilling time

Servings: 5

Ingredients:

- 1 ½ pounds green beans, trimmed
- 2 medium tomatoes, diced
- 2 bell peppers, seeded and diced
- 4 tablespoons shallots, chopped
- 1/2 cup pine nuts, roughly chopped
- 1/2 cup vegan mayonnaise
- 1 tablespoon deli mustard
- 2 tablespoons fresh basil, chopped
- 2 tablespoons fresh parsley, chopped
- 1/2 teaspoon red pepper flakes, crushed

- Sea salt and freshly ground black pepper, to taste

Directions:

1. Boil the green beans in a large saucepan of salted water until they are just tender or about 2 minutes.

2. Drain and let the beans cool completely; then, transfer them to a salad bowl. Toss the beans with the remaining ingredients.

3. Taste and adjust the seasonings. Bon appétit!

Nutrition: Calories: 308; Fat: 26.2g; Carbs: 16.6g; Protein: 5.8g

Cannellini Bean Soup with Kale

Preparation time: 10 minutes

Cooking Time: 25 minutes

Servings: 5

Ingredients:

- 1 tablespoon olive oil
- 1/2 teaspoon ginger, minced
- 1/2 teaspoon cumin seeds
- 1 red onion, chopped
- 1 carrot, trimmed and chopped
- 1 parsnip, trimmed and chopped
- 2 garlic cloves, minced
- 5 cups vegetable broth
- 12 ounces Cannellini beans, drained
- 2 cups kale, torn into pieces
- Sea salt and ground black pepper, to taste

Directions:

1. In a heavy-bottomed pot, heat the olive over medium-high heat. Now, sauté the ginger and cumin for 1 minute or so.

2. Now, add in the onion, carrot and parsnip; continue sautéing an additional 3 minutes or until the vegetables are just tender.

3. Add in the garlic and continue to sauté for 1 minute or until aromatic.

4. Then, pour in the vegetable broth and bring to a boil. Immediately reduce the heat to a simmer and let it cook for 10 minutes.

5. Fold in the Cannellini beans and kale; continue to simmer until the kale wilts and everything is thoroughly heated. Season with salt and pepper to taste.

6. Ladle into individual bowls and serve hot. Bon appétit!

Nutrition: Calories: 188; Fat: 4.7g; Carbs: 24.5g; Protein: 11.1g

Hearty Cream of Mushroom Soup

Preparation time: 10 minutes

Cooking Time: 15 minutes

Servings: 5

Ingredients:

- 2 tablespoons soy butter
- 1 large shallot, chopped
- 20 ounces Cremini mushrooms, sliced
- 2 cloves garlic, minced
- 4 tablespoons flaxseed meal
- 5 cups vegetable broth

- 1 1/3 cups full-fat coconut milk

- 1 bay leaf

- Sea salt and ground black pepper, to taste

Directions:

1. In a stockpot, melt the vegan butter over medium-high heat. Once hot, cook the shallot for about 3 minutes until tender and fragrant.

2. Add in the mushrooms and garlic and continue cooking until the mushrooms have softened. Add in the flaxseed meal and continue to cook for 1 minute or so.

3. Add in the remaining ingredients. Let it simmer, covered and continue to cook for 5 to 6 minutes more until your soup has thickened slightly.

4. Bon appétit!

Nutrition: Calories: 308; Fat: 25.5g; Carbs: 11.8g; Protein: 11.6g

Authentic Italian Panzanella Salad

Preparation time: 10 minutes

Cooking Time: 35 minutes

Servings: 3

Ingredients:

- 3 cups artisan bread, broken into 1-inch cubes

- 3/4-pound asparagus, trimmed and cut into bite-sized pieces

- 4 tablespoons extra-virgin olive oil

- 1 red onion, chopped

- 2 tablespoons fresh lime juice

- 1 teaspoon deli mustard

- 2 medium heirloom tomatoes, diced

- 2 cups arugula

- 2 cups baby spinach

- 2 Italian peppers, seeded and sliced

- Sea salt and ground black pepper, to taste

Directions:

1. Arrange the bread cubes on a parchment-lined baking sheet. Bake in the preheated oven at 310 degrees F for about 20 minutes, rotating the baking sheet twice during the baking time; reserve.

2. Turn the oven to 420 degrees F and toss the asparagus with 1 tablespoon of olive oil. Roast the asparagus for about 15 minutes or until crisp-tender.

3. Toss the remaining Ingredients in a salad bowl; top with the roasted asparagus and toasted bread.

4. Bon appétit!

Nutrition: Calories: 334; Fat: 20.4g; Carbs: 33.3g; Protein: 8.3g

Quinoa and Black Bean Salad

Preparation time: 10 minutes

Cooking Time: 15 minutes + chilling time

Servings: 4

Ingredients:

- 2 cups water

- 1 cup quinoa, rinsed

- 16 ounces canned black beans, drained

- 2 Roma tomatoes, sliced

- 1 red onion, thinly sliced
- 1 cucumber, seeded and chopped
- 2 cloves garlic, pressed or minced
- 2 Italian peppers, seeded and sliced
- 2 tablespoons fresh parsley, chopped
- 2 tablespoons fresh cilantro, chopped
- 1/4 cup olive oil
- 1 lemon, freshly squeezed
- 1 tablespoon apple cider vinegar
- 1/2 teaspoon dried dill weed
- 1/2 teaspoon dried oregano
- Sea salt and ground black pepper, to taste

Directions:

1. Place the water and quinoa in a saucepan and bring it to a rolling boil. Immediately turn the heat to a simmer.

2. Let it simmer for about 13 minutes until the quinoa has absorbed all of the water; fluff the quinoa with a fork and let it cool completely. Then, transfer the quinoa to a salad bowl.

3. Add the remaining Ingredients to the salad bowl and toss to combine well. Bon appétit!

Nutrition: Calories: 433; Fat: 17.3g; Carbs: 57g; Protein: 15.1g

Rich Bulgur Salad with Herbs

Preparation time: 10 minutes

Cooking Time: 20 minutes + chilling time

Servings: 4

Ingredients:

- 2 cups water
- 1 cup bulgur
- 12 ounces canned chickpeas, drained
- 1 Persian cucumber, thinly sliced
- 2 bell peppers, seeded and thinly sliced
- 1 jalapeno pepper, seeded and thinly sliced
- 2 Roma tomatoes, sliced
- 1 onion, thinly sliced
- 2 tablespoons fresh basil, chopped
- 2 tablespoons fresh parsley, chopped
- 2 tablespoons fresh mint, chopped
- 2 tablespoons fresh chives, chopped
- 4 tablespoons olive oil
- 1 tablespoon balsamic vinegar
- 1 tablespoon lemon juice
- 1 teaspoon fresh garlic, pressed
- Sea salt and freshly ground black pepper, to taste
- 2 tablespoons nutritional yeast
- 1/2 cup Kalamata olives, sliced

Directions:

1. In a saucepan, bring the water and bulgur to a boil. Immediately turn the heat to a simmer and let it cook for about 20 minutes or until the bulgur is tender and water is almost absorbed. Fluff with a fork and spread on a large tray to let cool.

2. Place the bulgur in a salad bowl followed by the chickpeas, cucumber, peppers, tomatoes, onion, basil, parsley, mint and chives.

3. In a small mixing dish, whisk the olive oil, balsamic vinegar, lemon juice, garlic, salt and black pepper. Dress the salad and toss to combine.

4. Sprinkle nutritional yeast over the top, garnish with olives and serve at room temperature. Bon appétit!

Nutrition: Calories: 408; Fat: 18.3g; Carbs: 51.8g; Protein: 13.1g

Classic Roasted Pepper Salad

Preparation time: 10 minutes

Cooking Time: 15 minutes + chilling time

Servings: 3

Ingredients:

- 6 bell peppers

- 3 tablespoons extra-virgin olive oil

- 3 teaspoons red wine vinegar

- 3 garlic cloves, finely chopped

- 2 tablespoons fresh parsley, chopped

- Sea salt and freshly cracked black pepper, to taste

- 1/2 teaspoon red pepper flakes

- 6 tablespoons pine nuts, roughly chopped

Directions:

1. Broil the peppers on a parchment-lined baking sheet for about 10 minutes, rotating the pan halfway through the cooking time, until they are charred on all sides.

2. Then, cover the peppers with a plastic wrap to steam. Discard the skin, seeds and cores.

3. Slice the peppers into strips and toss them with the remaining ingredients. Place in your refrigerator until ready to serve. Bon appétit!

Nutrition: Calories: 178; Fat: 14.4g; Carbs: 11.8g; Protein: 2.4g

Hearty Winter Quinoa Soup

Preparation time: 10 minutes

Cooking Time: 25 minutes

Servings: 4

Ingredients:

- 2 tablespoons olive oil

- 1 onion, chopped

- 2 carrots, peeled and chopped

- 1 parsnip, chopped

- 1 celery stalk, chopped

- 1 cup yellow squash, chopped

- 4 garlic cloves, pressed or minced

- 4 cups roasted vegetable broth

- 2 medium tomatoes, crushed

- 1 cup quinoa

- Sea salt and ground black pepper, to taste

- 1 bay laurel

- 2 cup Swiss chard, tough ribs removed and torn into pieces

- 2 tablespoons Italian parsley, chopped

Directions:

1. In a heavy-bottomed pot, heat the olive over medium-high heat. Now, sauté the onion, carrot, parsnip, celery and yellow squash for about 3 minutes or until the vegetables are just tender.

2. Add in the garlic and continue to sauté for 1 minute or until aromatic.

3. Then, stir in the vegetable broth, tomatoes, quinoa, salt, pepper and bay laurel; bring to a boil. Immediately reduce the heat to a simmer and let it cook for 13 minutes.

4. Fold in the Swiss chard; continue to simmer until the chard wilts.

5. Ladle into individual bowls and serve garnished with the fresh parsley. Bon appétit!

Nutrition: Calories: 328; Fat: 11.1g; Carbs: 44.1g; Protein: 13.3g

Green Lentil Salad

Preparation time: 10 minutes

Cooking Time: 20 minutes + chilling time

Servings: 5

Ingredients:

- 1 ½ cups green lentils, rinsed

- 2 cups arugula

- 2 cups Romaine lettuce, torn into pieces

- 1 cup baby spinach

- 1/4 cup fresh basil, chopped

- 1/2 cup shallots, chopped

- 2 garlic cloves, finely chopped

- 1/4 cup oil-packed sun-dried tomatoes, rinsed and chopped

- 5 tablespoons extra-virgin olive oil

- 3 tablespoons fresh lemon juice

- Sea salt and ground black pepper, to taste

Directions:

1. In a large-sized saucepan, bring 4 ½ cups of the water and red lentils to a boil.

2. Immediately turn the heat to a simmer and continue to cook your lentils for a further 15 to 17 minutes or until they've softened but not mushy. Drain and let it cool completely.

3. Transfer the lentils to a salad bowl; toss the lentils with the remaining Ingredients until well combined.

4. Serve chilled or at room temperature. Bon appétit!

Nutrition: Calories: 349; Fat: 15.1g; Carbs: 40.9g; Protein: 15.4g

Acorn Squash, Chickpea and Couscous Soup

Preparation time: 10 minutes

Cooking Time: 20 minutes

Servings: 4

Ingredients:

- 2 tablespoons olive oil

- 1 shallot, chopped

- 1 carrot, trimmed and chopped

- 2 cups acorn squash, chopped

- 1 stalk celery, chopped

- 1 teaspoon garlic, finely chopped

- 1 teaspoon dried rosemary, chopped
- 1 teaspoon dried thyme, chopped
- 2 cups cream of onion soup
- 2 cups water
- 1 cup dry couscous
- Sea salt and ground black pepper, to taste
- 1/2 teaspoon red pepper flakes
- 6 ounces canned chickpeas, drained
- 2 tablespoons fresh lemon juice

Directions:

1. In a heavy-bottomed pot, heat the olive over medium-high heat. Now, sauté the shallot, carrot, acorn squash and celery for about 3 minutes or until the vegetables are just tender.

2. Add in the garlic, rosemary and thyme and continue to sauté for 1 minute or until aromatic.

3. Then, stir in the soup, water, couscous, salt, black pepper and red pepper flakes; bring to a boil. Immediately reduce the heat to a simmer and let it cook for 12 minutes.

4. Fold in the canned chickpeas; continue to simmer until heated through or about 5 minutes more.

5. Ladle into individual bowls and drizzle with the lemon juice over the top. Bon appétit!

Nutrition: Calories: 378; Fat: 11g; Carbs: 60.1g; Protein: 10.9g

Cabbage Soup with Garlic Crostini

Preparation time: 10 minutes

Cooking Time: 1 hour

Servings: 4

Ingredients:

Soup:

- 2 tablespoons olive oil
- 1 medium leek, chopped
- 1 cup turnip, chopped
- 1 parsnip, chopped
- 1 carrot, chopped
- 2 cups cabbage, shredded
- 2 garlic cloves, finely chopped
- 4 cups vegetable broth
- 2 bay leaves
- Sea salt and ground black pepper, to taste
- 1/4 teaspoon cumin seeds
- 1/2 teaspoon mustard seeds
- 1 teaspoon dried basil
- 2 tomatoes, pureed

Crostini:

- 8 slices of baguette
- 2 heads garlic
- 4 tablespoons extra-virgin olive oil

Directions:

1. In a soup pot, heat 2 tablespoons of the olive over medium-high heat. Now, sauté the leek, turnip, parsnip and

carrot for about 4 minutes or until the vegetables are crisp-tender.

2. Add in the garlic and cabbage and continue to sauté for 1 minute or until aromatic.

3. Then, stir in the vegetable broth, bay leaves, salt, black pepper, cumin seeds, mustard seeds, dried basil and pureed tomatoes; bring to a boil. Immediately reduce the heat to a simmer and let it cook for about 20 minutes.

4. Meanwhile, preheat your oven to 375 degrees F. Now, roast the garlic and baguette slices for about 15 minutes. Remove the crostini from the oven.

5. Continue baking the garlic for 45 minutes more or until very tender. Allow the garlic to cool.

6. Now, cut each head of the garlic using a sharp serrated knife in order to separate all the cloves.

7. Squeeze the roasted garlic cloves out of their skins. Mash the garlic pulp with 4 tablespoons of the extra-virgin olive oil.

8. Spread the roasted garlic mixture evenly on the tops of the crostini. Serve with the warm soup. Bon appétit!

Nutrition: Calories: 408; Fat: 23.1g; Carbs: 37.6g; Protein: 11.8g

Cream of Green Bean Soup

Preparation time: 10 minutes

Cooking Time: 35 minutes

Servings: 4

Ingredients:

- 1 tablespoon sesame oil

- 1 onion, chopped

- 1 green pepper, seeded and chopped

- 2 russet potatoes, peeled and diced

- 2 garlic cloves, chopped

- 4 cups vegetable broth

- 1-pound green beans, trimmed

- Sea salt and ground black pepper, to season

- 1 cup full-fat coconut milk

Directions:

1. In a heavy-bottomed pot, heat the sesame over medium-high heat. Now, sauté the onion, peppers and potatoes for about 5 minutes, stirring periodically.

2. Add in the garlic and continue sautéing for 1 minute or until fragrant.

3. Then, stir in the vegetable broth, green beans, salt and black pepper; bring to a boil. Immediately reduce the heat to a simmer and let it cook for 20 minutes.

4. Puree the green bean mixture using an immersion blender until creamy and uniform.

5. Return the pureed mixture to the pot. Fold in the coconut milk and continue to simmer until heated through or about 5 minutes longer.

6. Ladle into individual bowls and serve hot. Bon appétit!

Nutrition: Calories: 410; Fat: 19.6g; Carbs: 50.6g; Protein: 13.3g

Traditional French Onion Soup

Preparation time: 10 minutes

Cooking Time: 1 hour 30 minutes

Servings: 4

Ingredients:

- 2 tablespoons olive oil
- 2 large yellow onions, thinly sliced
- 2 thyme sprigs, chopped
- 2 rosemary sprigs, chopped
- 2 teaspoons balsamic vinegar
- 4 cups vegetable stock
- Sea salt and ground black pepper, to taste

Directions:

1. In a or Dutch oven, heat the olive oil over a moderate heat. Now, cook the onions with thyme, rosemary and 1 teaspoon of the sea salt for about 2 minutes.

2. Now, turn the heat to medium-low and continue cooking until the onions caramelize or about 50 minutes.

3. Add in the balsamic vinegar and continue to cook for a further 15 more. Add in the stock, salt and black pepper and continue simmering for 20 to 25 minutes.

4. Serve with toasted bread and enjoy!

Nutrition: Calories: 129; Fat: 8.6g; Carbs: 7.4g; Protein: 6.3g

Roasted Carrot Soup

Preparation time: 10 minutes

Cooking Time: 50 minutes

Servings: 4

Ingredients:

- 1 ½ pounds carrots
- 4 tablespoons olive oil
- 1 yellow onion, chopped
- 2 cloves garlic, minced
- 1/3 teaspoon ground cumin
- Sea salt and white pepper, to taste
- 1/2 teaspoon turmeric powder
- 4 cups vegetable stock
- 2 teaspoons lemon juice
- 2 tablespoons fresh cilantro, roughly chopped

Directions:

1. Start by preheating your oven to 400 degrees F. Place the carrots on a large parchment-lined baking sheet; toss the carrots with 2 tablespoons of the olive oil.

2. Roast the carrots for about 35 minutes or until they've softened.

3. In a heavy-bottomed pot, heat the remaining 2 tablespoons of the olive oil. Now, sauté the onion and garlic for about 3 minutes or until aromatic.

4. Add in the cumin, salt, pepper, turmeric, vegetable stock and roasted carrots. Continue to simmer for 12 minutes more.

5. Puree your soup with an immersion blender. Drizzle lemon juice over your soup and serve garnished with fresh cilantro leaves. Bon appétit!

Nutrition: Calories: 264; Fat: 18.6g; Carbs: 20.1g; Protein: 7.4g

Italian Penne Pasta Salad

Preparation time: 10 minutes

Cooking Time: 15 minutes + chilling time

Servings: 3

Ingredients:

- 9 ounces penne pasta
- 9 ounces canned Cannellini bean, drained
- 1 small onion, thinly sliced
- 1/3 cup Niçoise olives, pitted and sliced
- 2 Italian peppers, sliced
- 1 cup cherry tomatoes, halved
- 3 cups arugula
- Dressing:
- 3 tablespoons extra-virgin olive oil
- 1 teaspoon lemon zest
- 1 teaspoon garlic, minced
- 3 tablespoons balsamic vinegar
- 1 teaspoon Italian herb mix
- Sea salt and ground black pepper, to taste

Directions:

1. Cook the penne pasta according to the package Directions. Drain and rinse the pasta. Let it cool completely and then, transfer it to a salad bowl.

2. Then, add the beans, onion, olives, peppers, tomatoes and arugula to the salad bowl.

3. Mix all the dressing Ingredients until everything is well incorporated. Dress

your salad and serve well-chilled. Bon appétit!

Nutrition: Calories: 614; Fat: 18.1g; Carbs: 101g; Protein: 15.4g

Arugula with Fruits and Nuts

Preparation Time: 10 Minutes

Cooking Time: 0 Minutes

Servings: 1

Ingredients:

- ½ cup arugula
- ½ peach
- ½ red onion
- ¼ cup blueberries
- 5 walnuts, chopped
- 1 tbsp. extra-virgin olive oil
- 2 tbsp. red wine vinegar
- 1 spring of fresh basil

Directions:

1. Halve the peach and remove the seed. Heat a grill pan and grill it briefly on both sides. Cut the red onion into thin half-rings. Roughly chop the pecans.
2. Heat a pan and roast the pecans in it until they are fragrant.
3. Place the arugula on a plate and spread peaches, red onions, blueberries, and roasted pecans over it.
4. Put all the ingredients for the dressing in a food processor and mix to an even dressing. Drizzle the dressing over the salad.

Nutrition:

Calories: 160

Fat: 7g

Carbohydrate: 25g

Protein: 3g

Broccoli Salad

Preparation Time: 25 Minutes

Cooking Time: 0 Minutes

Servings: 2

Ingredients:

- 1 head of broccoli
- 1/2 red onion
- 2 carrots, grated
- ¼ cup red grapes
- 2 1/2 tbsp. Coconut yogurt
- 1 tbsp. Water
- 1 tsp. mustard
- 1 pinch salt

Directions:

1. Cut the broccoli into florets and cook for 8 minutes. Cut the red onion into thin half-rings. Halve the grapes. Mix coconut yogurt, water, and mustard with a pinch of salt to make the dressing.
2. Drain the broccoli and rinse with ice-cold water to stop the cooking process.
3. Mix the broccoli with the carrot, onion, and red grapes in a bowl. Serve the dressing separately on the side.

Nutrition:

Calories: 230

Fat: 18g

Carbohydrate: 35g

Protein: 10g

Brunoise Salad

Preparation Time: 10 Minutes

Cooking Time: 0 Minutes

Servings: 2

Ingredients:

- 1 tomato
- 1 zucchini
- ½ red bell pepper
- ½ yellow bell pepper
- ½ red onion
- 3 springs fresh parsley
- ½ lemon
- 2 tbsp. olive oil

Directions:

1. Finely dice tomatoes, zucchini, peppers, and red onions to get a brunoise. Mix all the cubes in a bowl. Chop parsley and mix in the salad. Squeeze the lemon over the salad and add the olive oil.
2. Season with salt and pepper.

Nutrition:

Calories: 84

Carbohydrate: 3g

Fat: 4g

Protein: 0g

Brussels Sprouts and Ricotta Salad

Preparation Time: 15 Minutes

Cooking Time: 0 Minutes

Servings: 2

Ingredients:

- 1 ½ cups Brussels sprouts, thinly sliced
- 1 green apple cut "à la julienne."
- ½ red onion
- 8 walnuts, chopped
- 1 tsp. extra-virgin olive oil
- 1 tbsp. lemon juice
- 1 tbsp. orange juice
- 4 oz. ricotta cheese

Directions:

1. Put the red onion in a cup and cover it with boiling water. Let it rest 10 minutes, then drain and pat with kitchen paper. Slice Brussels sprouts as thin as you can, cut the apple à la julienne (sticks).
2. Mix Brussels sprouts, onion, and apple and season them with oil, salt, pepper, lemon juice, and orange juice and spread it on a serving plate.
3. Spread small spoonful of ricotta cheese over Brussels sprouts mixture and top with chopped walnuts.

Nutrition:

Calories: 353,

Fat: 4.8g,

Carbohydrate: 28.1g,

Protein: 28.3g

Celery and Raisins Snack Salad

Preparation Time: 10 Minutes

Cooking Time: 0 Minutes

Servings: 4

Ingredients:

- ½ cup raisins
- 4 cups celery, sliced
- ¼ cup parsley, chopped
- ½ cup walnuts, chopped
- Juice of ½ lemon
- 2 tbsp. olive oil
- Salt and black pepper to taste

Directions:

1. In a salad bowl, mix celery with raisins, walnuts, parsley, lemon juice, oil, and black pepper, toss.
2. Divide into small cups and serve as a snack.

Nutrition:

Calories 120 kcal,

Fat 1g,

Carbohydrate 6g,

Protein 5g

Dijon Celery Salad

Preparation Time: 10 Minutes

Cooking Time: 0 Minutes

Servings: 4

Ingredients:

- ½ cup lemon juice
- 1/3 cup Dijon mustard
- 2/3 cup olive oil
- Black pepper to taste
- 2 apples, cored, peeled, and cubed
- 1 bunch celery roughly chopped
- ¾ cup walnuts, chopped

Directions:

1. In a salad bowl, mix celery and its leaves with apple pieces and walnuts.
2. Add black pepper, lemon juice, mustard, and olive oil, whisk well, add to your salad, toss, divide into small cups and serve.

Nutrition:

Calories 125 kcal,

Fat 2g,

Carbohydrate 7g,

Protein 7g

Fresh Endive Salad

Preparation Time: 10 Minutes

Cooking Time: 0 Minutes

Servings: 1

Ingredients:

- ½ red endive
- 1 orange
- 1 tomato
- 1/2 cucumber
- 1/2 red onion

Directions:

1. Cut off the hard stem of the endive and remove the leaves. Peel the orange and cut the pulp into wedges.
2. Cut the tomatoes and cucumbers into small pieces. Cut the red onion into thin half-rings.
3. Place the endive boats on a plate; spread the orange wedges, tomato, cucumber, and red onion over the boats. Drizzle some olive oil and fresh lemon juice and serve.

Nutrition:

Calories: 112

Fat: 11g

Carbohydrate: 2g

Protein: 0g

Fresh Salad with Orange Dressing

Preparation Time: 10 Minutes

Cooking Time: 0 Minutes

Servings: 2

Ingredients:

- ½ cup lettuce
- 1 yellow bell pepper
- 1 red pepper
- 4 oz. carrot, grated
- 10 almonds
- 4 tbsp. extra-virgin olive oil
- ½ cup orange juice
- 1 tbsp. apple cider vinegar

Directions:

1. Clean the peppers and cut them into long thin strips. Tear off the lettuce leaves and cut them into smaller pieces.
2. Mix the salad with the peppers and the carrots in a bowl. Roughly chop the almonds and sprinkle over the salad.
3. Mix all the ingredients for the dressing in a bowl. Pour over the salad just before serving.

Nutrition:

Calories: 150

Fat: 10g

Carbohydrate: 11g

Protein: 2g

Greek Salad Skewers

Preparation Time: 10 Minutes

Cooking Time: 0 Minutes

Servings: 2

Ingredients:

- 8 big black olives
- 8 cherry tomatoes
- 1 yellow pepper, cut into 8 squares
- ½ red onion, split into 8 wedges
- 1 cucumber, cut into 8 pieces
- 4 oz. feta, cut into 8 cubes
- 1 tbsp. extra-virgin olive oil
- Juice of 1/2 lemon
- 1 tsp. balsamic vinegar
- 1/2 tsp. garlic, crushed

Directions:

1. Put the salad ingredients on the skewers following this order: cherry

tomato, yellow pepper, red onion, cucumber, feta, black olive.
2. Repeat for each skewer and put on a serving plate.
3. As a dressing, put in a bowl: olive oil, a pinch of salt and pepper, lemon juice, balsamic vinegar, and crushed garlic. Whisk well and drizzle on the skewers.

Nutrition:

Calories: 236kcal

Fat: 21g

Carbohydrate: 14g

Protein: 7g

Moroccan Leeks Snack Salad

Preparation Time: 10 Minutes

Cooking Time: 0 Minutes

Servings: 4

Ingredients:

- 1 bunch radishes, sliced
- 3 cups leeks, chopped
- 1 ½ cups olives, pitted and sliced
- A pinch of turmeric powder
- 1 cup parsley, chopped
- 2 tbsp. extra-virgin olive oil

Directions:

1. In a bowl, mix radishes with leeks, olives, and parsley.
2. Add black pepper, oil, and turmeric, toss to coat, and serve.

Nutrition:

Calories 135kcal,

Fat 1g,

Carbohydrate18g,

Protein 9g

Mung Beans Snack Salad

Preparation Time: 10 Minutes

Cooking Time: 0 Minutes

Servings: 6

Ingredients:

- 2 cups tomatoes, chopped
- 2 cups cucumber, chopped
- 2 cups mung beans, sprouted
- 2 cups clover sprouts
- 1 tbsp. cumin, ground
- 1 cup dill, chopped
- 4 tbsp. lemon juice
- 1 avocado, pitted and roughly chopped
- 1 cucumber, roughly chopped

Directions:

1. In a salad bowl, mix tomatoes with 2 cups cucumber, greens, clover, and mung sprouts.
2. In your blender, mix cumin with dill, lemon juice, 1 cup of cucumber, and avocado, blend well, add this to your salad, toss well and serve.

Nutrition:

Calories 120 kcal,

Fat 3g,

Carbohydrate 10g,

Protein 6g

Rainbow Salad

Preparation Time: 10 Minutes

Cooking Time: 0 Minutes

Servings: 1

Ingredients:

- 1 cup lettuce
- 1/2 pieces avocado
- 1 egg
- 1/4 green pepper
- 1/4 red bell pepper
- 2 tomatoes
- ½ red onion
- ½ carrot, grated
- 2 tbsp. olive oil
- tbsp. red wine vinegar

Directions:

1. Boil the egg until done (6 minutes for soft boiled, 8 minutes for hard-boiled). Cool it under running water, peel it and cut into slices.
2. Remove the seeds from the peppers and cut them into thin strips. Cut the tomatoes into small cubes. Cut the red onion into thin half-rings.
3. Cut the avocado into thin slices.
4. Place the salad on a plate and distribute all the vegetables in colorful rows.
5. Drizzle the vegetables with olive oil and red wine vinegar. Season with salt and pepper.

Nutrition:

Calories: 40kcal

Fat: 1g

Carbohydrate: 5g

Protein: 2g

Roasted Butternut and Chickpeas Salad

Preparation Time: 10 Minutes

Cooking Time: 30 Minutes

Servings: 4

Ingredients:

- 1 cup chickpeas, drained
- 1 lb. butternut squash
- 2 cups kale
- 2 tsp. oil
- ½ lemon, juiced
- 2 cloves of garlic
- green apple
- ½ tsp. honey

Directions:

1. Heat the oven to 400°F.
2. Cut the squash into medium cubes, put them in a baking tray, add drained chickpeas, garlic, 1 tbsp. oil, salt, and pepper and mix. Cook for 25 minutes.
3. Mix the kale with the dressing: salt, pepper, lemon, olive oil, and honey so that while the squash is cooking, it becomes softer and more pleasant to eat.
4. When squash and chickpeas are done, put them aside 10 minutes, and in the meantime, chop the apple and mix it with kale.
5. Add squash and chickpeas on top and serve warm.

Nutrition:

Calories: 353,

Fat: 4.8g,

Carbohydrate: 28.1g,

Protein: 28.3g

Salad with Cranberries and Apple

Preparation Time: 50 Minutes

Cooking Time: 0 Minutes

Servings: 2

Ingredients:

- ½ cup arugula

- 1/2 apple
- 2 tbsp. cranberries
- 1/2 red onion
- 1/2 red bell pepper
- 10 Walnuts
- 1 tsp. mustard yellow
- 1 tsp. honey
- 3 tbsp. extra-virgin olive oil

Directions:

1. Cut half the red onion into thin rings. Cut the bell pepper into small cubes. Cut the apple into four pieces and remove the core. Then cut into thin wedges. Drizzle some lemon juice on the apple wedges so that they do not change color.
2. Roughly chop walnuts. Mix the ingredients for the dressing in a bowl. Season with salt and pepper. Spread the lettuce on a plate and season with red pepper, red onions, apple wedges, and walnuts.
3. Sprinkle bacon and cranberries over the salad. Drizzle the dressing over the salad and serve.

Nutrition:

Calories: 70

Fat: 3g

Carbohydrate: 6g

Protein: 7g

Sirt Fruit Salad

Preparation Time: 10 Minutes

Cooking Time: 0 Minutes

Servings: 1

Ingredients:

- 1/2 cup matcha green tea

- 1 tsp. honey
- 1 orange, halved
- 1 apple, cored and roughly chopped
- 10 red seedless grapes
- 10 blueberries

Directions:

1. Stir the honey into half a cup of green tea and let it chill.
2. When chilled, add the juice of half an orange.
3. Slice the other half and put in a bowl with the chopped apple, blueberries, and grapes.
4. Cover with tea and let rest in the fridge for 30 minutes before serving.

Nutrition:

Calories: 110

Fat: 0g

Carbohydrate: 17g

Protein: 2g.

Sprouts and Apples Snack Salad

Preparation Time: 10 Minutes

Cooking Time: 0 Minutes

Servings: 4

Ingredients:

- 1 lb. Brussels sprouts, shredded
- 1 cup walnuts, chopped
- 1 apple, cored and cubed
- 1 red onion, chopped
- 3 tbsp. red vinegar
- 1 tbsp. mustard
- ½ cup olive oil
- 1 garlic clove, crushed
- Black pepper to the taste

Directions:

1. In a salad bowl, mix sprouts with apple, onion, and walnuts.
2. In another bowl, mix vinegar with mustard, oil, garlic, and pepper, whisk well, add this to your salad, toss well and serve as a snack.

Nutrition:

Calories 120 kcal,

Fat 2g,

Carbohydrate 8g,

Protein 6g

Tomato and Avocado Salad

Preparation Time: 10 Minutes

Cooking Time: 0 Minutes

Servings: 1

Ingredients:

- 1 tomato
- 4 oz. cherry tomatoes
- 1/2 red onion
- 1 ripe avocado
- 1 tsp. fresh oregano
- 1 tbsp. extra-virgin olive oil
- 1 tsp. red wine vinegar
- 1 pinch Celtic sea salt

Directions:

1. Cut the tomato into thick slices. Cut half of the cherry tomatoes into slices and the remaining in half. Cut the red onion into super-thin half rings. (if you have it, use a mandolin for this)
2. Cut the avocado into 6 parts. Spread the tomatoes on a plate, place the avocado on top.
3. Sprinkle red onion and oregano and drizzle olive oil, vinegar, and a pinch of salt on the salad.

Nutrition:

Calories: 165

Fat: 14g

Carbohydrate: 7g

Protein: 5g

Avocado-Potato Salad

Preparation Time: 10 Minutes

Cooking Time: 0 Minutes

Servings: 2

Ingredients:

- 1 ripe avocado, mashed
- 6 Yukon gold or red potatoes
- 1/2 cup red onion, chopped
- 2 ribs of celery, chopped
- 1/2 cup sweet red bell pepper
- 1 handful parsley, chopped

Directions:

1. Steam and cook the potatoes until tender but not too soft. Stir thoroughly with all other ingredients.
2. Keep refrigerated until ready to serve.

Nutrition:

Calories: 213

Fat: 9g

Carbohydrate: 28g

Protein: 3g

Avocado with Raspberry Vinegar Salad

Preparation Time: 25 Minutes

Cooking Time: 0 Minutes

Servings: 2

Ingredients:

- 4 oz. raspberries
- 3 oz, red wine vinegar
- 1 tsp. extra-virgin olive oil
- 2 firm-ripe avocados
- 1 red endive

Directions:

1. Place half the raspberries in a bowl. Heat the vinegar in a saucepan until it starts to bubble, then pour it over the raspberries and leave to**o** steep for 5 minutes.
2. Strain the raspberries, pressing the fruit gently to extract all the juices but not the pulp.
3. Whisk the strained raspberry vinegar together with the oils and seasonings. Set aside.
4. Carefully halve each avocado and twist out the stone.
5. Peel away the skin and cut the flesh straight into the dressing.
6. Stir gently until the avocados are entirely covered in the dressing.
7. Cover tightly and chill in the fridge for about 2 hours.
8. Meanwhile, separate the radicchio leaves, rinse and drain them, then dry them on kitchen paper. Store in the fridge in a polythene bag.
9. To serve, place a few radicchios leaves on individual plates.
10. Spoon on the avocado, stir and trim with the remaining raspberries.

Nutrition:

Calories: 163

Fat: 4g

Carbohydrate: 15g

Protein: 14g

Bitter Greens, Mung Sprouts, Avocado, and Orange Salad

Preparation Time: 5 Minutes

Cooking Time: 0 Minutes

Servings: 4

Ingredients:

- 1 cup baby spinach leaves
- 1 stir bitter greens (arugula, dandelion, watercress, etc.)
- 1 cup Mung sprouts
- 1 orange, into wedges
- 1/2 cup diced avocado
- ¼ cup walnuts, soaked
- 2 tbsp. extra-virgin olive oil
- 1 tbsp. lemon juice
- 1 tsp. lemon zest
- Fresh cracked black pepper to taste
- 1 Tbsp. tahini
- 1/2 tsp. diced fresh ginger

Directions:

1. Mix spinach leaves, bitter greens, and Mung sprouts in a bowl. Add the orange and avocado. In another bowl, whisk the lemon juice, olive oil, lemon zest, salt, pepper, ginger, and tahini.
2. Pour the dressing over the salad and toss to coat. Trim with the chopped walnuts and serve immediately.

Nutrition:

Calories: 173

Fat: 4g

Carbohydrate: 15g

Protein: 9g

Veggie and Chorizo Stew

Preparation Time: 10 Minutes

Cooking Time: 30 Minutes

Servings: 4

Ingredients:

- 1 yellow onion, chopped
- 1 tbsp. coconut oil
- 2 chorizo sausages, skinless and thinly sliced
- 1 red bell pepper, chopped
- 1 carrot, thinly sliced
- 2 white potatoes, chopped
- 1 celery stick, chopped
- 1 tomato, chopped
- 2 garlic cloves, finely minced
- 2 cups chicken broth
- 1 tbsp. lemon juice
- Salt and black pepper to taste
- 1 zucchini, cut
- A handful parsley leaves, finely chopped

Directions:

1. Heat up a pan with the oil over medium-high heat, add chorizo, onion, celery and carrot, stir and cook for 3 minutes.
2. Add red bell pepper, tomatoes, garlic, and potato, stir and cook 1 minute.
3. Add lemon juice, stock, salt, and pepper, stir, bring to a boil, cover pan, reduce heat to medium and cook for 10 minutes.
4. Add zucchini, stir, cover again and cook for ten more minutes.
5. Uncover pan, cook the stew for 2 minutes more stirring often.
6. Add parsley, stir, take off heat, transfer to dishes and serve.

7. Enjoy!

Nutrition:

Calories: 420 Fat: 12g Carbs: 45g Protein: 33.2g Fiber: 11g Sugar: 0g

Green Pea Soup

Preparation Time: 5 Minutes

Cooking Time: 50 Minutes

Servings: 6

Ingredients:

- 1 (16-ounce) package dried green split peas, soaked overnight
- 5 cups vegetable broth or water
- 2 teaspoons garlic powder
- 2 teaspoons onion powder
- 1 teaspoon dried oregano
- 1 teaspoon dried thyme
- ¼ teaspoon freshly ground black pepper

Directions:

1. In a large stockpot, combine the split peas, broth, garlic powder, onion powder, oregano, thyme, and pepper. Bring to a boil over medium-high heat.
2. Cover, reduce the heat to medium-low, and simmer for 45 minutes, stirring every 5 to 10 minutes. Serve warm.

Nutrition:

Calories: 297;

Fat: 2g;

Carbohydrates: 48g;

Protein: 23g

Coconut Watercress Soup

Preparation Time: 10 Minutes

Cooking Time: 20 Minutes

Servings: 4

Ingredients:

- 1 teaspoon coconut oil
- 1 onion, diced
- 2 cups fresh or frozen peas
- 6 cups water, or vegetable stock
- 1 cup fresh watercress, chopped
- 1 tablespoon fresh mint, chopped
- Pinch sea salt
- Pinch freshly ground black pepper
- ¾ cup coconut milk

Directions:

1. Preparing the Ingredients.
2. Melt the coconut oil in a large pot over medium-high heat. Add the onion and cook until soft for about 5 minutes, then add the peas and water. Bring to a boil, lower the heat, then add the watercress, mint, salt, and pepper.
3. Cover and simmer for 5 minutes. Stir in the coconut milk.
4. Finish and serve
5. Purée the soup until smooth in a blender or with an immersion blender.
6. Try this soup with any other fresh, leafy green—anything from spinach to collard greens to arugula to Swiss chard.

Nutrition:

Calories: 178;

Fat: 10g;

Protein: 6g;

Carbohydrates: 18g

Beef Soup

Preparation Time: 15 Minutes

Cooking Time: 60 Minutes

Servings: 6

Ingredients:

- 1 lb. beef, ground
- 1 lb. sausage, sliced
- 4 cups beef stock
- 30 oz. canned tomatoes, diced
- 1 green bell pepper, chopped
- 3 zucchinis, chopped
- 1 cup celery, chopped
- 1 tsp. Italian seasoning
- ½ yellow onion, chopped
- ½ teaspoon oregano, dried
- ½ teaspoon basil, dried
- ¼ teaspoon garlic powder
- Salt and black pepper to the taste

Directions:

1. Cook until it browns and drains excess fat.
2. Add tomatoes, zucchini, bell pepper, celery, onion, Italian seasoning, basil, oregano, garlic powder, salt, pepper to the taste and the stock, stir, bring to a boil, reduce heat to medium-low and simmer for 1 hour.
3. Enjoy!

Nutrition:

Calories: 370

Fat: 17g

Carbs: 35g

Protein: 25g

Fiber: 10g

Sugar: 0g

Easy Borscht

Preparation Time: 30 Minutes

Cooking Time: 45 Minutes

Servings: 8

Ingredients:

- 6 cups shredded red cabbage
- 2 large potatoes, peeled and chopped
- 1 cup peeled julienned beets
- ¼ cup chopped fresh parsley
- 2 cloves garlic, crushed
- ¼ cup red-wine vinegar
- 1 onion, chopped
- 5 teaspoons chopped fresh dill
- 2 tablespoons maple syrup (optional)
- 1 teaspoon paprika
- Freshly ground pepper, to taste
- 2 cups water
- Fresh dill, for garnish

Directions:

1. Combine all the ingredients in a large pot, except the dill.
2. Bring to a boil, cover, reduce the heat, and cook over medium heat for 45 minutes.
3. Garnish with fresh dill and serve!

Nutrition:

Calories: 127;

Fat: 0.3.g;

Protein: 3.1g;

Carbohydrates: 29.5g

Potato and Corn Chowder

Preparation Time: 20 Minutes

Cooking Time: 30 Minutes

Servings: 4

Ingredients:

- 2 tablespoons low-sodium vegetables broth
- 1 medium yellow onion, diced

- 1 stalk celery, diced
- 1 small red bell pepper, diced
- 2 teaspoons minced fresh thyme leaves (about 4 sprigs)
- ½ teaspoon smoked paprika
- ½ teaspoon no-salt-added Old Bay seasoning
- 1 jalapeño pepper, deseeded and minced
- 1 clove garlic, minced
- 1 pound (454 g) new potatoes, diced
- 3 cups fresh corn kernels (about 4 fresh cobs)
- Salt, to taste (optional)
- Ground black or white pepper, to taste
- 4 cup low-sodium vegetable broth
- 2 teaspoons white wine vinegar
- Chopped chives, for garnish

Directions:

1. Heat the vegetables broth in a large pot over medium heat. Add the onions and sauté for 4 minutes or until translucent.
2. Add the red bell pepper, celery, paprika, thyme, jalapeño, and Old Bay seasoning. Sauté for 1 minutes or until the vegetables are tender.
3. Add the garlic and sauté for another 1 minutes or until fragrant.
4. Add the corn, potatoes, vegetable broth, salt (if desired), and pepper. Stir to mix well. Bring to a boil, then reduce the heat to low and simmer for 25 minutes or until the potatoes are soft.
5. Pour half of the soup in a blender, then process until the soup is creamy and smooth. Pour the puréed soup back to the pot and add the white wine vinegar. Stir to mix well.
6. Spread the chopped chives on top and serve.

Nutrition:

Calories: 733;

Fat: 8.5g

Carbohydrates: 148.5g;

Protein: 20.4g

Pumpkin Soup

Preparation Time: 20 Minutes

Cooking Time: 1 Hour 10 Minutes

Servings: 8

Ingredients:

- 3 pounds of quartered seeded sugar pumpkin
- 3 cups of vegetable broth
- 2 chopped large shallots
- 3 chopped fresh sage leaves
- ¼ cup of Greek yogurt
- 6 springs of thyme
- 1 tablespoon of grated gigger
- 1/8 teaspoon of nutmeg
- 1 teaspoon of sea salt
- Pinch of ground pepper
- 1 tablespoon of butter
- 1 ½ tablespoons of olive oil

Directions:

1. Preheat your oven to 450ºF. Spread some oil on a baking sheet.
2. Put pieces of pumpkin on the baking sheet. Drizzle them with olive oil, season with ground pepper and ¼ teaspoon of sea salt. Put thyme sprigs on top.
3. Roast for 1 hour, stirring halfway. Let it cool and remove the skin.
4. Put a large stockpot on medium heat, pour olive oil, and warm it. Add chopped shallots and cook for 5 minutes, stirring frequently, until tender.

5. Mix in vegetable broth, pumpkin, sage, and ginger. Season with the remaining salt and ground pepper to taste.
6. Bring the mixture to a boil, then remove from the heat.
7. Puree with a blender until smooth consistency. Pour in Greek yogurt and blend repeatedly.
8. Serve with some Greek yogurt and enjoy!

Nutrition:

Calories: 145;

Fat: 8g;

Carbohydrates: 16g;

Protein: 3.5g

Cannellini Pesto Spaghetti

Preparation Time: 5 Minutes

Cooking Time: 10 Minutes

Servings: 4

Ingredients:

- 12 ounces whole-grain spaghetti, cooked, drained, and kept warm, ½ cup cooking liquid reserved
- 1 cup pesto
- 2 cups cooked cannellini beans, drained and rinsed

Directions:

1. Put the cooked spaghetti in a large bowl and add the pesto.
2. Add the reserved cooking liquid and beans and toss well to serve.

Nutrition:

Calories: 549;

Protein: 18.3g;

81

Carbohydrates: 45g;

Fats: 35g

Classic Tomato Soup

Preparation Time: 10 Minutes

Cooking Time: 60 Minutes

Servings: 6

Ingredients:

- 3 pounds of halved tomatoes
- 1 cup of canned crush tomatoes
- 2–3 chopped carrots
- 2 chopped yellow onions
- 5 minced garlic cloves
- 2 ounces of basil leaves
- 2 teaspoons of thyme leaves
- 1 teaspoon of dry oregano
- ½ teaspoon of ground cumin
- ½ teaspoon of paprika
- 2 ½ cups of water
- Fresh lime juice, to taste
- Extra virgin olive oil
- Salt, to taste
- Black Pepper, to taste

Directions:

1. Preheat your oven to 450ºF. Spread some oil inside a baking sheet.
2. Mix carrots with tomatoes in a large bowl. Add some oil, salt, black pepper, and toss.
3. Put the vegetable mixture on the baking sheet in a single layer. Roast for 30 minutes, then set aside for 10 minutes.
4. Transfer the roasted vegetables in a food processor or a blender, add just a little water, and blend.
5. Place a large stockpot on medium-high heat, pour 2 tablespoons of olive oil, and warm it. Add chopped onions and simmer for 3 minutes, then add minced garlic and cook until golden.

6. Pour the blended mixture into the stockpot. Add in 2 ½ cups of water, canned tomatoes, thyme, basil, and other seasonings. Bring it to a boil, reduce to low heat, and cover. Simmer for about 20 minutes.
7. Serve with a splash of lime juice and enjoy!

Nutrition:

Calories: 104;

Fats: 0.8g;

Carbohydrates: 23.4g;

Protein: 4.3g

Scallion and Mint Soup

Preparation Time: 5 Minutes

Cooking Time: 15 Minutes

Servings: 4

Ingredients:

- 6 cups vegetable broth
- ¼ cup fresh mint leaves, roughly chopped
- ¼ cup chopped scallions, white and green parts
- 3 garlic cloves, minced
- 3 tablespoons freshly squeezed lime juice

Directions:

1. In a large stockpot, combine the broth, mint, scallions, garlic, and lime juice. Bring to a boil over medium-high heat.
2. Cover, reduce the heat to low, simmer for 15 minutes, and serve.

Nutrition:

Calories: 55;

Protein: 5g;

Carbohydrates: 5g;

Fat: 2g

Kale and Lentils Stew

Preparation Time: 10 Minutes

Cooking Time: 50 Minutes

Servings: 8

Ingredients:

- 6 cups (2 pounds) brown or green dry lentils
- 8 cups vegetable broth or water
- 4 cups kale, stemmed and chopped into 2-inch pieces
- 2 large carrots, diced
- 1 tablespoon smoked paprika
- 2 teaspoons onion powder
- 2 teaspoons garlic powder
- 1 teaspoon red pepper flakes
- 1 teaspoon dried oregano
- 1 teaspoon dried thyme

Directions:

1. In a large stockpot, combine the lentils, broth, kale, carrots, paprika, onion powder, garlic powder, red pepper flakes, oregano, and thyme. Bring to a boil over medium-high heat.
2. Cover, reduce the heat to medium-low, and simmer for 45 minutes, stirring every 5 to 10 minutes. Serve warm.

Nutrition:

Calories: 467;

Fat: 3g;

Carbohydrates: 78g;

Protein: 32g

Lentil Soup with Swiss Chard

Preparation Time: 10 Minutes

Cooking Time: 25 Minutes

Servings: 5

Ingredients:

- 2 tablespoons olive oil
- 1 white onion, chopped
- 1 teaspoon garlic, minced
- 2 large carrots, chopped
- 1 parsnip, chopped
- 2 stalks celery, chopped
- 2 bay leaves
- 1/2 teaspoon dried thyme
- 1/4 teaspoon ground cumin
- 6 cups roasted vegetable broth
- 1 ¼ cups brown lentils, soaked overnight and rinsed
- 2 cups Swiss chard, torn into pieces

Directions:

1. In a heavy-bottomed pot, heat the olive oil over a moderate heat. Now, sauté the vegetables along with the spices for about 3 minutes until they are just tender.
2. Add in the vegetable broth and lentils, bringing it to a boil. Immediately turn the heat to a simmer and add in the bay leaves. Let it cook for about 15 minutes or until lentils are tender.
3. Add in the Swiss chard, cover and let it simmer for 5 minutes more or until the chard wilts.
4. Serve in individual bowls and enjoy!

Nutrition:

Calories: 148;

Fat: 7.2g;

Carbohydrates: 14.6g;

Protein: 7.7g

Spicy Farro Soup

Preparation Time: 10 Minutes

Cooking Time: 30 Minutes

Servings: 4

Ingredients:

- 2 tablespoons olive oil
- 1 medium-sized leek, chopped
- 1 medium-sized turnip, sliced
- 2 Italian peppers, seeded and chopped
- 1 jalapeno pepper, minced
- 2 potatoes, peeled and diced
- 2 cups vegetable broth
- 1 cup farro, rinsed
- 1/2 teaspoon granulated garlic
- 1/2 teaspoon turmeric powder
- 1 bay laurel
- 2 cups spinach, turn into pieces

Directions:

1. In a heavy-bottomed pot, heat the olive oil over a moderate heat. Now, sauté the leek, turnip, peppers and potatoes for about 5 minutes until they are crisp-tender.
2. Add in the vegetable broth, farro, granulated garlic, turmeric and bay laurel; bring it to a boil.
3. Immediately turn the heat to a simmer. Let it cook for about 25 minutes or until farro and potatoes have softened.
4. Add in the spinach and remove the pot from the heat; let the spinach sit in the residual heat until it wilts. Bon appétit!

Nutrition:

Calories: 298;

Fat: 8.9g;

Protein: 11.7g;

Carbohydrates: 44.6g

Cannellini Soup with Kale

Preparation Time: 5 Minutes

Cooking Time: 25 Minutes

Servings: 5

Ingredients:

- 1 tablespoon olive oil
- 1/2 teaspoon ginger, minced
- 1/2 teaspoon cumin seeds
- 1 red onion, chopped
- 1 carrot, trimmed and chopped
- 1 parsnip, trimmed and chopped
- 2 garlic cloves, minced
- 6 cups vegetable broth
- 12 ounces Cannellini beans, drained
- 2 cups kale, torn into pieces
- Sea salt and ground black pepper, to taste

Directions:

1. In a heavy-bottomed pot, heat the olive over medium-high heat. Now, sauté the ginger and cumin for 1 minute or so.
2. Now, add in the onion, carrot and parsnip; continue sautéing an additional 3 minutes or until the vegetables are just tender.
3. Add in the garlic and continue to sauté for 1 minute or until aromatic.
4. Then, pour in the vegetable broth and bring to a boil. Immediately reduce the heat to a simmer and let it cook for 10 minutes.
5. Fold in the Cannellini beans and kale; continue to simmer until the kale wilts and everything is thoroughly heated. Season with salt and pepper to taste.
6. Ladle into individual bowls and serve hot. Bon appétit

Nutrition:

Calories: 188;

Fat: 4.7g

Carbohydrates: 24.5g;

Protein: 11g

Chickpea Noodle Soup

Preparation Time: 10 Minutes

Cooking Time: 25 Minutes

Servings: 6

Ingredients:

- 6 ounces dried soba noodles
- 4 cups vegetable broth, divided
- 2 cups diced onions
- 1 cup chopped carrots
- 1 cup chopped celery
- 3 garlic cloves, finely diced
- ½ teaspoon dried parsley
- ½ teaspoon dried sage
- ½ teaspoon dried thyme
- ½ teaspoon freshly ground black or white pepper
- (15-ounce) can chickpeas, drained and rinsed
- ¼ cup chopped fresh parsley, for garnish (optional)

Directions:

1. In a large saucepan, bring 4 cups water to a boil over high heat. Add the soba noodles and cook, stirring occasionally, until just tender, 4 to 5 minutes. Drain in a colander and rinse well under cold water. Set aside.
2. In the same saucepan, heat ¼ cup of broth over medium-high heat. Add the onions, carrots, celery, garlic, parsley, sage, thyme, and pepper and sauté for 5 minutes, or until the carrots are fork-tender.

3. Add the chickpeas and remaining 3¾ cups of broth and bring to a boil. Lower the heat to low, cover, and simmer for 15 minutes.
4. Serve garnished with the parsley, if desired.

Nutrition:

Calories: 266;

Total fat: 3g;

Carbohydrates: 53g;

Protein: 12g

Greens and Grains Soup

Preparation Time: 5 Minutes

Cooking Time: 35 Minutes

Servings: 6

Ingredients:

- 2 cups sliced onions
- 1 cup diced carrots
- 1 cup diced celery
- 1 cup dry farro
- teaspoon dried basil
- 1 teaspoon dried oregano
- ½ teaspoon dried rosemary
- ½ teaspoon dried thyme
- 1 (15-ounce) can diced tomatoes
- 1 (15-ounce) can white kidney beans, drained and rinsed
- 6 ounces arugula
- tablespoons lemon juice

Directions:

1. In a large saucepan, combine the onions, carrots, and celery and dry sauté over medium-high heat, stirring occasionally, until the carrots are softened, about 5 minutes.

2. Add the farro and stir until coated. Add the basil, oregano, rosemary, thyme, and 4 cups water and bring to a boil. Lower the heat to low, cover, and simmer for 30 minutes.
3. Add the tomatoes and beans, raise the heat to medium-high, and bring back to a boil.
4. Add the arugula and lemon juice and cook, stirring, until the arugula is a deep green and lightly wilted, 1 to 2 minutes more.
5. Remove from the heat and serve.

Nutrition:

Calories: 183;

Protein: 9g;

Carbohydrates: 38g;

Fats: 1g

Vegan Pho

Preparation Time: 10 Minutes

Cooking Time: 15 Minutes

Servings: 6

Ingredients:

- 1 package of wide rice noodles, cooked
- 1 medium white onion, peeled, quartered
- 2 teaspoons minced garlic
- 1 inch of ginger, sliced into coins
- 8 cups vegetable broth
- 1 whole cloves
- 2 tablespoons soy sauce
- 1 whole star anise
- 1 cinnamon stick
- 3 cups of water

For Toppings:

- Basil as needed for topping
- Chopped green onions as needed for topping
- Ming beans as needed for topping
- Hot sauce as needed for topping
- Lime wedges for serving

Directions:

1. Take a large pot, place it over medium-high heat, add all the ingredients for soup in it, except for soy sauce and broth, and bring it to boil.
2. Then switch heat to medium-low level, simmer the soup for 30 minutes and then stir in soy sauce.
3. When done, distribute cooked noodles into bowls, top with soup, then top with toppings and serve.

Nutrition:

Calories: 31;

 Fats: 0g;

Carbohydrates: 7g;

Protein: 2g

Creamy Spinach Rotini Soup

Preparation Time: 5 Minutes

Cooking Time: 15 Minutes

Servings: 4

Ingredients:

- 1 teaspoon extra-virgin olive oil
- 1 cup chopped mushrooms
- ¼ teaspoon plus a pinch salt
- 4 garlic cloves, minced, or 1 teaspoon garlic powder
- 2 peeled carrots or ½ red bell pepper, chopped
- 6 cups vegetable broth or water
- Pinch freshly ground black pepper
- 1 cup rotini or gnocchi

- ¾ cup unsweetened nondairy milk
- ¼ cup nutritional yeast
- 2 cups chopped fresh spinach
- ¼ cup pitted black olives or sun-dried tomatoes, chopped
- Herbed Croutons, for topping (optional)

Directions:

1. Heat the olive oil in a large soup pot over medium-high heat.
2. Add the mushrooms and a pinch of salt. Sauté for about 4 minutes until the mushrooms soften. Add the garlic (if using fresh) and carrots, then sauté for 1 minute. Add the vegetable broth, then add the remaining ¼ teaspoon of salt, and pepper (plus the garlic powder if using). Bring to boil and add the pasta. Cook for about 10 minutes until the pasta is cooked.
3. Finish and Serve
4. Turn off the heat and stir in the milk, nutritional yeast, spinach, and olives. Top with croutons (if using). Leftovers will keep in an airtight container for up to 1 week in the refrigerator, or up to 1 month in the freezer.

Nutrition:

Calories: 207;

Fat: 5g;

Carbohydrates: 34g;

Protein: 11g

Hot and Sour Tofu Soup

Preparation Time: 10 Minutes

Cooking Time: 15 Minutes

Servings: 3

Ingredients:

- 6 to 7 ounces firm or extra-firm tofu
- 1 teaspoon extra-virgin olive oil
- 1 cup sliced mushrooms
- 1 cup finely chopped cabbage
- 1 garlic clove, minced
- ½-inch piece fresh ginger, peeled and minced
- Salt
- 4 cups water or Vegetable Broth
- 2 tablespoons rice vinegar or apple cider vinegar
- 2 tablespoons soy sauce
- 1 teaspoon toasted sesame oil
- 1 teaspoon sugar
- Pinch red pepper flakes
- 1 scallion, white and light green parts only, chopped

Directions:

1. Press your tofu before you start: Put it between several layers of paper towels and place a heavy pan or book (with a waterproof cover or protected with plastic wrap) on top. Let it stand for 30 minutes. Discard the paper towels. Cut the tofu into ½-inch cubes.
2. In a large soup pot, heat the olive oil over medium-high heat.
3. Add the mushrooms, cabbage, garlic, ginger, and a pinch of salt. Sauté for 7 to 8 minutes until the vegetables are softened.
4. Add the water, vinegar, soy sauce, sesame oil, sugar, red pepper flakes, and tofu.
5. Bring to a boil, then turn the heat to low.
6. Finish and Serve
7. Simmer the soup for 5 to 10 minutes.
8. Serve with the scallion sprinkled on top.

Nutrition:

Calories: 161;

Protein: 13g;

Carbohydrates: 10g;

Fat: 9g

Winter Quinoa Soup

Preparation Time: 10 Minutes

Cooking Time: 25 Minutes

Servings: 4

Ingredients:

- 2 tablespoons olive oil
- 1 onion, chopped
- 2 carrots, peeled and chopped
- 1 parsnip, chopped
- 1 celery stalk, chopped
- 1 cup yellow squash, chopped
- 4 garlic cloves, pressed or minced
- 4 cups roasted vegetable broth
- 2 medium tomatoes, crushed
- 1 cup quinoa
- Sea salt and ground black pepper, to taste
- 1 bay laurel
- 2 cup Swiss chard, tough ribs removed and torn into pieces
- 2 tablespoons Italian parsley, chopped

Directions:

1. In a heavy-bottomed pot, heat the olive over medium-high heat. Now, sauté the onion, carrot, parsnip, celery and yellow squash for about 3 minutes or until the vegetables are just tender.
2. Add in the garlic and continue to sauté for 1 minute or until aromatic.
3. Then, stir in the vegetable broth, tomatoes, quinoa, salt, pepper and bay laurel; bring to a boil. Immediately reduce the heat to a simmer and let it cook for 1minutes.
4. Fold in the Swiss chard; continue to simmer until the chard wilts.
5. Ladle into individual bowls and serve garnished with the fresh parsley. Bon appétit!

Nutrition:

Calories: 328;

Fat: 11.1g;

Carbohydrates: 44g;

Protein: 13.3g

Veggie Noodle Soup

Preparation Time: 10minutes

Cooking time: 15minutes

Servings: 4

Ingredients:

- 4 celery stalks, chopped into bite-size pieces
- 4 carrots, chopped into bite-size pieces
- 2 sweet potatoes
- 1 sweet onion, chopped into bite-size pieces
- 1 cup broccoli florets
- 1 tomato, diced
- 2 garlic cloves, minced
- 1 bay leaf
- 1 teaspoon dried oregano
- 1 teaspoon dried thyme
- 1 teaspoon dried basil
- 1 to 2 teaspoons salt
- Pinch freshly ground black pepper
- 1 cup dried pasta (I prefer a small pasta shape)
- 4 cups DIY Vegetable Stock, or store-bought stock, plus more as needed

- 1 to 11/2 cups water, plus more as needed
- Chopped fresh parsley, for garnishing (optional)
- Lemon zest, for garnishing (optional)
- Crackers, for serving (optional)

Directions:

1. In your Instant Pot, combine the celery, carrots, sweet potatoes, onion, broccoli, tomato, garlic, bay leaf, oregano, thyme, basil, salt, pepper, pasta, stock, and water, making sure all the good stuff is submerged (add more water or stock, if needed). Close the lid and cooker to High Pressure for 4 minutes (3 minutes at sea level).

2. Once the cook time is complete, release naturally the pressure for 5 minutes; quick release any remaining pressure.

3. Gently remove the lid and stir the soup. Remove and discard the bay leaf and enjoy garnished as desired!

Nutrition:

Calories: 197

Total fat: 3g

Saturated fat: 2g

Sodium: 754mg

Carbs: 43g

Fiber: 6g

Protein: 6g

Carrot Ginger Soup

Preparation Time: 10minutes

Cooking time: 15minutes

Servings: 3

Ingredients:

- 7 carrots, chopped
- 1-inch piece fresh ginger, peeled and chopped
- 1/2 sweet onion, chopped
- 1.1/4 cups Vegetable Stock
- 1/2 teaspoon salt
- 1/2 teaspoon sweet paprika
- Freshly ground black pepper
- Cashew Sour Cream, for garnishing (optional)
- Fresh herbs, for garnishing (optional)

Directions:

1. In your Instant Pot, combine the carrots, ginger, onion, stock, salt, and paprika. Season to taste with pepper. Shut down the lid and cook.

2. Once the cook time is processed, let the pressure release naturally for 5 minutes; quick release any remaining pressure.

3. Carefully remove the lid, blend the soup until completely smooth. Taste and season with more salt and pepper, as needed. Serve with garnishes of choice.

Nutrition:

Calories: 127

Total fat: 3g

Saturated fat: 2g

Sodium: 654mg

Carbs: 43g

Fiber: 6g

Protein: 6g

Creamy Tomato Basil SOUP

Preparation Time: 5minutes

Cooking time: 15minutes

Servings: 4

Ingredients:

- 2 tablespoons vegan butter
- 1 small sweet onion, chopped
- 2 garlic cloves, minced
- 1 large carrot, chopped
- 1 celery stalk, chopped
- 3 cups DIY Vegetable Stock, or store-bought stock
- 3 pounds tomatoes, quartered
- 1/4 cup fresh basil
- 1/4 cup nutritional yeast
- Salt
- Freshly ground black pepper
- 1 cup nondairy milk

Directions:

1. On your Instant Pot, select Sauté Low. When the display reads "Hot," add the butter to melt. Add the onion and garlic. Sauté for 3 to 4 minutes, stirring frequently. Add the carrot and celery and cook for 1 to 2 minutes more. Continue to stir frequently so nothing sticks.

2. Stir in the stock (now is your chance to reincorporate any veggies stuck to the bottom).

3. Add the tomatoes, basil, yeast, and a pinch or two of salt. Stir one last time. Shut down the lid and cook.

4. Once the cook time is processed, let the pressure release for 5 to 10 minutes; quick release any remaining pressure.

5. Carefully remove the lid. Blend the soup to your preferred consistency. Stir in the milk. Garnish with the remaining fresh basil.

Nutrition:

Calories: 137

Total fat: 3g

Saturated fat: 2g

Sodium: 554mg

Carbs: 43g

Fiber: 7g

Protein: 8g

Cream of Mushroom Soup

Preparation Time: 10minutes

Cooking time: 30minutes

Servings: 4

Ingredients:

- 2 tablespoons vegan butter
- 1 small sweet onion, chopped
- 11/2 pounds white button mushrooms, sliced
- 2 garlic cloves, minced
- 2 teaspoons dried thyme
- 1 teaspoon sea salt

- 1.3/4 cups DIY Vegetable Stock, or store-bought stock
- 1/2 cup silken tofu
- Chopped fresh thyme, for garnishing (optional)

Directions:

1. On your Instant Pot, select Sauté Low. When the display reads "Hot," add the butter to melt. Add the onion. Sauté for 1 to 2 minutes. Add the mushrooms, garlic, dried thyme, and salt.

2. Stir in the stock. Shut down the lid and cook.

3. While the soup cooks, place the tofu in a food processor or blender and process until smooth. Set aside.

4. Once the cook time is processed, let the pressure release naturally for 10 minutes; quick release any remaining pressure.

5. Carefully remove the lid. Using an immersion blender, blend the soup until completely creamy. Stir in the tofu, garnish as desired, and it's ready!

Nutrition:

Calories: 127

Total fat: 3g

Saturated fat: 4g

Sodium: 354mg

Carbs: 23g

Fiber: 7g

Protein: 8g

Potato Leek Soup

Preparation Time: 10minutes

Cooking time: 30minutes

Servings: 5

Ingredients:

- 3 tablespoons vegan butter
- 2 large leeks
- 2 garlic cloves, minced
- 4 cups Vegetable Stock
- 1 pound Yukon Gold potatoes, cubed
- 1 bay leaf
- 1/2 teaspoon salt
- 2/4 cup soy milk
- 1/3 cup extra-virgin olive oil
- Freshly ground white pepper

Directions:

1. On your Instant Pot, select Sauté Low. When the display reads "Hot," add the butter and leeks. Cook until soft, stirring occasionally. Add the garlic. Cook for 30 to 45 seconds, stirring frequently, until fragrant.

2. Pour in the stock and add the potatoes, bay leaf, and salt. Stir to combine. Shut down the lid. Using the Manual function, set the cooker to High Pressure for 5 minutes (4 minutes at sea level).

3. Once the cook time is processed, let the pressure release naturally for 15 minutes; quick release any remaining pressure.

4. While waiting for the pressure to release, in a blender, combine the soy milk and olive oil. Blend until combined, about 1 minute. This is an easy dairy-free substitute for heavy cream.

5. Carefully remove the lid, remove and discard the bay leaf, and stir in the "cream." Using an immersion blender, purée the soup until smooth.

Nutrition:

Calories: 117

Total fat: 6g

Saturated fat: 5g

Sodium: 254mg

Carbs: 23g

Fiber: 7g

Protein: 7g

Cozy Wild Rice Soup

Preparation Time: 10minutes

Cooking time: 50minutes

Servings: 4

Ingredients:

- 8 tablespoons vegan butter, divided
- 5 carrots, sliced, with thicker end cut into half-moons
- 5 celery stalks, sliced
- 1 small sweet onion, diced
- 4 garlic cloves, minced
- 8 ounces baby belle mushrooms, sliced
- 2 bay leaves
- 1/2 teaspoon paprika
- 1/2 teaspoon dried thyme
- 1/2 teaspoon salt
- 4 cups Vegetable Stock, or store-bought stock
- 1 cup wild rice
- 1/2 cup all-purpose flour
- 1 cup nondairy milk
- Freshly ground black pepper

Directions:

1. On your Instant Pot, select Sauté Low. When the display reads "Hot," add 2 tablespoons of butter to melt. Add the carrots, celery, onion, garlic, mushrooms, bay leaves, paprika, thyme, and salt.

2. Stir in the stock and wild rice. Shut down the lid and set the cooker to High Pressure for 35 minutes.

3. When there are just a few minutes of cook time remaining, in a small pan over medium-low heat on your stovetop, melt the remaining 6 tablespoons of butter. Whisk in the flour and cook for 3 to 4 minutes.

4. Once the cook time is processed, quick release the pressure.

5. Gently remove the lid, and remove and discard the bay leaves.

Nutrition:

Calories: 157

Total fat: 4g

Saturated fat: 7g

Sodium: 154mg

Carbs: 23g

Fiber: 8g

Protein: 7g

Curried Squash Soup

Preparation Time: 10minutes

Cooking time: 41minutes

Servings: 6

Ingredients:

- 1 tablespoon olive oil
- 1 onion, chopped
- 2 garlic cloves, chopped
- 1 tablespoon curry powder
- 1 (2- to 3-pound) butternut squash, peeled and cubed
- 4 cups DIY *Vegetable Stock*, or store-bought stock
- 1 teaspoon salt
- 1 (14-ounce) can lite coconut milk

Directions:

1. On your Instant Pot, select Sauté Low. When the display reads "Hot," add the oil and heat until it shimmers. Add the onion and cook in a low heat.

2. Add the squash, stock, and salt. Shut down the lid and set the cooker to High Pressure for 30 minutes

3. Once the cook time is processed, quick release the pressure.

4. Carefully remove the lid. Using an immersion blender, blend the soup until completely smooth. Stir in the coconut milk, saving a little bit for topping when served.

Nutrition:

Calories: 127

Total fat: 5g

Saturated fat: 5g

Sodium: 124mg

Carbs: 13g

Fiber: 9g

Protein: 7g

Minestrone Soup

Preparation Time: 5minutes

Cooking time: 15minutes

Servings: 7

Ingredients:

- 2 tablespoons olive oil
- 2 celery stalks, sliced
- 1 sweet onion, diced
- 1 large carrot, sliced, with thicker end cut into half-moons
- 2 garlic cloves, minced
- 1 teaspoon dried oregano
- 1 teaspoon dried basil
- 1/2 to 1 teaspoon salt, plus more as needed
- 1 bay leaf
- 1 zucchini, roughly diced
- 1 (28-ounce) can diced tomatoes
- 1 (16-ounce) can kidney beans, drained and rinsed
- 1 cup small dried pasta
- 6 cups store-bought stock
- 2 to 3 cups fresh baby spinach
- Freshly ground black pepper

Directions:

1. On your Instant Pot, select Sauté Low. When the display reads "Hot," add the oil, celery, onion, and carrot. Attach the garlic and cook for another minute or so, stirring frequently. Turn off the Instant Pot and add the oregano, basil, salt, and bay leaf. Stir and let sit for 30 seconds to 1 minute.

2. Add the zucchini, tomatoes, kidney beans, pasta, and stock. Shut down the lid and set the cooker to High Pressure for 4 minutes (3 minutes at sea level).

3. Once the cook time is processed, quick release the pressure.

4. Carefully remove the lid, and remove and discard the bay leaf. Stir in the spinach and let it get all nice and wilt. Taste and season with more salt, as needed, and pepper. Serve hot.

Nutrition:

Calories: 127

Total fat: 7g

Saturated fat: 5g

Sodium: 124mg

Carbs: 17g

Fiber: 8g

Protein: 7g

Carrot-Ginger Soup

Preparation Time: 5minutes

Cooking time: 60minutes

Servings: 5

Ingredients:

- 2 (10-ounce) packages frozen carrots

- 2 cans diced tomatoes

- 1 medium yellow onion, diced

- 1-piece fresh ginger

- 1.1/2 teaspoons minced garlic (3 cloves)

- Zest and juice of 1 lemon

- 2 vegetable bouillon cubes

- 3.1/2 cups water

- 2 tablespoons vegan sour cream

- Pinch salt

- Freshly ground black pepper

Directions:

1. Combine the carrots, diced tomatoes, onion, ginger, garlic, lemon zest and juice, bouillon cubes, and water in a slow cooker; mix well

2. Shut down and cook on low heat.

3. Purée using an immersion blender (or with a regular blender, working in batches).

4. Stir in the vegan sour cream and season with salt and pepper.

Nutrition:

Calories: 137

Total fat: 6g

Saturated fat: 9g

Sodium: 138mg

Carbs: 18g

Fiber: 8g

Protein: 6g

Avocado, Spinach and Kale Soup

Preparation time: 10 minutes

Cooking time: 0 minutes

Servings: 4

Ingredients:

- 2 avocados, pitted, peeled and cut in halves
- 4 cups vegetable stock
- 2 tablespoons cilantro, chopped
- Juice of 1 lime
- 1 teaspoon rosemary, dried
- 1/2 cup spinach leaves
- 1/2 cup kale, torn
- Salt and black pepper to the taste

Directions

1. In a blender, combine the avocados with the stock and the other ingredients, pulse well, divide into bowls and serve for lunch.

Nutrition:

Calories: 124

 Total fat: 9g

Saturated fat: 6g

Sodium: 158mg

Carbs: 18g

Fiber: 8g

Protein: 6g

Spinach and Broccoli Soup

Preparation time: 10 minutes

Cooking time: 20 minutes

Servings: 4

Ingredients:

- 3 shallots, chopped
- 1 tablespoon olive oil
- 2 garlic cloves, minced
- 1/2-pound broccoli florets
- 1/2-pound baby spinach
- Salt and black pepper to the taste
- 4 cups veggie stock
- 1 teaspoon turmeric powder
- 1 tablespoon lime juice

Directions:

2. Heat up a pot with the oil over medium high heat; add the shallots and the garlic and sauté for 5 minutes.

3. Add the broccoli, spinach and the other ingredients toss bring to a simmer and cook over medium heat for 15 minutes.

4. Ladle into soup bowls and serve.

Nutrition:

Calories: 124

 Total fat: 9g

Saturated fat: 6g

Sodium: 158mg

Carbs: 18g

Fiber: 8g

Protein: 6g

Zucchini and Cauliflower Soup

Preparation time: 10 minutes

Cooking time: 25 minutes

Servings: 4

Ingredients:

- 4 scallions, chopped
- 1 teaspoon ginger, grated
- 2 tablespoons olive oil
- 1-pound zucchinis, sliced
- 2 cups cauliflower florets
- Salt and black pepper to the taste
- 6 cups veggie stock
- 1 garlic clove, minced
- 1 tablespoon lemon juice
- 1 cup coconut cream

Directions:

1. Heat up a pot with the oil over medium heat; add the scallions, ginger and the garlic and sauté for 5 minutes.
2. Add the rest of the ingredients, bring to a simmer and cook over medium heat for 20 minutes.
3. Blend everything using an immersion blender, ladle into soup bowls and serve.

Nutrition:

Calories: 114

Total fat: 8g

Saturated fat: 6g

Sodium: 128mg

Carbs: 18g

Fiber: 8g

Protein: 6g

Mushrooms and Chard Soup

Preparation time: 10 minutes

Cooking time: 30 minutes

Servings: 4

Ingredients:

- 3 cups Swiss chard, chopped
- 6 cups vegetable stock
- 1 cup mushrooms, sliced
- 2 garlic cloves, minced
- 1 tablespoon olive oil
- 2 scallions, chopped
- 2 tablespoons balsamic vinegar
- 1/4 cup basil, chopped
- Salt and black pepper to the taste
- 1 tablespoon cilantro, chopped

Directions:

1. Heat up a pot with the oil over medium high heat; add the scallions and the garlic and sauté for 5 minutes.
2. Add the mushrooms and sauté for another 5 minutes.
3. Add the rest of the ingredients, toss, bring to a simmer and cook over medium heat for 20 minutes more.
4. Ladle the soup into bowls and serve.

Nutrition:

Calories: 124

Total fat: 4g

Saturated fat: 3g

Sodium: 188mg

Carbs: 18g

Fiber: 8g

Protein: 6g

Tomato, Green Beans and Chard Soup

Preparation time: 10 minutes

Cooking time: 35 minutes

Servings: 4

Ingredients:

- 2 scallions, chopped
- 1 cup Swiss chard, chopped
- 1 tablespoon olive oil
- 1 red bell pepper, chopped
- Salt and black pepper to the taste
- 1 cup tomatoes, cubed
- 1 cup green beans, chopped
- 6 cups vegetable stock
- 2 tablespoons tomato pasta
- 2 garlic cloves, minced
- 2 teaspoons thyme, chopped
- 1/2 Teaspoon red pepper flakes

Directions:

1. Heat up a pot with the oil over medium heat; add the scallions, garlic and the pepper flakes and sauté for 5 minutes.

2. Add the chard and the other ingredients toss bring to a simmer and cook over medium heat for 30 minutes more.

3. Ladle the soup into bowls and serve for lunch.

Nutrition:

Calories: 119

Total fat: 8g

Saturated fat: 6g

Sodium: 136mg

Carbs: 17g

Fiber: 7g

Protein: 4g

Eggplant and Peppers Soup

Preparation time: 10 minutes

Cooking time: 40 minutes

Servings: 4

Ingredients:

- 2 red bell peppers, chopped
- 3 scallions, chopped
- 3 garlic cloves, minced
- 2 tablespoon olive oil
- Salt and black pepper to the taste
- 5 cups vegetable stock
- 1 bay leaf
- 1/2 cup coconut cream
- 1-pound eggplants, roughly cubed
- 2 tablespoons basil, chopped

Directions:

1. Heat up a pot with the oil over medium heat; add the scallions and the garlic and sauté for 5 minutes.

2. Add the peppers and the eggplants and sauté for 5 minutes more.

3. Add the remaining ingredients, toss, bring to a simmer, cook for 30 minutes, ladle into bowls and serve for lunch.

Nutrition:

Calories: 119

Total fat: 8g

Saturated fat: 6g

Sodium: 116mg

Carbs: 17g

Fiber: 9g

Protein: 6g

Cauliflower and Artichokes Soup

Preparation time: 10 minutes

Cooking time: 25 minutes

Servings: 4

Ingredients:

- 1 pound cauliflower florets
- 1 cup canned artichoke hearts
- 2 scallions, chopped
- 2 tablespoons olive oil
- 2 garlic cloves, minced
- 6 cups vegetable stock
- Salt and black pepper to the taste
- 2/3 cup coconut cream
- 2 tablespoons cilantro, chopped

Directions:

1. Heat up a pot with the oil over medium heat; add the scallions and the garlic and sauté for 5 minutes.

2. Add the cauliflower and the other ingredients toss bring to a simmer and cook over medium heat for 20 minutes more.

3. Blend the soup using an immersion blender, divide it into bowls and serve.

Nutrition:

Calories: 124

Total fat: 9g

Saturated fat: 8g

Sodium: 168mg

Carbs: 18g

Fiber: 8g

Protein: 6g

Rich Beans Soup

Preparation time: 10 minutes

Cooking time: 7 minutes

Servings: 4

Ingredients:

- 1 pound navy beans
- 1 yellow onion, chopped
- 4 garlic cloves, crushed
- 2 quarts veggie stock
- A pinch of sea salt
- Black pepper to the taste
- 2 potatoes, peeled and cubed

- 2 teaspoons dill, dried
- 1 cup sun-dried tomatoes, chopped
- 1-pound carrots, sliced
- 4 tablespoons parsley, minced

Directions:

1. Put the stock in your slow cooker.
2. Add beans, onion, garlic, potatoes, tomatoes, carrots, dill, salt and pepper, stir, cover and cook on low for 7 hours.
3. Stir your soup, add parsley, divide into bowls and serve.

Nutrition:

Calories: 134

Total fat: 8g

Saturated fat: 5g

Sodium: 168mg

Carbs: 13g

Fiber: 8g

Protein: 6g

Mushroom Soup (Instant Pot)

Preparation time: 10 minutes

Cooking time: 7 minutes

Servings: 4

Ingredients:

- 1 onion (small, diced)
- 1 cup white button mushrooms (chopped)
- 1 cup Portobello mushrooms (stems removed, chopped)
- 2 cloves garlic (minced)
- 1/4 cup white wine
- 2 1/2 cups mushroom stock
- 2 tsp. salt and pepper
- 1 tsp. fresh thyme
- Cashew Cream:
- 1/2 cup raw cashews (soaked)
- 1/2 cup mushroom stock

Directions:

1. Add the onions and mushrooms to the instant pot, stirring every now and then, and set on "Sauté" mode for about 10 minutes (until the mushrooms have shrunk in size).
2. Add the garlic and sauté for 2 more minutes.
3. Add the wine and stir in until it evaporates and the smell of wine isn't as strong.
4. Add the salt, pepper, thyme, and mushroom stock, and stir. Cancel the sauté mode.
5. Put the lid on and put it on manual, setting the time to 5 minutes.
6. Add cashews and water into a blender, and blend until smooth. Release the pressure from the pot, remove the lid, and transfer to the blender and blend until smooth.

Nutrition:

Calories: 134

Total fat: 9g

Saturated fat: 5g

Sodium: 118mg

Carbs: 16g

Fiber: 8g

Protein: 6g

Indian Chana Chaat Salad

Preparation time: 10 minutes

Cooking Time: 45 minutes + chilling time

Servings: 4

Ingredients:

- 1-pound dry chickpeas, soaked overnight
- 2 San Marzano tomatoes, diced
- 1 Persian cucumber, sliced
- 1 onion, chopped
- 1 bell pepper, seeded and thinly sliced
- 1 green chili, seeded and thinly sliced
- 2 handfuls baby spinach
- 1/2 teaspoon Kashmiri chili powder
- 4 curry leaves, chopped
- 1 tablespoon chaat masala
- 2 tablespoons fresh lemon juice, or to taste
- 4 tablespoons olive oil
- 1 teaspoon agave syrup
- 1/2 teaspoon mustard seeds
- 1/2 teaspoon coriander seeds
- 2 tablespoons sesame seeds, lightly toasted
- 2 tablespoons fresh cilantro, roughly chopped

Directions:

1. Drain the chickpeas and transfer them to a large saucepan. Cover the chickpeas with water by 2 inches and bring it to a boil.

2. Immediately turn the heat to a simmer and continue to cook for approximately 40 minutes.

3. Toss the chickpeas with the tomatoes, cucumber, onion, peppers, spinach, chili powder, curry leaves and chaat masala.

4. In a small mixing dish, thoroughly combine the lemon juice, olive oil, agave syrup, mustard seeds and coriander seeds.

5. Garnish with sesame seeds and fresh cilantro. Bon appétit!

Nutrition:

Calories: 604;

Fat: 23.1g;

Carbs: 80g;

Protein: 25.3g

Thai-Style Tempeh and Noodle Salad

Preparation time: 10 minutes

Cooking Time: 45 minutes

Servings: 3

Ingredients:

- 6 ounces tempeh
- 4 tablespoons rice vinegar
- 4 tablespoons soy sauce
- 2 garlic cloves, minced
- 1 small-sized lime, freshly juiced
- 5 ounces rice noodles

- 1 carrot, julienned

- 1 shallot, chopped

- 3 handfuls Chinese cabbage, thinly sliced

- 3 handfuls kale, torn into pieces

- 1 bell pepper, seeded and thinly sliced

- 1 bird's eye chili, minced

- 1/4 cup peanut butter

- 2 tablespoons agave syrup

Directions:

1. Place the tempeh, 2 tablespoons of the rice vinegar, soy sauce, garlic and lime juice in a ceramic dish; let it marinate for about 40 minutes.

2. Meanwhile, cook the rice noodles according to the package Directions. Drain your noodles and transfer them to a salad bowl.

3. Add the carrot, shallot, cabbage, kale and peppers to the salad bowl. Add in the peanut butter, the remaining 2 tablespoons of the rice vinegar and agave syrup and toss to combine well.

4. Top with the marinated tempeh and serve immediately. Enjoy!

Nutrition:

Calories: 494;

Fat: 14.5g;

Carbs: 75g;

Protein: 18.7g

Chapter 7: Main Recipes

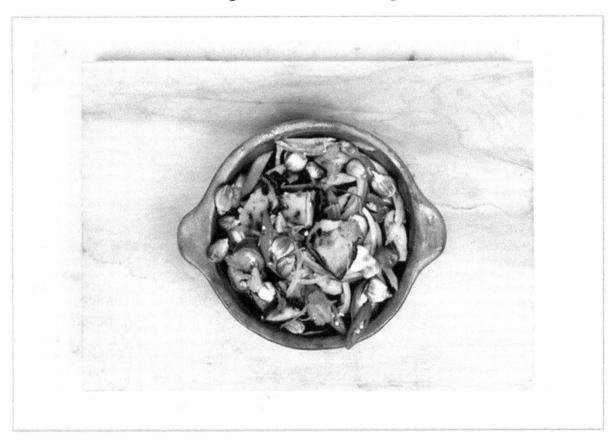

Black Bean Burgers

Preparation Time: 5 Minutes

Cooking Time: 20 Minutes

Servings: 4

Ingredients:

- 1 onion, diced
- 1/2 cup corn nibs
- 2 cloves garlic, minced
- 1/2 teaspoon oregano, dried
- 1/2 cup flour
- 1 jalapeno pepper, small
- 2 cups black beans, mashed & canned
- 1/4 cup breadcrumbs (vegan)
- 2 teaspoons parsley, minced
- 1/4 teaspoon cumin
- 1 tablespoon olive oil
- 2 teaspoons chili powder
- 1/2 red pepper, diced
- Sea salt to taste

Directions:

1. Set your flour on a plate, and then get out your garlic, onion, peppers and oregano, throwing it in a pan.
2. Cook over medium-high heat, and then cook until the onions are translucent.
3. Place the peppers in, and sauté until tender.
4. Cook for two minutes, and then set it to the side.
5. Use a potato masher to mash your black beans, and then stir in the vegetables, cumin, breadcrumbs, parsley, salt and chili powder, and then divide it into six patties.
6. Coat each side, and then cook until it's fried on each side.

Nutrition:

Calories: 211

Carbs: 12g

Fat: 7g

Protein: 12g

Dijon Maple Burgers

Preparation Time: 10 Minutes

Cooking Time: 40 Minutes

Servings: 12

Ingredients:

- 1 red bell pepper
- 19 ounces can chickpeas, rinsed & drained
- 1 cup almonds, ground
- 2 teaspoons Dijon mustard
- 1 teaspoon oregano
- 1/2 teaspoon sage
- 1 cup spinach, fresh
- 1 – 1/2 cups rolled oats
- 1 clove garlic, pressed
- 1/2 lemon, juiced
- 2 teaspoons maple syrup, pure

Directions:

1. Get out a baking sheet. Line it with parchment paper.
2. Cut your red pepper in half and then take the seeds out. Place it on your baking sheet, and roast in the oven while you prepare your other *Ingredients:*
3. Process your chickpeas, almonds, mustard and maple syrup together in a food processor.
4. Add in your lemon juice, oregano, sage, garlic and spinach, processing again. Make sure it's combined, but don't puree it.
5. Once your red bell pepper is softened, which should roughly take ten minutes,

add this to the processor as well. Add in your oats, mixing well.

Nutrition:

Calories: 209

Carbs: 11g

Fat: 5g

Protein: 9g

Hearty Black Lentil Curry

Preparation Time: 15 Minutes

Cooking Time: 6 Hours

Servings: 7

Ingredients:

- 1 cup of black lentils, rinsed and soaked overnight
- 14 ounces of chopped tomatoes
- 2 large white onions, peeled and sliced
- 1 1/2 teaspoon of minced garlic
- 1 teaspoon of grated ginger
- 1 red chili
- 1 teaspoon of salt
- 1/4 teaspoon of red chili powder
- 1 teaspoon of paprika
- 1 teaspoon of ground turmeric
- 2 teaspoons of ground cumin
- 2 teaspoons of ground coriander
- 1/2 cup of chopped coriander
- 4-ounce of vegetarian butter
- 1 fluid of ounce water
- 2 fluid of ounce vegetarian double cream

Directions:

1. Place a large pan over a moderate heat, add butter and let heat until melt.
2. Add the onion and garlic and ginger and let cook for 10 to 15 minutes or until onions are caramelized.

3. Then stir in salt, red chili powder, paprika, turmeric, cumin, ground coriander, and water.
4. Transfer this mixture to a 6-quarts slow cooker and add tomatoes and red chili.
5. Drain lentils, add to slow cooker and stir until just mix.
6. Plug in slow cooker; adjust cooking time to 6 hours and let cook on low heat setting.
7. When the lentils are done, stir in cream and adjust the seasoning.
8. Serve with boiled rice or whole wheat bread.

Nutrition:

Calories: 171

Carbs: 10g

Fat: 7g

Protein: 12g

Flavorful Refried Beans

Preparation Time: 15 Minutes

Cooking Time: 8 Hours

Servings: 8

Ingredients:

- 3 cups of pinto beans, rinsed
- 1 small jalapeno pepper, seeded and chopped
- 1 medium-sized white onion, peeled and sliced
- 2 tablespoons of minced garlic
- 5 teaspoons of salt
- 2 teaspoons of ground black pepper
- 1/4 teaspoon of ground cumin
- 9 cups of water

Directions:

1. Using a 6-quarts slow cooker, place all the *Ingredients:* and stir until it mixes properly.
2. Cover the top, plug in the slow cooker; adjust the cooking time to 6 hours, let it cook on high heat setting and add more water if the beans get too dry.
3. When the beans are done, drain them and reserve the liquid.
4. Mash the beans using a potato masher and pour in the reserved cooking liquid until it reaches your desired mixture.
5. Serve immediately.

Nutrition:

Calories: 198

Carbs: 22g

Fat: 7g

Protein: 19g

Smoky Red Beans and Rice

Preparation Time: 15 Minutes

Cooking Time: 5 Hours

Servings: 8

Ingredients:

- 30 ounces of cooked red beans
- 1 cup of brown rice, uncooked
- 1 cup of chopped green pepper
- 1 cup of chopped celery
- 1 cup of chopped white onion
- 1 1/2 teaspoon of minced garlic
- 1/2 teaspoon of salt
- 1/4 teaspoon of cayenne pepper
- 1 teaspoon of smoked paprika
- 2 teaspoons of dried thyme
- 1 bay leaf
- 2 1/3 cups of vegetable broth

Directions:

1. Using a 6-quarts slow cooker, all the Ingredients are except for the rice, salt, and cayenne pepper.
2. Stir until it mixes appropriately and then cover the top.
3. Plug in the slow cooker; adjust the cooking time to 4 hours, and steam on a low heat setting.
4. Then pour in and stir the rice, salt, cayenne pepper and continue cooking for an additional 2 hours at a high heat setting.

Nutrition:

Calories: 234

Carbs: 13g

Fat: 7g

Protein: 19g

Spicy Black-Eyed Peas

Preparation Time: 15 Minutes

Cooking Time: 60 Minutes

Servings: 8

Ingredients:

- 32-ounce black-eyed peas, uncooked
- 1 cup of chopped orange bell pepper
- 1 cup of chopped celery
- 8-ounce of chipotle peppers, chopped
- 1 cup of chopped carrot
- 1 cup of chopped white onion
- 1 teaspoon of minced garlic
- 3/4 teaspoon of salt
- 1/2 teaspoon of ground black pepper
- 2 teaspoons of liquid smoke flavoring
- 2 teaspoons of ground cumin
- 1 tablespoon of adobo sauce
- 2 tablespoons of olive oil
- 1 tablespoon of apple cider vinegar
- 4 cups of vegetable broth

Directions:

1. Place a medium-sized non-stick skillet pan over an average temperature of heat; add the bell peppers, carrot, onion, garlic, oil and vinegar.
2. Stir until it mixes properly and let it cook for 5 to 8 minutes or until it gets translucent.
3. Transfer this mixture to a 6-quarts slow cooker and add the peas, chipotle pepper, adobo sauce and the vegetable broth.
4. Stir until mixes properly and cover the top.
5. Plug in the slow cooker; adjust the cooking time to 8 hours and let it cook on the low heat setting or until peas are soft.

Nutrition:

Calories: 211

Carbs: 22g

Fat: 7g

Protein: 19g

Creamy Artichoke Soup

Preparation Time: 5 Minutes

Cooking Time: 40 Minutes

Servings: 4

Ingredients:

- 1 can artichoke hearts, drained
- 3 cups vegetable broth
- 2 tablespoon lemon juice
- 1 small onion, finely cut
- 2 cloves garlic, crushed
- 3 tablespoons olive oil
- 2 tablespoon flour
- 1/2 cup vegan cream

Directions:

1. Gently sauté the onion and garlic in some olive oil.
2. Add the flour, whisking constantly, and then add the hot vegetable broth slowly, while still whisking. Cook for about 5 minutes.
3. Blend the artichoke, lemon juice, salt and pepper until smooth. Add the puree to the broth mix, stir well, and then stir in the cream.
4. Cook until heated through. Garnish with a swirl of vegan cream or a sliver of artichoke.

Nutrition:

Calories: 211

Carbs: 12g

Fat: 7g

Protein: 11g

Super Rad-ish Avocado Salad

Preparation Time: 10 Minutes

Cooking Time: 25 Minutes

Servings: 2

Ingredients:

- 6 shredded carrots
- 6 ounces diced radishes
- 1 diced avocado
- 1/3 cup ponzu

Directions:

1. Bring all the above ingredients together in a serving bowl and toss.
2. Enjoy!

Nutrition:

Calories: 211

Carbs: 9g

Fat: 7g

Protein: 12g

Beauty School Ginger Cucumbers

Preparation Time: 10 Minutes

Cooking Time: 5 Minutes

Servings: 2

Ingredients:

- 1 sliced cucumber
- 3 teaspoon rice wine vinegar
- 1 1/2 tablespoon sugar
- 1 teaspoon minced ginger

Directions:

1. Bring all of the above ingredients together in a mixing bowl, and toss the ingredients well.
2. Enjoy!

Nutrition:

Calories: 210

Carbs: 14g

Fat: 7g

Protein: 19g

Mushroom Salad

Preparation Time: 10 Minutes

Cooking Time: 20 Minutes

Servings: 2

Ingredients:

- 1 tablespoon butter
- 1/2-pound cremini mushrooms, chopped
- 2 tablespoons extra-virgin olive oil
- Salt and black pepper to taste
- 2 bunches arugula

- 4 slices prosciutto
- 1 tablespoon apple cider vinegar
- 4 sundried tomatoes in oil, drained and chopped
- Fresh parsley leaves, chopped

Directions:

1. Heat a pan with butter and half of the oil.
2. Add the mushrooms, salt, and pepper. Stir-fry for 3 minutes. Reduce heat. Stir again, and cook for 3 minutes more.
3. Add rest of the oil and vinegar. Stir and cook for 1 minute.
4. Place arugula on a platter, add prosciutto on top, add the mushroom mixture, sundried tomatoes, more salt and pepper, parsley, and serve.

Nutrition:

Calories: 191

Carbs: 6g

Fat: 7g

Protein: 17g

Red Quinoa and Black Bean Soup

Preparation Time: 5 Minutes

Cooking Time: 40 Minutes

Servings: 6

Ingredients:

- 1/4 cup red quinoa
- 4 minced garlic cloves
- 1/2 tablespoon coconut oil
- 1 diced jalapeno
- 3 cups diced onion
- 2 teaspoon cumin
- 1 chopped sweet potato
- 1 teaspoon coriander
- 1 teaspoon chili powder

- 5 cups vegetable broth
- 15 ounces' black beans
- 1/2 teaspoon cayenne pepper
- 2 cups spinach

Directions:

1. Begin by bringing the quinoa into a saucepan to boil with two cups of water. Allow the quinoa to simmer for twenty minutes. Next, remove the quinoa from the heat.
2. To the side, heat the oil, the onion, and the garlic together in a large soup pot.
3. Add the jalapeno and the sweet potato and sauté for an additional seven minutes.
4. Next, add all the spices and the broth and bring the soup to a simmer for twenty-five minutes. The potatoes should be soft.
5. Before serving, add the quinoa, the black beans, and the spinach to the mix. Season, and serve warm. Enjoy.

Nutrition:

Calories: 211

Carbs: 22g

Fat: 7g

Protein: 19g

October Potato Soup

Preparation Time: 5 Minutes

Cooking Time: 20 Minutes

Servings: 3

Ingredients:

- 4 minced garlic cloves
- 2 teaspoon coconut oil
- 3 diced celery stalks
- 1 diced onion

- 2 teaspoon yellow mustard seeds
- 5 diced Yukon potatoes
- 6 cups vegetable broth
- 1 teaspoon oregano
- 1 teaspoon paprika
- 1/2 teaspoon cayenne pepper
- 1 teaspoon chili powder
- Salt and pepper to taste

Directions:

1. Begin by sautéing the garlic and the mustard seeds together in the oil in a large soup pot.
2. Next, add the onion and sauté the mixture for another five minutes.
3. Add the celery, the broth, the potatoes, and all the spices, and continue to stir.
4. Allow the soup to simmer for thirty minutes without a cover.
5. Next, Position about three cups of the soup in a blender, and puree the soup until you've reached a smooth consistency. Pour this back into the big soup pot, stir, and serve warm. Enjoy.

Nutrition:

Calories: 203

Carbs: 12g

Fat: 7g

Protein: 9g

Rice with Asparagus and Cauliflower

Preparation Time: 5 Minutes

Cooking Time: 20 Minutes

Servings: 2

Ingredients:

- 3 ounces' asparagus
- 3 ounces' cauliflower, chopped
- 2 ounces' tomato sauce

- 1/2 cup of brown rice
- 3/4 cup of water
- 1/3 teaspoon salt
- 1/4 teaspoon ground black pepper
- 1/4 teaspoon garlic powder
- 1 tablespoon olive oil

Directions:

1. Take a medium saucepan, place it over medium heat, add oil, add asparagus and cauliflower and then sauté for 5 to 7 minutes until golden brown.
2. Season with garlic powder, salt, and black pepper, stir in tomato sauce, and then cook for 1 minute.
3. Add rice, pour in water, stir until mixed, cover with a lid and cook for 10 to 12 minutes until rice has absorbed all the liquid and become tender.
4. When done, remove the pan from heat, fluff rice with a fork, and then serve.

Nutrition:

Calories: 257

Carbs: 4g

Fat: 4g

Protein: 40g

Spaghetti with Tomato Sauce

Preparation Time: 5 Minutes

Cooking Time: 15 Minutes

Servings: 2

Ingredients:

- 4 ounces' spaghetti
- 2 green onions, greens, and whites separated
- 1/8 teaspoon coconut sugar

- 3 ounces' tomato sauce
- 1 tablespoon olive oil
- 1/3 teaspoon salt
- 1/4 teaspoon ground black pepper

Directions:

1. Prepare the spaghetti, and for this, cook it according to the *Directions* on the packet and then set aside.
2. Then take a skillet pan, place it over medium heat, add oil and when hot, add white parts of green onions and cook for 2 minutes until tender.
3. Add tomato sauce, season with salt and black pepper and bring it to a boil.
4. Switch heat to medium-low level, simmer sauce for 1 minute, then add the cooked spaghetti and toss until mixed.
5. Divide spaghetti between two plates, and then serve.

Nutrition:

Calories: 265

Carbs: 8g

Fat: 2g

Protein: 7g

Crispy Cauliflower

Preparation Time: 5 Minutes

Cooking Time: 15 Minutes

Servings: 2

Ingredients:

- 6 ounces of cauliflower florets
- 1/2 of zucchini, sliced
- 1/2 teaspoon of sea salt
- 1/2 tablespoon curry powder
- 1/4 teaspoon maple syrup
- 2 tablespoons olive oil

Directions:

1. Switch on the oven, then set it to 450 degrees F and let it preheat.
2. Meanwhile, take a medium bowl, add cauliflower florets and zucchini slices, add remaining ingredients reserving 1 tablespoon oil, and toss until well coated.
3. Take a medium skillet pan, place it over medium-high heat, add remaining oil and wait until it gets hot.
4. Spread cauliflower and zucchini in a single layer and sauté for 5 minutes, tossing frequently.
5. Then transfer the pan into the oven and then bake for 8 to 10 minutes until vegetables have turned golden brown and thoroughly cooked, stirring halfway.

Nutrition:

Calories: 161

Carbs: 2g

Fat: 2g

Protein: 7g

Avocado Toast with Chickpeas

Preparation Time: 5 Minutes

Cooking Time: 5 Minutes

Servings: 2

Ingredients:

- 1/2 of avocado, peeled, pitted
- 4 tablespoons canned chickpeas, liquid reserved
- 1 tablespoon lime juice
- 1 teaspoon apple cider vinegar
- 2 slices of bread, toasted
- 1/4 teaspoon salt
- 1/4 teaspoon paprika
- 1 teaspoon olive oil

Directions:

1. Take a medium skillet pan, place it over medium heat, add oil and when hot, add chickpeas and cook for 2 minutes.
2. Sprinkle 1/8 teaspoon each salt and paprika over chickpeas, toss to coat, and then remove the pan from heat.
3. Place avocado in a bowl, mash by using a fork, drizzle with lime juice and vinegar and stir until well mixed.
4. Spread mashed avocado over bread slices, scatter chickpeas on top and then serve.

Nutrition:

Calories: 235

Carbs: 5g

Fat: 5g

Protein: 31g

Green Onion Soup

Preparation Time: 5 Minutes

Cooking Time: 12 Minutes

Servings: 2

Ingredients:

- 6 green onions, chopped
- 7 ounces diced potatoes
- 1/3 teaspoon salt
- 2 tablespoons olive oil
- 1/4 cup vegetable broth
- 1/4 teaspoon ground white pepper
- 1/4 teaspoon ground coriander

Directions:

1. Take a small pan, place potato in it, cover with water, and then place the pan over medium heat.

2. Boil the potato until cooked and tender, and when done, drain the potatoes and set aside until required.
3. Return saucepan over low heat, add oil and add green onions and cook for 5 minutes until cooked.
4. Season with salt, pepper, and coriander, add potatoes, pour in vegetable broth, stir until mixed and bring it to simmer.
5. Then remove the pan from heat and blend the mixture by using an immersion blender until creamy.
6. Taste to adjust seasoning, then ladle soup into bowls and then serve.

Nutrition:

Calories: 191

Carbs: 1g

Fat: 1g

Protein: 15g

Potato Soup

Preparation Time: 5 Minutes

Cooking Time: 12 Minutes

Servings: 2

Ingredients:

- 2 potatoes, peeled, cubed
- 1/3 teaspoon salt
- 1/2 cup vegetable broth
- 3/4 cup of water
- 1/8 teaspoon ground black pepper
- 1 tablespoon Cajun seasoning

Directions:

1. Take a small pan, place potato cubes in it, cover with water and vegetable broth, and then place the pan over medium heat.
2. Boil the potato until cooked and tender, and when done, remove the pan from

heat and blend the mixture by using an immersion blender until creamy.
3. Return pan over medium-low heat, add remaining *Ingredients:* stir until mixed and bring it to a simmer.
4. Taste to adjust seasoning, then ladle soup into bowls and then serve.

Nutrition:

Calories: 203

Carbs: 5g

Fat: 6g

Protein: 37g

Teriyaki Eggplant

Preparation Time: 5 Minutes

Cooking Time: 15 Minutes

Servings: 2

Ingredients:

- 1/2-pound eggplant
- 1 green onion, chopped
- 1/2 teaspoon grated ginger
- 1/2 teaspoon minced garlic
- 1/3 cup soy sauce
- 1 tablespoon coconut sugar
- 1/2 tablespoon apple cider vinegar
- 1 tablespoon olive oil

Directions:

1. Prepare vegan teriyaki sauce and for this, take a medium bowl, add ginger, garlic, soy sauce, vinegar, and sugar in it and then whisk until sugar has dissolved completely.
2. Cut eggplant into cubes, add them into vegan teriyaki sauce, toss until well coated and marinate for 10 minutes.
3. When ready to cook, take a grill pan, place it over medium-high heat, grease

it with oil, and when hot, add marinated eggplant.

4. Cook for 3 to 4 minutes per side until nicely browned and beginning to charred, drizzling with excess marinade frequently and transfer to a plate.
5. Sprinkle green onion on top of the eggplant and then serve.

Nutrition:

Calories: 132

Carbs: 4g

Fat: 4g

Protein: 13g

Broccoli Stir-Fry with Sesame Seeds

Preparation Time: 10 Minutes

Cooking Time: 8 Minutes

Servings: 4

Ingredients:

- Two tablespoons extra-virgin olive oil (optional)
- One tablespoon grated fresh ginger
- cups broccoli florets
- ¼teaspoon sea salt (optional)
- Two garlic cloves, minced
- Two tablespoons toasted sesame seeds

Directions:

1. Heat the olive oil (if desired) in a large nonstick skillet over medium-high heat until shimmering.
2. Fold in the ginger, broccoli, and sea salt (if desired) and stir-fry for 5 to 7 minutes, or until the broccoli is browned.
3. Cook the garlic until tender, about 30 seconds.
4. Sprinkle with the sesame seeds and serve warm.

Nutrition:

Calories: 135

Fat: 10.9g

Carbs: 9.7g

Protein: 4.1g

Fiber: 3.3g

Moroccan Couscous

Preparation time: 5minutes

Cooking time: 5minutes

Servings: 4

Ingredients:

- 1 cup couscous
- 1.1/2 cups water
- 1.1/2 teaspoons orange
- 3/4 cup freshly squeezed orange juice
- 4 or 5 garlic cloves, minced or pressed
- 2 tablespoons raisins
- 2 tablespoons pure maple syrup or agave nectar
- 2.1/4 teaspoons ground cumin
- 2.1/4 teaspoons ground cinnamon
- 1/4 teaspoon paprika
- 2.1/2 tablespoons minced fresh mint
- 2 teaspoons freshly squeezed lemon juice
- 1/2 teaspoon sea salt

Directions:

1. Merge the couscous and water. Add the orange zest and juice, garlic, raisins,

112

maple syrup, cumin, cinnamon, and paprika and stir. Bring the mixture to a boil over medium-high heat.

2. Remove the couscous from the heat and stir well. Cover with a tight-fitting lid and set aside until all of the liquids are absorbed and the couscous is tender and fluffy. Gently stir in the mint, lemon juice, and salt. Serve warm or cold.

Nutrition:

Calories: 637

Total fat: 7g

Protein: 52g

Sodium: 246

Fat: 19g

Moroccan Tempeh

Preparation time: 15minutes

Cooking time: 20minutes

Servings: 4

Ingredients:

- 1-pound plain tempeh
- 1 cup water
- 1/4 cup tamari, shout, or soy sauce
- 1.1/2 cups gluten-free all-purpose flour
- 1/2 cup cornmeal
- 1/4 cup sesame seeds
- 1 teaspoon paprika
- 1 teaspoon sea salt
- 1 teaspoon freshly ground black pepper
- 1 cup plain unsweetened nondairy milk
- 1/2 cup sunflower oil

Directions:

1. Gently slice the tempeh into 8 rectangular cutlets that are approximately 21/2 by 4 inches in size and 1/2 inch thick, or half their original thickness. Evenly pour the water and tamari on top.

2. Mix the flour, cornmeal, sesame seeds, paprika, salt, and pepper. Pour the milk into another shallow bowl.

3. In the now-empty skillet, heat the oil over medium-high heat. While it is heating, dip a tempeh cutlet in the milk, and then in the flour coating. Then dip the tempeh in the milk again, then in the flour coating a second time to form an even, thick layer of coating on all sides. Repeat with all the tempeh cutlets.

4. Working in batches, pan-fry the cutlets for about 2 minutes on each side until golden brown. Remove and drain on paper towels.

5. Place each tempeh cutlet on a plate, drizzle with the sauce, and serve immediately.

Nutrition:

Calories: 437

Total fat: 7g

Protein: 32g

Sodium: 446

Fat: 19g

Red Tofu Curry

Preparation time: 15 minutes

Cooking time: 65 minutes

Servings: 4

Ingredients:

- 1 1/2 tablespoon canola oil
- 1 package extra-firm tofu
- 3 cups baby carrots
- 2 cups peeled red
- 2 onions,
- 3 teaspoons garlic
- 1 piece ginger
- 1.1/2 cups water
- 1 cup canned unsweetened coconut milk
- 1.1/2 tablespoons red curry paste
- 1 vegetable bouillon cube
- 1/2 teaspoon salt
- Cooked rice, for serving
- Fresh cilantro, for garnish

Directions:

1. Heat the oil in a skillet. Place the tofu and brown.
2. Merge all the ingredients and mix well.
3. Cook on low heat
4. Present over rice and garnished with cilantro.

Nutrition:

Calories: 617

Total fat: 2g

Protein: 32g

Sodium: 563mg

Fiber: 10g

Spicy Tomato-Lentil Stew

Preparation time: 15 minutes

Cooking time: 60 minutes

Servings: 5

Ingredients:

- 2 cups dry brown
- 1 can crushed tomatoes
- 1 can diced tomatoes
- 2 cups peeled potatoes
- 1 yellow onion
- 1/2 cup carrot
- 1/2 cup celery
- 2 tablespoons hot sauce
- 2 teaspoons garlic
- 2 teaspoons cumin
- 1 teaspoon chili
- 1/2 teaspoon coriander
- 1/4 teaspoon paprika
- 1 1/4 bay leaf
- pepper
- 4 bouillon cubes

Directions:

1. Merge all the ingredients and mix well.
2. Cook on low heat
3. Ready to serve.

Nutrition:

Calories: 517

Total fat: 2g

Protein: 32g

Sodium: 1,063mg

Fiber: 38g

Mixed-Bean Chili

Preparation time: 10minutes

Cooking time: 60 minutes

Servings: 4

Ingredients:

- 5 (15-ounce) cans your choice beans, drained and rinsed
- 1 (15-ounce) can diced tomatoes, with juice
- 1 (6-ounce) can tomato paste
- 1 cup water
- 1 green bell pepper, diced
- 2 cups stemmed and chopped kale
- 1/2 medium yellow onion, diced
- 2 tablespoons ground cumin
- 1 tablespoon chili powder
- 1 teaspoon minced garlic (2 cloves)
- 1 teaspoon cayenne pepper
- Pinch salt

Directions:

1. Place the beans, diced tomatoes, tomato paste, water, bell pepper, kale, onion, cumin, chili powder, garlic, and cayenne pepper in a slow cooker.
2. Season with salt and serve.

Nutrition:

Calories: 417

Total fat: 2g

Protein: 72g

Sodium: 463mg

Fiber: 10g

Butternut Squash Soup

Preparation time: 10minutes

Cooking time: 70 minutes

Servings: 4

Ingredients:

- 2 (10-ounce) packages frozen butternut squash
- 6 cups water
- 1 medium yellow onion, chopped
- 1 teaspoon minced garlic (2 cloves)
- 5 vegetable bouillon cubes
- 2 bay leaves
- 1/4 teaspoon freshly ground black pepper
- 1/8 teaspoon cayenne pepper
- 1 (8-ounce) package vegan cream cheese, cut into chunks

Directions:

1. Combine the butternut squash, water, onion, garlic, bouillon cubes, bay leaves, black pepper, and cayenne pepper in a slow cooker. Stir to mix.
2. Cook on low heat.
3. Remove the bay leaves.
4. Purée half of the soup using a blender.
5. Stir in the cream cheese. Cover and cook on low for 30 minutes longer.

Nutrition:

Calories: 617

Total fat: 2g

Protein: 82g

Sodium: 563mg

Fiber: 10g

Split-Pea Soup

Preparation time: 10minutes

Cooking time: 65 minutes

Servings: 5

Ingredients:

- 1-pound dried green split peas, rinsed
- 6 cups water
- 3 carrots, diced
- 3 celery stalks, diced
- 1 medium russet potato, peeled and diced
- 1 small yellow onion, diced
- 1.1/2 teaspoons minced garlic (3 cloves)
- 5 vegetable bouillon cubes
- 1 bay leaf
- Freshly ground black pepper

Directions:

1. Combine the split peas, water, carrots, celery, potato, onion, garlic, bouillon cubes, and bay leaf in a slow cooker; mix well.

2. Cook on low heat, and season with pepper.

Nutrition:

Calories: 817

Total fat: 2g

Protein: 82g

Sodium: 363mg

Fiber: 10g

Tomato Bisque

Preparation time: 10minutes

Cooking time: 65 minutes

Servings: 4

Ingredients:

- 2 (28-ounce) cans crushed tomatoes
- 1 (28-ounce) can whole peeled tomatoes, with juice
- 1 (15-ounce) can white beans, drained and rinsed
- 1/2 cup cashew pieces
- 2 vegetable bouillon cubes
- 1 tablespoon dried basil
- 2 teaspoons minced garlic (4 cloves)
- 3 cups water
- Pinch salt
- Freshly ground black pepper

Directions:

1. Combine the crushed tomatoes, whole peeled tomatoes, white beans, cashew pieces, bouillon cubes, dried basil, garlic, and water in a slow cooker.

2. Cook on low heat.

3. Blend the soup until smooth. Season with salt and pepper.

Nutrition:

Calories: 817

Total fat: 2g

Protein: 82g

Sodium:

Cheesy Potato-Broccoli Soup

Preparation time: 15minutes

Cooking time: 70minutes

Servings: 4

Ingredients:

- 2 pounds red or Yukon potatoes, chopped
- 1 (10-ounce) bag frozen broccoli
- 2 cups unsweetened nondairy milk
- 1 small yellow onion, chopped
- 1.1/2 teaspoons minced garlic (3 cloves)
- 3 vegetable bouillon cubes
- 4 cups water
- 1 cup melts able vegan Cheddar-cheese shreds (such as Diana or Follow Your Heart)
- Pinch salt
- Freshly ground black pepper

Directions:

1. Combine the potatoes, broccoli, nondairy milk, onion, garlic, bouillon cubes, and water in a slow cooker; mix well.

2. Cook on low heat.

3. Forty-five minutes before serving, use an immersion blender (or a regular blender, working in batches) to blend the soup until it's nice and creamy.

4. Stir in the vegan cheese, cover, and cook for another 45 minutes.

5. Season with salt and pepper.

Nutrition:

Calories: 517

Total fat: 2g

Protein: 92g

Sodium:

Vegetable Stew

Preparation time: 15minutes

Cooking time: 65minutes

Servings: 4

Ingredients:

- 1 (28-ounce) can diced tomatoes, with juice
- 1 can white beans
- 1 cup diced green beans
- 2 medium potatoes, diced
- 1 cup frozen carrots and peas mix
- 1 small yellow onion, diced
- 1 (1-inch) piece ginger, peeled and minced
- 1 teaspoon minced garlic (2 cloves)
- 3 cups Vegetable Broth
- 2 teaspoons ground cumin

- 1/2 teaspoon red pepper flakes
- Juice of 1/2 lemon
- 1 cup dried pasta
- Pinch salt
- Freshly ground black pepper
- Pesto, for serving

Directions:

1. Combine the diced tomatoes, white beans, green beans, potatoes, carrots and peas mix, onion, ginger, garlic, vegetable broth, cumin, red pepper flakes, and lemon juice in a slow cooker.

2. Cook on low heat.

3. Pour with salt and pepper and serve with a dollop of pesto.

Nutrition:

Calories: 617

Total fat: 2g

Protein: 92g

Sodium: 356

Fat: 16g

Frijoles De La Olla

Preparation time: 15minutes

Cooking time: 65minutes

Servings: 4

Ingredients:

- 1-pound dry pinto beans, rinsed
- 1 small yellow onion, diced
- 1 jalapeño pepper, seeded and finely chopped

- 1.1/2 teaspoons minced garlic (3 cloves)
- 1 tablespoon ground cumin
- 1/2 teaspoon Mexican oregano (optional)
- 1 teaspoon red pepper flakes (optional)
- 4 cups water
- 2 tablespoons salt

Directions:

1. Place the beans, onion, jalapeño, garlic, cumin, oregano (if using), red pepper flakes (if using), water, and salt in a slow cooker.

2. Cook on low heat.

Nutrition

Total fat: 2g

Protein: 82g

Sodium: 346

Fat: 16g

Vegetable Hominy Soup

Preparation time: 15minutes

Cooking time: 30minutes

Servings: 4

Ingredients:

- 1 (28-ounce) can hominy, drained
- 1 (28-ounce) can diced tomatoes with green chills
- 5 medium red or Yukon potatoes, diced
- 1 large yellow onion, diced
- 2 cups chopped carrots

- 2 celery stalks, chopped
- 2 teaspoons minced garlic (4 cloves)
- 2 tablespoons chopped cilantro
- 1.1/2 tablespoons ground cumin
- 1.1/2 tablespoons seasoned salt
- 1 tablespoon chili powder
- 1 bay leaf
- 4 vegetable bouillon cubes
- 5 cups water
- Pinch salt
- Freshly ground black pepper

Directions:

1. Combine the hominy, diced tomatoes, potatoes, onion, carrots, celery, garlic, cilantro, cumin, seasoned salt, chili powder, bay leaf, vegetable bouillon, and water in a slow cooker; mix well. Cook on low heat.
2. . Remove the bay leaf. Season with salt and pepper.

Nutrition:

Calories: 417

Total fat: 2g

Protein: 72g

Sodium: 346

Fat: 16g

Lentil-Quinoa Chili

Preparation time: 15minutes

Cooking time: 30minutes

Servings: 4

Ingredients:

- 1/2 cup dry green lentils
- 1 can black beans
- 1/3 cup uncooked quinoa, rinsed
- 1 small yellow onion, diced
- 2 medium carrots, diced
- 2 teaspoons ground cumin
- 2 teaspoons chili powder
- 1.1/2 teaspoons minced garlic (3 cloves)
- 1 teaspoon dried oregano
- 3 vegetable bouillon cubes
- 1 bay leaf
- 4 cups water
- Pinch salt

Directions:

1. Place the lentils, black beans, quinoa, onion, carrots, cumin, chili powder, garlic, oregano, bouillon cubes, bay leaf, and water in a slow cooker; mix well.
2. Cook on low heat.
3. Remove the bay leaf, season with salt, and serve.

Nutrition:

Calories: 617

Total fat: 2g

Protein: 72g

Sodium: 346

Fat: 16g

Eggplant Curry

Preparation time: 15minutes

Cooking time: 35minutes

Servings: 5

Ingredients:

- 5 cups chopped eggplant
- 4 cups chopped zucchini
- 2 cups stemmed and chopped kale
- 1 (15-ounce) can full-fat coconut milk
- 1 (14.5-ounce) can diced tomatoes, drained
- 1 (6-ounce) can tomato paste
- 1 medium yellow onion, chopped
- 2 teaspoons minced garlic (4 cloves)
- 1 tablespoon curry powder
- 1 tablespoon gram masala
- 1/4 teaspoon cayenne pepper
- 1/4 teaspoon ground cumin
- 1 teaspoon salt
- Cooked rice, for serving

Directions:

1. Combine the eggplant, zucchini, kale, coconut milk, diced tomatoes, tomato paste, onion, garlic, curry powder, gram masala, cayenne pepper, cumin, and salt in a slow cooker; mix well.

2. Cook on low heat.

Nutrition:

Calories: 417

Total fat: 2g

Protein: 72g

Sodium: 346

Fat: 19g

Meaty Chili

Preparation time: 15minutes

Cooking time: 40minutes

Servings: 5

Ingredients:

- 1 tablespoon olive oil
- 2 packages of faux-ground-beef veggie crumble (such as Beyond Meat)
- 1 large red onion, chopped
- 1 large jalapeño pepper, seeded and chopped
- 2 1/2 teaspoons minced garlic
- 1 can diced tomatoes
- 1 can kidney beans
- 1 can black beans
- 1/2 cup frozen corn
- 1/4 cup chili powder
- 2 tablespoons ground cumin
- 1 teaspoon smoked paprika
- 1 vegetable bouillon cube
- 1.1/2 cups water

Directions:

1. Heat the olive oil in a sauté pan over medium-high heat. Add the veggie crumbles, onion, jalapeño, and garlic, and cook for 3 to 4 minutes, stirring occasionally.

2. Combine the veggie-crumble mixture, diced tomatoes, kidney beans, black beans, frozen corn, chili powder, cumin, smoked paprika, bouillon cube, and water in a slow cooker; mix well.

3. Cook on low heat.

Nutrition:

Calories: 547

Total fat: 8g

Protein: 62g

Sodium: 346

Fat: 19g

Sweet Potato Bisque

Preparation time: 15minutes

Cooking time: 45minutes

Servings: 4

Ingredients:

- 2 sweet potatoes, peeled and sliced
- 2 cups frozen butternut squash
- 2 (14.5-ounce) cans full-fat coconut milk
- 1 medium yellow onion, sliced
- 1 teaspoon minced garlic (2 cloves)
- 1 tablespoon dried basil
- 1 tablespoon chili powder
- 1 tablespoon ground cumin
- 1/2 cup water
- Pinch salt
- Freshly ground black pepper

Directions:

1. Combine the sweet potatoes, butternut squash, coconut milk, onion, garlic, dried basil, chili powder, cumin, and water in a slow cooker; mix well.

2. Cook on low heat.

3. Blend the soup until it's nice and creamy.

4. Season with salt and pepper.

Nutrition:

Calories: 447

Total fat: 8g

Protein: 72g

Sodium: 346

Fat: 19g

Chickpea Medley

Preparation time: 5minutes

Cooking time: 15minutes

Servings: 4

Ingredients:

- 2 tablespoons tahini
- 2 tablespoons coconut amines
- 1 (15-ounce) can chickpeas or 1.1/2 cups cooked chickpeas, rinsed and drained
- 1 cup finely chopped lightly packed spinach
- Carrot, peeled and grated

Directions:

1. Merge together the tahini and coconut amines in a bowl.

2. Add the chickpeas, spinach, and carrot to the bowl. Stir well and serve at room temperature.

3. *Simple Swap*: Coconut amines are almost like a sweeter, mellower version of soy sauce. However, if you want to use regular soy sauce or tamari, just use 11/2 tablespoons and add a dash of maple syrup or agave nectar to balance out the saltiness.

Nutrition:

Calories: 437

Total fat: 8g

Protein: 92g

Sodium: 246

Fat: 19g

Pasta with Lemon and Artichokes

Preparation time: 10minutes

Cooking time: 20minutes

Servings: 4

Ingredients:

- 16 ounces linguine or angel hair pasta
- 1/4 cup extra-virgin olive oil
- 8 garlic cloves, finely minced or pressed
- 2 (15-ounce) jars water-packed artichoke hearts, drained and quartered
- 2 tablespoons freshly squeezed lemon juice
- 1/4 cup thinly sliced fresh basil
- 1 teaspoon sea salt
- Freshly ground black pepper

Directions:

1. Use a large pot of water to a boil over high heat and cook the pasta until al dente according to the directions on the package.

2. While the pasta is cooking, heat the oil in a skillet over medium heat and cook the garlic, stirring often, for 1 to 2 minutes until it just begins to brown. Toss the garlic with the artichokes in a large bowl.

3. When the pasta is done, drain it and add it to the artichoke mixture, then add the lemon juice, basil, salt, and pepper. Gently stir and serve.

Nutrition:

Calories: 237

Total fat: 7g

Protein: 52g

Sodium: 346

Fat: 19g

Roasted Pine Nut Orzo

Preparation time: 10minutes

Cooking time: 15minutes

Servings: 3

Ingredients:

- 16 ounces orzo
- 1 cup diced roasted red peppers
- 1/4 cup pitted, chopped Klamath olives
- 4 garlic cloves, minced or pressed
- 3 tablespoons olive oil
- 1.1/2 tablespoons squeezed lemon juice
- 2 teaspoons balsamic vinegar

- 1 teaspoon sea salt

- 1/4 cup pine nuts

- 1/4 cup packed thinly sliced or torn fresh basil

Directions:

1. Use a large pot of water to a boil over medium-high heat and add the orzo. Cook, stirring often, for 10 minutes, or until the orzo has a chewy and firm texture. Drain well.

2. While the orzo is cooking, in a large bowl, combine the peppers, olives, garlic, olive oil, lemon juice, vinegar, and salt. Stir well.

3. In a dry skillet toasts the pine nuts over medium-low heat until aromatic and lightly browned, shaking the pan often so that they cook evenly

4. Upon reaching the desired texture and add it to the sauce mixture within a minute or so, to avoid clumping.

Nutrition:

Calories: 537

Total fat: 7g

Protein: 72g

Sodium: 246

Fat: 19g

Banana and Almond Butter Oats

Preparation Time: 10 minutes
Cooking time: 5 minutes
Servings: 2
Ingredients:

- 1 cup gluten-free moved oats

- 1 cup almond milk

- 1 cup of water

- 1 teaspoon cinnamon

- 2 tablespoons almond spread

- 1 banana, cut

Directions:

1. Mix the water and almond milk to a bubble in a little pot. Add the oats and diminish to a stew.

2. Cook until oats have consumed all fluid. Blend in cinnamon. Top with almond spread and banana and serve.

Nutrition:

Calories: 112;

Fat: 10g;

Protein: 9g;

Carbohydrates: 54g;

Fiber: 15g;

Sugar: 5g;

Sodium: 180mg

Greek Flatbreads

Preparation time: 15minutes

Cooking time: 10minutes

Servings: 4

Ingredients:

- 4 *Pita Bread* rounds or store-bought pita rounds

- 2 cups baby spinach leaves

- 1 cup sliced grape tomatoes

- 1/2 cup pitted, halved Klamath olives

- 1/2 cup thinly sliced red onion
- 1/3 cup thinly sliced fresh basil
- 1/4 cup sliced Greek pepperoncini (optional)
- 3 tablespoons extra-virgin olive oil (optional)

Directions:

1. Preheat the oven to 350°F.
2. Set the pita rounds on the oven rack and bake for 5 to 10 minutes until lightly browned and crisp.
3. Place a pita on each plate. Spread the hummus evenly over each. Evenly distribute the spinach, tomatoes, olives, onion, basil, and pepperoncini (if using) on top. Drizzle with olive oil (if using), then cut into quarters and serve immediately.

Nutrition:

Calories: 437

Total fat: 7g

Protein: 82g

Sodium: 346

Fat: 19g

Mediterranean Macro Plate

Preparation time: 10minutes

Cooking time: 10minutes

Servings: 4

Ingredients:

- 6 cups cauliflower florets
- 8 ounces firm or extra-firm tofu
- Olive oil cooking spray

- 1 tablespoon herbs de Provence
- Sea salt
- 1 recipe Full Madams
- *1* recipe Happy Hummus
- 6 cups sliced cucumber

Directions:

1. Spout an inch of water into a large pot and insert a steamer rack. Bring the water to a boil, add the cauliflower, cover, and cook over medium heat until tender, about 10 minutes.
2. While the cauliflower is cooking, cut the tofu into 1-inch cubes. Heat a large skillet over medium-high heat. Spray with cooking spray and lay the tofu in a single layer in the skillet. Sprinkle evenly with the herbs de Provence and salt. Cook for 4 minutes, or until the undersides are golden brown. Spray with cooking spray, flip, and cook for an additional 3 to 4 minutes until golden brown on the other side. Remove from the heat.
3. Divide the full me dames and hummus among 6 plates. Add a scoop of tofu and cauliflower to each plate and divide the cucumber for dipping into the hummus. Serve immediately.

Nutrition:

Calories: 537

Total fat: 7g

Protein: 82g

Sodium: 446

Fat: 19g

The Athena Pizza

Preparation time: 10minutes

Cooking time: 15minutes

Servings: 3

Ingredients:

- 4 *Pita Bread* rounds or store-bought pita bread
- 6 cups lightly packed stemmed and thinly sliced kale
- 2 tablespoons freshly squeezed lemon juice
- 1 tablespoon extra-virgin olive oil
- 4 garlic cloves, finely minced or pressed
- 1/4 teaspoon sea salt
- 1 recipe Macadamia-Rosemary Cheese
- 1 cup halved grape or cherry tomatoes
- 1/2 cup pitted, chopped Klamath olives

Directions:

1. Preheat the oven to 400°F.
2. Arrange the pita bread rounds in a single layer on two large rimmed baking sheets. Bake for 5 to 10 minutes until golden brown and crisp. Remove and set aside.
3. In a large bowl, mix the kale, lemon juice, and olive oil. Using your hands, work the lemon and oil into the kale, squeezing firmly, so that the kale becomes soft and tenderized, as well as a darker shade of green. Stir in the garlic and salt.
4. . Assemble the pizzas by spreading each pita with a generous coating of macadamia cheese and topping evenly

with the kale salad, tomatoes, and olives.

Nutrition:

Calories: 537

Total fat: 7g

Protein: 82g

Sodium: 446

Fat: 19g

Bream

Preparation time: 10minutes

Cooking time: 60minutes

Servings: 4

Ingredients:

- Olive oil cooking spray
- 2 medium zucchinis, cut into 1/2inch-thick rounds
- 2 gold potatoes, thinly sliced
- 4 tomatoes, sliced
- 1.3/4 cups tomato sauce
- 10 garlic cloves cut into large chunks
- 1.1/2 tablespoons olive oil
- 4 teaspoons dried basil
- 2 teaspoons dried oregano
- Teaspoon sea salt

Directions:

1. In a large bowl, combine the zucchini, potatoes, tomatoes, tomato sauce, garlic, olive oil, basil, oregano, and salt and stir well. Pour the vegetable into the dish.

2. Bake for 30 minutes, stir well, and bake for another 30 minutes, or until the potatoes are tender. Stir again and serve.

Nutrition:

Calories: 337

Total fat: 8

Protein: 82g

Sodium: 346

Fat: 19g

Green-Glory Soup (Instant Pot)

Preparation time: 10 minutes

Cooking time: 15 minutes

Servings: 4

Ingredients:

- 1 head cauliflower (florets)
- 1 onion (diced)
- 2 cloves garlic (minced)
- 1 cup spinach (fresh or frozen)
- 1 bay leaf (crumbled)
- 1 cup coconut milk
- 4 cups vegetable stock
- Salt and pepper to taste
- Herbs for garnish (optional)
- 1/2 cup coconut oil

Directions:

1. In a pressure pot on "sauté" mode, sauté onions and garlic until onions are browned. Once cooked, add the cauliflower and bay leaf and cook for about 5 minutes, stirring occasionally.

2. Add the spinach and continue cooking and stirring for 5 minutes.

3. Pour in the vegetable stock and set the timer for 10 minutes on high pressure to let the mix come to a boil; then allow quick pressure release and add the coconut milk.

4. Season with garnishes of choice as well as salt and pepper. Turn off the pot and mix the soup until it becomes thick and creamy with a hand blender.

Nutrition:

Calories: 114

Total fat: 9g

Saturated fat: 5g

Sodium: 128mg

Carbs: 19g

Fiber: 8g

Protein: 6g

Veggie Soup (Instant Pot)

Preparation time: 5 minutes

Cooking time: 10 minutes

Servings: 4

Ingredients:

- 2 tbsp. olive oil
- 1 onion (medium, chopped)
- 3 tbsp. parsley (fresh, minced)
- 1 clove of garlic (minced)
- 3 (14.5 oz.) cans vegetable broth
- 4 cups tomatoes (chopped)
- 1 cup celery (chopped)

- 1 cup carrots (sliced)
- 1 zucchini (halved and sliced)
- 2 tsp. basil (dried, crushed)
- 1/2 tsp. salt
- 1/2 tsp. Italian seasoning
- 1 tsp. red pepper flakes (crushed)
- 5 cups kale leaves (chopped)

Directions:

1. Heat pot on "sauté" mode until it says "hot"; then adds the oil.
2. Attach the onion, and cook until it is tender. Add the parsley and garlic, stirring constantly for 30 seconds; then add the vegetable broth.
3. Stir in the celery, tomato, zucchini, carrots, Italian seasoning, and red pepper to the pot and turn off the heat. Close the lid.
4. Turn the steam option to "sealing," selecting high pressure for 6 minutes. When done, turn the cooker off again, choosing the quick pressure release option; then select "sauté."
5. Add kale, stirring for 3 minutes or so until the soup comes to a boil. Turn the cooker off and serve.

Nutrition:

Calories: 134

Total fat: 9g

Saturated fat: 5g

Sodium: 138mg

Carbs: 26g

Fiber: 8g

Protein: 6g

Creamy Italian Herb Soup

Preparation time: 10 minutes

Cooking time: 30 minutes

Servings: 4

Ingredients:

- 2 cans full fat coconut milk
- 1/2 cup coconut cream
- 1/4 cup fresh parsley
- 1 cup broccoli florets
- 1 cup veggie broth
- 1 tbsp. olive oil
- 1 tsp. nutritional yeast
- 1 finely chopped onion
- 2 cloves minced garlic
- 1 cup fresh Italian herbs (basil, oregano, rosemary, thyme, and sage)
- Salt and black pepper to taste

Directions:

1. Caramelize onion and garlic in a large cooking pan over medium heat.
2. Add Italian herbs, stir, and adding coconut milk while stirring.
3. Add remaining ingredients with salt and pepper to taste and cook for 30 minutes.
4. You can blend it after cooking or eat it when it's the right temperature.
5. If you want to store and freeze, you have to blend it.

6. Either transfers it directly to a heat safe blender, or let it cool, then blends until smooth.

Nutrition:

Calories: 124

Total fat: 9g

Saturated fat: 5g

Sodium: 118mg

Carbs: 16g

Fiber: 8g

Protein: 6g

Cauliflower Soup (Instant Pot)

Preparation time: 10 minutes

Cooking time: 30 minutes

Servings: 4

Ingredients:

- 3 cups vegetable stock
- 2 tsp. thyme powder
- 1/2 tsp. match green tea powder
- 1 head cauliflower (about 2.5 cups, florets)
- 1 tbsp. olive oil
- 5 garlic cloves (minced)
- Salt and pepper to taste

Directions:

1. In an instant pressure pot, add the vegetable stock, thyme, and match powder on medium heat. Bring to a boil.

2. Add the cauliflower and set timer for 10 minutes on high pressure, allowing for quick pressure release when finished.

3. In a saucepan, add garlic and olive oil until tender and you can smell it; then add it to the pot along with salt and cook for 1 to 2 minutes.

4. Turn off the heat and. blend the soup and creamy with a blender.

Nutrition:

Calories: 114

Total fat: 9g

Saturated fat: 5g

Sodium: 128mg

Carbs: 18g

Fiber: 8g

Protein: 6g

Lasagna Soup

Preparation time: 5 minutes

Cooking time: 30 minutes

Servings: 5

Ingredients:

- Vegetable broth – 2 cups
- Portobello mushrooms, gills removed and finely diced – 8 ounces
- Onion powder – 1 teaspoon
- Crushed tomatoes – 28 ounces
- Diced tomatoes – 28 ounces
- Olive oil – 2 tablespoons
- Garlic, minced – 4 cloves
- Basil, fresh, chopped - .33 cup

- Nutritional yeast – 2 tablespoons
- Sea salt – 1 teaspoon
- Lentil Lasagna noodles (Explore Cuisine) – 8 ounces
- Vegan mozzarella shreds - .66 cup
- Thyme, dried – 1 teaspoon

Directions:

1. Pour the olive oil and allow it to heat over medium-high. Add in the diced mushrooms and cook while stirring regularly for eight minutes. Pour the diced tomatoes, garlic, and basil into the pot and continue to cook for four minutes.

2. Into the soup pot, add the crushed tomatoes, onion powder, thyme, nutritional yeast, and vegetable broth. Bring this mixture to a boil. Crack the lasagna noodles into small pieces and add them into the pot. Reduce the heat, fit on a lid, and allow the soup to simmer on low for twenty minutes.

3. Serve the soup topped with the vegan mozzarella shreds.

Nutrition:

Calories: 134

Total fat: 9g

Saturated fat: 5g

Sodium: 118mg

Carbs: 19g

Fiber: 9g

Protein: 6g

Tabbouleh Salad

Preparation time: 5minutes

Cooking time: 12minutes

Servings: 4

Ingredients:

- 1/4 cup olive oil
- 2 tablespoons freshly squeezed lemon juice
- 2 garlic cloves, minced
- Pinch salt
- Pinch freshly ground black pepper
- 2 tomatoes, diced
- 1/2 cup chopped fresh parsley
- Cup dry bulgur wheat, cooked according to the package directions

Directions:

1. Merge together the olive oil, lemon juice, garlic, salt, and pepper. Gently stir in the tomatoes and parsley.

2. Attach the bulgur and toss to combine everything thoroughly. Taste and season with salt and pepper as needed.

Nutrition:

Calories: 110

Fats: 12.1g,

Carbs: 15.6g

Fiber: 7.5g

Sugar: 17.1g

Proteins: 7.6g

Sodium: 121mg

Caesar Salad

Preparation time: 10minutes

Cooking time: 0minutes

Servings: 4

Ingredients:

- 2 cups chopped romaine lettuce
- 2 **tablespoons** Caesar Dressing
- 1 serving *Herbed Croutons* or store-bought croutons
- Vegan cheese, grated (optional)
- Make it a meal
- 1/2 cup cooked pasta
- 1/2 cup canned chickpeas
- 2 additional tablespoons *Caesar Dressing*

Directions:

1. To make the Caesar salad
2. Merge together the lettuce, dressing, croutons, and cheese (if using).
3. To make it a meal
4. Add the pasta, chickpeas, and additional dressing. Toss to coat.

Nutrition:

Calories: 120

Fats: 13.1g,

Carbs: 12.6g

Fiber: 7.5g

Sugar: 17.1g

Proteins: 7.6g

Sodium: 121mg

Greek Potato Salad

Preparation time: 10minutes

Cooking time: 20minutes

Servings: 3

Ingredients:

- 6 potatoes, scrubbed or peeled and chopped
- Salt
- 1/4 cup olive oil
- 2 tablespoons apple cider vinegar
- 2 tablespoons freshly squeezed lemon juice
- 1 teaspoon dried herbs
- 1/2 cucumber, chopped
- 1/4 red onion, diced
- 1/4 cup chopped pitted black olives
- Freshly ground black pepper

Directions:

1. Set the potatoes in a pot, add a pinch of salt, and pour in enough water to cover. Boil the water. Cook the potatoes for 15 to 20 minutes, until soft. Drain and set aside to cool. (Alternatively, put the potatoes in a large microwave-safe dish with a bit of water. Cover and heat on high power for 10 minutes.)
2. In a large bowl, whisk together the olive oil, vinegar, lemon juice, and dried herbs. Toss the cucumber, red onion, and olives with the dressing.
3. Add the cooked, cooled potatoes, and toss to combine. Taste and season with salt and pepper as needed.

Nutrition:

Calories: 110

Fats: 17.1g,

Carbs: 19.6g

Fiber: 7.5g

Sugar: 17.1g

Proteins: 7.6g

Sodium: 121mg

Pesto and White Bean Pasta Salad

Preparation time: 15minutes

Cooking time: 10minutes

Servings: 4

Ingredients:

- 1.1/2 cups canned cannellini beans
- 1/2 cup Spinach Pesto
- 1 cup chopped tomato or red bell pepper
- 1/4 red onion, finely diced
- 1/2 cup chopped pitted black olives

Directions:

1. In a large bowl, combine the pasta, beans, and pesto. Toss to combine.
2. Add the tomato, red onion, and olives, tossing thoroughly.

Nutrition:

Calories: 110

Fats: 17.1g,

Carbs: 19.6g

Fiber: 7.5g

Sugar: 17.1g

Proteins: 7.6g

Sodium: 121mg

Mediterranean Orzo and Chickpea Salad

Preparation time: 15minutes

Cooking time: 8minutes

Servings: 4

Ingredients:

- 1/4 cup olive oil
- 2 tablespoons freshly squeezed lemon juice
- Pinch salt
- 1.1/2 cups canned chickpeas, drained and rinsed
- 2 cups orzo or other small pasta shape, cooked according to the package directions, drained, and rinsed with cold water to cool
- 2 cups raw spinach, finely chopped
- 1 cup chopped cucumber
- 1/4 red onion, finely diced

Directions:

1. In a large bowl, whisk together the olive oil, lemon juice, and salt. Add the chickpeas and cooked orzo, and toss to coat.
2. Stir in the spinach, cucumber, and red onion.

Nutrition:

Calories: 110

Fats: 17.1g,

Carbs: 19.6g

Fiber: 7.5g

Sugar: 17.1g

Proteins: 7.6g

Sodium: 121mg

Vegetable Stir-Fry

Preparation Time: 10minutes

Cooking time: 15minutes

Servings: 4

Ingredients:

- Zucchini (.50)
- Red Bell Pepper (.50)
- Broccoli (.50)
- Red Cabbage (1 C.)
- Brown Rice (.50 C.)
- Tamari Sauce (2 T.)
- Red Chili Pepper (1)
- Fresh Parsley (.25 t.)
- Garlic (4)
- Olive Oil (2 T.)
- Optional: Sesame Seeds

Directions:

1. To begin, you will want to cook your brown rice according to the directions that are placed on the package. Once this step is done, place the brown rice in a bowl and put it to the side.

2. Next, you will want to take a frying pan and place some water in the bottom. Bring the pan over medium heat and then add in your chopped vegetables.

Once in place, cook the vegetables for five minutes or until they are tender.

3. When the vegetables are cooked through, you will then want to add in the parsley, cayenne powder, and the garlic. You will want to cook this mixture for a minute or so. Be sure you stir the ingredients so that nothing sticks to the bottom of your pan.

4. Now, add in the rice and tamari to your pan. You will cook this mixture for a few more minutes or until everything is warmed through.

5. For extra flavor, try adding sesame seeds before you enjoy your lunch! If you have any left-overs, you can keep this stir-fry in a sealed container for about five days in your fridge.

Nutrition:

Calories: 280

Protein: 10g

Fat: 12g

Carbs: 38g

Fibers: 6g

Broccoli Over Orzo

Preparation Time: 10minutes

Cooking time: 25minutes

Servings: 3

Ingredients:

- Olive Oil (3 t.)
- Smashed Garlic Cloves (4)
- Broccoli Florets (2 C.)
- Orzo Pasta (4.50 Oz.)

- Salt (.25 t.)
- Pepper (.25 t.)

Directions:

1. Start off by preparing your broccoli. You can do this by trimming the stems off and slicing the broccoli into small, bite-size pieces. If you want, go ahead and season with salt.

2. Next, you will want to steam your broccoli over a little bit of water until it is cooked through. Once the broccoli is cooked, chop it up into even smaller pieces.

3. When the broccoli is done, cook your pasta according to the directions provided on the box. Once this is done, drain the water and then place the pasta back into the pot.

4. With the pasta and broccoli done, place it back into the pot with the garlic. Stir everything together well and cook until the garlic turns a nice golden color. Be sure to stir everything to combine your meal well. Serve warm and enjoy a simple dinner!

Nutrition:

Calories: 230

Protein: 10g

Fat: 5g

Carbs: 39g

Fibers: 5g

Miso Spaghetti Squash

Preparation Time: 5minutes

Cooking time: 50minutes

Servings: 4

Ingredients:

- 1 (3-pound) spaghetti squash
- 1 tablespoon hot water
- 1 tablespoon unseasoned rice vinegar
- 1 tablespoon white miso

Directions:

1. Preheat the oven.

2. Peel the squash, cut-side down, on the prepared baking sheet. Bake for 35 to 40 minutes, until tender.

3. Cool until the squash is easy to handle. With a fork, scrape out the flesh, which will be stringy, like spaghetti. Transfer to a large bowl.

4. In a small bowl, combine the hot water, vinegar, and miso with a whisk or fork. Pour over the squash. Gently toss with tongs to coat the squash.

5. Divide the squash evenly among 4 single-serving containers. Let cool before sealing the lids.

6. Storage: Place in the refrigerator for up to 1 week or freeze for up to 4 months. To thaw, refrigerate overnight. Reheat in a microwave for 2 to 3 minutes.

Nutrition:

Calories: 120

Protein: 10g

Fat: 16g

Carbs: 79g

Fibers: 5g

Garlic and Herb Oodles

Preparation Time: 5minutes

Cooking time: 2minutes

Servings: 3

Ingredients:

- 1 teaspoon extra-virgin olive oil or 2 tablespoons vegetable broth
- 1 teaspoon minced garlic (about 1 clove)
- 4 medium zucchinis, spiraled
- 1/2 teaspoon dried basil
- 1/2 teaspoon dried oregano
- 1/41/4 to 1/2 teaspoon red pepper flakes, to taste
- 1/4 teaspoon salt (optional)
- 1/4 teaspoon freshly ground black pepper

Directions:

1. Heat the olive oil. Add the garlic, zucchini, basil, oregano, red pepper flakes, salt (if using), and black pepper. Sauté for 1 to 2 minutes, until barely tender.
2. Divide the oodles evenly among 4 storage containers. Let cool before sealing the lids.

Nutrition:

Calories: 120

Protein: 10g

Fat: 44g

Carbs: 32g

Fibers: 5g

Baked Brussels Sprouts

Preparation Time: 10minutes

Cooking time: 40minutes

Servings: 4

Ingredients:

- 1 pound Brussels sprouts
- 2 teaspoons extra-virgin olive or canola oil
- 4 teaspoons minced garlic (about 4 cloves)
- 1 teaspoon dried oregano
- 1/2 teaspoon dried rosemary
- 1/2 teaspoon salt
- 1/4 teaspoon freshly ground black pepper
- 1 tablespoon balsamic vinegar

Directions:

1. . Preheat the oven to 400ºF.
2. Trim and halve the Brussels sprouts. Transfer to a large bowl. Toss with the olive oil, garlic, oregano, rosemary, salt, and pepper to coat well.
3. Transfer to the prepared baking sheet. Bake for 35 to 40 minutes, shaking the pan occasionally to help with even browning, until crisp on the outside and tender on the inside.
4. Remove from the oven and transfer to a large bowl. Stir in the balsamic vinegar, coating well.
5. Divide the Brussels sprouts evenly among 4 single-serving containers. Let cool before sealing the lids.

Nutrition:

Calories: 128

Protein: 10g

Fat: 50g

Carbs: 23g

Fibers: 5g

Roasted Herb Carrots

Preparation Time: 10minutes

Cooking time: 25minutes

Servings: 4

Ingredients:

- 2 1/2 pounds carrots, quartered
- 2 tablespoons olive oil or avocado oil
- 1/4 cup Clean Ranch Seasoning, or store-bought light or low-sodium ranch dressing mix
- Salt
- Freshly ground black pepper

Directions:

1. Preheat the oven to 425°F. Line a baking sheet with aluminum foil.
2. On the prepared baking sheet, toss the carrots with the olive oil. Sprinkle with the ranch seasoning and season with salt and pepper. Shake the pan so the carrots are in a single layer.
3. 3.
4. Roast for 25 minutes, or until browned and bubbly.
5. 4.
6. Let cool and portion the carrots into 4 single-serving 24-ounce meal prep containers. Refrigerate for up to 5 days.

Nutrition:

Calories: 191;

Fat: 7g;

Protein: 2g;

Total carbs: 31g;

Net carbs: 22g;

Fiber: 7g;

Sugar: 14g;

Sodium: 234mg

Gluten-Free, Vegan Banana Pancakes

Preparation Time: 10 minutes

Cooking time: 5 minutes

Servings: 2-3

Ingredients:

- 1 cup generally useful, gluten-free flour
- 1/2 tsp. preparing powder
- 1/2 tsp. cinnamon dash ocean salt
- 1 tsp. apple juice vinegar
- 2/3 cup almond milk
- 1 ready banana
- 1 teaspoon vanilla
- 1 tbsp. + 2 tsp. dissolved coconut oil, isolated

Directions:

1. Mix the flour, preparing powder, cinnamon, and ocean salt together.
2. Mix the vinegar to the almond milk and whisk together till foam. Include the almond/vinegar blend to a blender, alongside the banana, vanilla, and 1 tbsp. coconut oil. Mix till smooth.

3. Mix the fluid blend into the flour blend till consolidated.

4. Warm 2 tsp. coconut oil in a nonstick skillet. Include the hitter, storing 1/4 cup at once. Give the hotcakes a chance to cook till air pockets structure on the top; at that point, flip and keep cooking till flapjacks are cooked through. Rehash with all outstanding hitter.

5. Serve flapjacks with new berries.

Nutrition:

Calories: 122;

Fat: 19g;

Protein: 13g;

Carbohydrates: 54g;

Fiber: 25g;

Sugar: 10g;

Sodium: 124mg

Apple Cinnamon Oatmeal

Preparation Time: 5 minutes
Cooking time: 0 minutes
Servings: 2
Ingredients:

- 1 cup gluten-free moved oats
- 1 cup of water
- 3/4 cup almond milk
- 3/4 cup diced apples
- 1/2 teaspoon cinnamon or pumpkin pie zest
- 2 tbsp. maple syrup
- 1/4 cup slashed crude pecan pieces

Directions:

1. Add the oats, water, almond milk, apples, cinnamon, and syrup in a medium pot or pan. Heat to the point of boiling and lower to a stew. Cook until oats have assimilated. The fluid and apples are delicate (around 10-15 minutes).

2. Divide oats into two dishes and top with crude pecan pieces. Appreciate.

Nutrition:

Calories: 122;

Fat: 2g;

Protein: 43g;

Carbohydrates: 64g;

Fiber: 95g;

Sugar: 17g;

Sodium: 224mg

Pumpkin Spice Overnight Oats

Preparation Time: 5 minutes
Cooking time: 0minutes
Servings: 1
Ingredients:

- 1/2 t. vanilla
- 3/4 t. pumpkin spice
- 3 to 4 drops liquid stevia
- 1 tbsp. chia seed
- 2 tbsp. canned pumpkin puree
- 1/2 c. hemp hearts
- 1/3 c. of the following:
- Brewed coffee

- Almond milk unsweetened vanilla silk

Directions:

1. In a bowl with a lid, add all the ingredients, mixing until well-combined.

2. Cover and refrigerate overnight or 8 hours.

3. Remove from the fridge and add additional milk until the oats reach your desired consistency.

4. Divide into 2 bowls and enjoy.

Nutrition:

Calories: 132

Proteins: 6.5 g

Carbohydrates: 4.9 g

Fats: 1 g

Crab with Spicy Seeds

Preparation time: 5 minutes

Cooking time: 20 minutes

Servings: 6

Ingredients:

- 1 cup sunflower seeds

- Seeds for cupping cups

- 1/2 cup chia seeds

- 1/2 cup sesame (I used a mixture of black and white sesame)

- 1 copper (starch) seeds

- 1 cup of water 1 1/2

- Selected 1 tablespoon dried herbs

- 1 tea spoon of peppers standard, (optional)

Directions:

1. Preheat the oven to 170° C.

2. Mix all ingredients and let the seeds float in water for 10-15 minutes.

3. Mix well, then divide the mixture into two baking trays and lightly grease. The ideal thickness is about 3-4 mm. They are very thin, the cakes are very weak, very thick, and more like granular cakes.

4. Bake every time (partially change the dishes) or until golden and crispy. If you do not feel an explosion after an hour, return to the oven for another 5-10 minutes.

5. Remove from the oven, cool and press into rough places. Storage in stored containers.

Nutrition:

Calories: 5

Fat: 19 g

Protein: 18g

Sodium: 101mg

Fiber: 6 g

Carbohydrates: 187g

Sugar: 1.4 g

Sweet Potato Slaw in Wonton Cups

Preparation time: 15 minutes

Cooking time: 20minutes

Servings: 5

Ingredients:

- 1 cup water

- 2 cups sliced green cabbage (roughly 1 small head)

- 1 cup shredded sweet potato

- 1/2 sweet onion, sliced

- 2 tablespoons lite soy sauce

- 1 tablespoon hoisin sauce

- 11/2 tablespoons freshly squeezed lime juice

- 11/2 teaspoons sesame oil

- Zest of 1 lime

- 1/2 teaspoon ground ginger, plus more to taste

- 3 scallions, green and light green parts, sliced

Directions:

1. Preheat the oven to 350°F. Lightly coat a muffin tin with the nonstick spray.

2. Place one wonton wrapper in each well of the prepared tin, pressing down to create a cup shape. Bake for 5 to 6 minutes, or until the cups are crispy and lightly browned. Set aside to cool.

Nutrition:

Calories: 5

Fat: 19 g

Protein: 17g

Sodium: 11mg

Fiber: 8 g

Carbohydrates: 54g

Sugar: 1.4 g

Mediterranean Cod Stew

Preparation Time: 10 minutes

Cooking time: 20minutes

Servings: 6

Ingredients:

- 2 tablespoons olive oil

- 2 cups chopped onion (about 1 medium onion)

- 2 garlic cloves, minced (about 1 teaspoon)

- 3/4 teaspoon smoked paprika

- 1 can diced tomatoes,

- 1 jar roasted red peppers

- 1 cup sliced olives, green or black

- 3/4 cup dry red wine

- 1/4 teaspoon black pepper

- 1/4 teaspoon kosher

- 1.1/2 pounds cod fillets,

- 3 cups sliced mushrooms

Directions:

1. Heat the pot and heat the oil. Attach the onion and cook.

2. Attach the garlic and smoked paprika and cook.

3. Mix in the tomatoes with their juices, roasted peppers, olives, wine, pepper, and salt, and turn the heat up to medium-high. Bring to a boil. Add the cod and mushrooms, and reduce the heat to medium.

4. Cook in a low heat and, stir for a few times, until the cod is cooked through and flakes easily, and serve.

Nutrition:

Calories: 223

Total Fat: 4g

Saturated Fat: 9g

Cholesterol: 7

 Sodium: 45mg

Total Carbohydrates: 8g

Fiber: 3g; Protein: 6g

Steamed Mussels in White Wine Sauce

Preparation Time: 5 minutes
Cooking time: 10minutes
Servings: 4
Ingredients:

- 2 pounds small mussels
- 1 tablespoon extra-virgin olive oil
- 1 cup sliced red onion
- 3 garlic cloves, sliced
- 1 cup dry white wine
- 2 (1/4-inch-thick) lemon slices
- 1/4 teaspoon freshly ground black pepper
- 1/4 teaspoon kosher or sea salt
- Fresh lemon wedges, for serving (optional)

Directions:

1. In a large colander in the sink, run cold water over the mussels (but don't let the mussels sit in standing water). All the shells should be closed tight; discard any shells that are a little bit open or any shells that are cracked. Leave the mussels in the colander until you're ready to use them.

2. Heat the oil in a skillet. Attach the onion and cook,

3. Add the mussels and cover. Cook in a low heat.

4. All the shells should now be wide open. Using a slotted spoon, discard any mussels that are still closed. Spoon the opened mussels into a shallow serving bowl, and pour the broth over the top. Serve with additional fresh lemon slices, if desired.

Nutrition:

Calories: 123

Total Fat: 7g

Saturated Fat: 9g

Cholesterol: 15

 Sodium: 45mg

Total Carbohydrates: 8g

Fiber: 3g; Protein: 6g

Orange and Garlic Shrimp

Preparation Time: 10 minutes
Cooking time: 20minutes
Servings: 5
Ingredients:

- 1 large orange
- 3 tablespoons extra-virgin olive oil, divided

- 1 tablespoon chopped fresh rosemary
- 1 tablespoon chopped fresh thyme (about 6 sprigs) or 1 teaspoon dried thyme
- 3 garlic cloves, minced (about 1 1/2 teaspoons)
- 1/4 teaspoon freshly ground black pepper
- 1/4 teaspoon kosher or sea salt
- 1 1/2 pounds fresh raw shrimp, (or frozen and thawed raw shrimp) shells and tails removed

Directions:

1. Zest the entire orange using a Micro plane or citrus grater.

2. Using a zip-top bag, merge the orange zest and 2 tablespoons of oil with the rosemary, thyme, garlic, pepper, and salt. Attach the shrimp, seal the bag, and gently massage the shrimp.

3. . Heat a grill, grill pan, or a large skillet over medium heat. Brush on or swirl in the remaining 1 tablespoon of oil. Add half the shrimp, and cook for 4 to 6 minutes, or until the shrimp turn pink and white, flipping halfway through if on the grill or stirring every minute if in a pan.

4. While the shrimp cook, peel the orange and cut the flesh into bite-size pieces. Serve immediately or refrigerate and serve cold.

Nutrition:

Calories: 223

Total Fat: 7g

Saturated Fat: 10g

Cholesterol: 45

Sodium: =15mg

Total Carbohydrates: 8g

Fiber: 3g; Protein: 6g

Roasted Shrimp-Gnocchi Bake

Preparation Time: 10 minutes
Cooking time: 20minutes
Servings: 6
Ingredients:

- 1 cup tomato
- 2 tablespoons extra-virgin olive oil
- 2 garlic cloves, minced
- 1/2 teaspoon black pepper
- 1/4 teaspoon crushed red pepper
- 1 jar red peppers
- 1-pound fresh raw shrimp
- 1-pound frozen gnocchi
- 1/2 cup cubed feta cheese
- 1/3 cup fresh torn basil leaves

Directions:

1. Preheat the oven to 425°F.

2. In a baking dish, mix the tomatoes, oil, garlic, black pepper, and crushed red pepper. Roast in the oven for 10 minutes.

3. Stir in the roasted peppers and shrimp. Roast for 10 more minutes, until the shrimp turn pink and white.

4. While the shrimp cooks, cook the gnocchi on the stove top according

to the package directions. Drain in a colander and keep warm.

5. Remove the dish from the oven. Mix in the cooked gnocchi, feta, and basil, and serve.

Nutrition:

Calories: 223

Total Fat: 7g

Saturated Fat: 16g

Cholesterol: 25

 Sodium: =10mg

Total Carbohydrates: 8g

Fiber: 3g; Protein: 6g

Spicy Shrimp Puttanesca

Preparation Time: 5 minutes
Cooking time: 15minutes
Servings: 4
Ingredients:

- 2 tablespoons extra-virgin olive oil

- 3 anchovy fillets, drained and chopped (half a 2-ounce tin), or 11/2 teaspoons anchovy paste

- 3 garlic cloves, minced (about 11/2 teaspoons)

- 1/2 teaspoon crushed red pepper

- 1 (14.5-ounce) can low-sodium or no-salt-added diced tomatoes, untrained

- 1 (2.25-ounce) can sliced black olives, drained (about 1/2 cup)

- 2 tablespoons capers

- 1 tablespoon chopped fresh oregano or 1 teaspoon dried oregano

- 1-pound fresh raw shrimp (or frozen and thawed shrimp), shells and tails removed

Directions:

1. In a large skillet over medium heat, heat the oil. Mix in the anchovies, garlic, and crushed red pepper. Cook for 3 minutes, stirring frequently and mashing up the anchovies with a wooden spoon, until they have melted into the oil.

2. Stir in the tomatoes with their juices, olives, capers, and oregano. Turn up the heat to medium-high, and bring to a simmer.

3. When the sauce is lightly bubbling, stir in the shrimp. Reduce the heat, and cook the shrimp and serve.

Nutrition:

Calories: 423

Total Fat: 7g

Saturated Fat: 16g

Cholesterol: 25

 Sodium: =55mg

Total Carbohydrates: 34g

Fiber: 3g;

Protein: 6g

Burrito & Cauliflower Rice Bowl

Preparation Time: 15 minutes

Cooking Time: 10 minutes

Servings: 4

Ingredients:

- 1 cup cooked tofu cubes

- 12 oz. frozen cauliflower rice
- 4 teaspoons olive oil
- 1 teaspoon unsalted taco seasoning
- 1 cup red cabbage, sliced thinly
- 1/2 cup salsa
- 1/4 cup fresh cilantro, chopped
- 1 cup avocado, diced

Directions:

1. Prepare cauliflower rice according to directions in the package.
2. Toss cauliflower rice in olive oil and taco seasoning.
3. Divide among 4 food containers with lid.
4. Top with tofu, cabbage, salsa and cilantro.
5. Seal the container and chill in the refrigerator until ready to serve.
6. Before serving, add avocado slices.

Nutrition:

Calories 298

Total Fat 20 g

Saturated Fat 3 g

Cholesterol 0 mg

Sodium 680 mg

Total Carbohydrate 15 g

Dietary Fiber 6 g

Total Sugars 5 g

Protein 15 g

Super food Buddha Bowl

Preparation Time: 10 minutes

Cooking Time: 10 minutes

Servings: 4

Ingredients:

- 8 oz. microwavable quinoa
- 2 tablespoons lemon juice
- 1/2 cup hummus
- Water
- 5 oz. baby kale
- 8 oz. cooked baby beets, sliced
- 1 cup frozen shelled edam me (thawed)
- 1/4 cup sunflower seeds, toasted
- 1 avocado, sliced
- 1 cup pecans
- 2 tablespoons flaxseeds

Directions:

1. Cook quinoa according to directions in the packaging.
2. Set aside and let cool.
3. In a bowl, mix the lemon juice and hummus.
4. Add water to achieve desired consistency.
5. Divide mixture into 4 condiment containers.
6. Cover containers with lids and put in the refrigerator.
7. Divide the baby kale into 4 food containers with lids.
8. Top with quinoa, beets, Edam me and sunflower seeds.
9. Place in the refrigerator until it's ready.

Nutrition:

Calories 381

Total Fat 19 g

Saturated Fat 2 g

Cholesterol 0 mg

Sodium 188 mg

Total Carbohydrate 43 g

Dietary Fiber 13 g

Total Sugars 8 g

Protein 16 g

Potassium 1,066 mg

Grilled Summer Veggies

Preparation Time: 15 minutes

Cooking Time: 6 minutes

Servings: 6

Ingredients:

- 2 teaspoons cider vinegar
- 1 tablespoon olive oil
- 1/4 teaspoon fresh thyme, chopped
- 1 teaspoon fresh parsley, chopped
- 1/4 teaspoon fresh rosemary, chopped
- Salt and pepper to taste
- 1 onion, sliced into wedges
- 2 red bell peppers, sliced
- 3 tomatoes, sliced in half
- 6 large mushrooms, stems removed
- 1 eggplant, sliced crosswise
- 3 tablespoons olive oil
- 1 tablespoon cider vinegar

Directions:

1. Merge the vinegar, oil, thyme, parsley, rosemary, salt and pepper to make the dressing.
2. In a bowl, mix the onion, red bell pepper, tomatoes, mushrooms and eggplant.
3. Toss in remaining olive oil and cider vinegar.
4. Grill over medium heat for 3 minutes.
5. Turn the vegetables and grill for another 3 minutes.
6. Arrange grilled vegetables in a food container.
7. Drizzle with the herbed mixture when ready to serve.

Nutrition:

Calories 127

Total Fat 9 g

Saturated Fat 1 g

Cholesterol 0 mg

Sodium 55 mg

Total Carbohydrate 11 g

Dietary Fiber 5 g

Total Sugars 5 g

Protein 3 g

Potassium 464 mg

"Cheesy" Spinach Rolls

Preparation Time: 20 minutes

Cooking Time: 15 minutes

Servings: 6

Ingredients:

- 18 spinach leaves
- 18 vegan spring roll wrappers
- 6 slices cheese, cut into 18 smaller strips

Water

- 1 cup vegetable oil
- 6 cups cauliflower rice
- 3 cups tomato, cubed
- 3 cups cucumber, cubed
- 1 tablespoon olive oil
- 1 teaspoon balsamic vinegar

Directions:

1. Add one spinach leaf over each wrapper.
2. Add a small strip of vegan cheese on top of each spinach leaf.
3. Roll the wrapper and seal the edges with water.
4. In a pan over medium high heat, add the vegetable oil.
5. Cook the rolls until golden brown.
6. Drain in paper towels.
7. Divide cauliflower rice into 6 food containers.
8. Add 3 cheesy spinach rolls in each food container.
9. Toss cucumber and tomato in olive oil and vinegar.

Nutrition:

Calories 746

Total Fat 38.5g

Saturated Fat 10.1g

Cholesterol 33mg

Sodium 557mg

Total Carbohydrate 86.2g

Dietary Fiber 3.8g

Total Sugars 2.6g

Protein 18g

Potassium 364mg

Pesto Pasta

Preparation Time: 10 minutes

Cooking Time: 8 minutes

Servings: 2

Ingredients:

- 1 cup fresh basil leaves
- 4 cloves garlic
- 2 tablespoons walnut
- 2 tablespoons olive oil
- 1 tablespoon vegan Parmesan cheese
- 2 cups cooked penne pasta
- 2 tablespoons black olives, sliced

Directions:

1. Put the basil leaves, garlic, walnut, olive oil and Parmesan cheese in a food processor.
2. Pulse until smooth.
3. Divide pasta into 2 food containers.
4. Spread the basil sauce on top.
5. Top with black olives.
6. Store until ready to serve.

Nutrition:

Calories 374

Total Fat 21.1g

Saturated Fat 2.6g

Cholesterol 47mg

Sodium 92mg

Total Carbohydrate 38.6g

Dietary Fiber 1.1g

Total Sugars 0.2g

Protein 10g

Potassium 215mg

Tofu Sharma Rice

Preparation Time: 15 minutes

Cooking Time: 15 minutes

Servings: 4

Ingredients:

- 4 cups cooked brown rice
- 4 cups cooked tofu, sliced into small cubes
- 4 cups cucumber, cubed
- 4 cups tomatoes, cubed
- 4 cups white onion, cubed
- 2 cups cabbage, shredded
- 1/2 cup vegan mayo
- 1/8 cup garlic, minced
- Garlic salt to taste
- Hot sauce

Directions:

1. Add brown rice into 4 food containers.
2. Arrange tofu, cucumber, tomatoes, white onion and cabbage on top.
3. In a bowl, mix the mayo, garlic, and garlic salt.
4. Drizzle top with garlic sauce and hot sauce before serving.

Nutrition:

Calories 667

Total Fat 12.6g

Saturated Fat 2.2g

Cholesterol 0mg

Sodium 95mg

Total Carbohydrate 116.5g

Dietary Fiber 9.9g

Total Sugars 9.4g

Protein 26.1g

Potassium 1138mg

Risotto with Tomato & Herbs

Preparation Time: 10 minutes

Cooking Time: 20 minutes

Servings: 32

Ingredients:

- 2 oz. Arborio rice
- 1 teaspoon dried garlic, minced
- 3 tablespoons dried onion, minced
- 1 tablespoon dried Italian seasoning, crushed
- 3/4 cup snipped dried tomatoes

Directions:

1. Make the dry risotto mix by combining all the ingredients except broth in a large bowl.

2. Divide the mixture into eight resalable plastic bags. Seal the bag.

3. Store at room temperature for up to 3 months.

4. When ready to serve, pour the broth in a pot.

5. Add the contents of 1 plastic bag of dry risotto mix.

6. Bring to a boil and then reduce heat.

7. Bring with vegetables.

Nutrition:

Calories 80

Total Fat 0 g

Saturated Fat 0 g

Cholesterol 0 mg

Sodium 276 mg

Total Carbohydrate 17 g

Dietary Fiber 2 g

Total Sugars 0 g

Protein 3 g

Potassium 320 mg

Vegan Tacos

Preparation Time: 20 minutes

Cooking Time: 10 minutes

Servings: 4

Ingredients:

- 1/2 teaspoon onion powder
- 1/2 teaspoon garlic powder
- 1 teaspoon chili powder
- 2 tablespoons tamari
- 16 oz. tofu, drained and crumbled
- 1 tablespoon olive oil
- 1 ripe avocado
- 1 tablespoon vegan mayonnaise
- 1 teaspoon lime juice
- Salt to taste
- 8 corn tortillas, warmed
- 1/2 cup fresh salsa
- 2 cups iceberg lettuce, shredded
- Pickled radishes

Directions:

1. Merge all the ingredients in a bowl.

2. Marinate the tofu in the mixture for 10 minutes.

3. Pour the oil in a pan over medium heat.

4. Cook the tofu mixture for 10 minutes.

5. In another bowl, mash the avocado and mix with mayo, lime juice and salt.

6. Stuff each corn tortilla with tofu mixture, mashed avocado, salsa and lettuce.

7. Serve with pickled radishes.

Nutrition:

Calories 360

Total Fat 21 g

Saturated Fat 3 g

Cholesterol 0 mg

Sodium 610 mg

Total Carbohydrate 33 g

Dietary Fiber 8 g

Total Sugars 4 g

Protein 17 g

Potassium 553 mg

Spinach with Walnuts & Avocado

Preparation Time: 5 minutes

Cooking Time: 0 minute

Servings: 1

Ingredients:

- 3 cups baby spinach
- 1/2 cup strawberries, sliced
- 1 tablespoon white onion, chopped
- 2 tablespoons vinaigrette
- 1/4 medium avocado, diced
- 2 tablespoons walnut, toasted

Directions:

1. Put the spinach, strawberries and onion in a glass jar with lid.
2. Drizzle dressing on top.
3. Top with avocado and walnuts.
4. Shut down the lid and refrigerate until ready to serve.

Nutrition:

Calories 296

Total Fat 18 g

Saturated Fat 2 g

Cholesterol 0 mg

Sodium 195 mg

Total Carbohydrate 27 g

Dietary Fiber 10 g

Total Sugars 11 g

Protein 8 g

Potassium 103 mg

Roasted Veggies in Lemon Sauce

Preparation Time: 15 minutes

Cooking Time: 20 minutes

Servings: 5

Ingredients:

- 2 cloves garlic, sliced
- 1 .1/2 cups broccoli florets
- 1 .1/2 cups cauliflower florets
- 1 tablespoon olive oil
- Salt to taste
- 1 teaspoon dried oregano, crushed
- 3/4 cup zucchini, diced
- 3/4 cup red bell pepper, diced
- 2 teaspoons lemon zest

Directions:

1. Preheat your oven to 425 degrees F.
2. Merge the garlic, broccoli and cauliflower.
3. Put in the oil and season with salt and oregano.
4. Roast in the oven for 10 minutes.

5. Attach the zucchini and bell pepper to the pan.

6. Stir well.

7. Roast for another 10 minutes.

8. Sprinkle lemon zest on top before serving.

9. Fill to a food container and reheat before serving.

Nutrition:

Calories 52

Total Fat 3 g

Saturated Fat 0 g

Cholesterol 0 mg

Sodium 134 mg

Total Carbohydrate 5 g

Dietary Fiber 2 g

Total Sugars 2 g

Protein 2 g

Potassium 270 mg

Tender Lamb Chops

Preparation Time: 10 Minutes

Cooking Time: 3 Hours

Servings: 4

Ingredients:

- 8 lamb chops
- ½ teaspoon dried thyme
- 1 onion, sliced
- 1 teaspoon dried oregano
- 2 garlic cloves, minced
- 4 baby carrots
- Pepper and salt

- 2 potatoes, cubed
- 8 small tomatoes, halved

Directions:

1. Add the onion, carrots, tomatoes and potatoes into a pot.
2. Combine together thyme, oregano, pepper, and salt. Rub over lamb chops.
3. Place lamb chops in the pot and top with garlic.
4. Pour ¼ cup water around the lamb chops.
5. Cover and cook on low flame for around 3 hours.
6. Uncover the pot and roast at high flame for 10 minutes.
7. Serve and enjoy.

Nutrition:

Calories 210

Fat 4.1 g

Carbohydrates 7.3 g

Protein 20.4 g

Beef Stroganoff

Preparation Time: 10 Minutes

Cooking Time: 4 Hours

Servings: 2

Ingredients:

- 1/2 lb. beef stew meat
- 10 oz mushroom soup, homemade
- 1 medium onion, chopped
- 1/2 cup sour cream
  - o oz mushrooms, sliced
- Pepper and salt

Directions:

1. Add all fixings excluding sour cream into a pot and mix well.
2. Cover and cook on low flame for 4 hours.
3. Add sour cream and stir well.
4. Serve and enjoy.

Nutrition:

Calories 470

Fat 25 g

Carbohydrates 8.6 g

Protein 49 g

Lamb & Couscous Salad

Preparation Time: 7 Minutes

Cooking Time: 25 Minutes

Servings: 2

Ingredients:

- 1/2 Cup Water
- 1/2 Tablespoon Garlic, Minced
- 1 1/4 lb. Lamb Loin Chops, Trimmed
- 1/4 Cup Couscous, Whole Wheat
- Pinch Sea Salt
- 1/2 Tablespoon Parsley, Fresh & Chopped Fine
- 1 Tomato, Chopped
- 1 Teaspoon Olive Oil
- 1 Small Cucumber, Chopped
- 1 1/2 Tablespoons Lemon Juice, Fresh
- 1/4 Cup Feta, Crumbled
- 1 Tablespoon Dill, Fresh & Chopped Fine

Directions:

1. Get out a saucepan and bring the water to a boil.
2. Get out a bowl and mix your garlic, salt and parsley. Press this mixture into the side of each lamb chop, and then heat your oil using medium-high heat in a skillet.
3. Add the lamb, cooking for six minutes per side. Place it to the side, and cover to help keep the lamb chops warm.
4. Stir the couscous into the water once it's started to boil, returning it to a boil before reducing it to low so that it simmers. Cover, and then cook for about two minutes more. Take away from heat, then allow it to stand uncovered for five minutes. Fluff using a fork, and then add in your tomatoes, lemon juice, feta and dill. Stir well. Serve on the side of your lamb chops.

Nutrition:

Calories: 232,

Fat: 7.9g,

Protein: 5.6g,

Carbohydrates: 31.2g

Smoky Pork & Cabbage

Preparation Time: 10 Minutes

Cooking Time: 3 Hours

Servings: 6

Ingredients:

3lb pork

1/2 cabbage head, chopped

1 cup water

1/3 cup liquid smoke

1 tablespoon kosher salt

Directions:

1. Rub the pork with kosher salt and place into a pot.

2. Pour liquid smoke over the pork. Add water.
3. Cover then cook on low flame for 2 hours.
4. Remove pork from the pot and add cabbage in the bottom.
5. Place pork on top of the cabbage.
6. Cover again and cook for 1 hour more.
7. Slice the pork and serve.

Nutrition:

Calories 484

Fat 21.5 g

Carbohydrates 4 g

Protein 36 g

Lemon Beef

Preparation Time: 10 Minutes

Cooking Time: 3 Hours

Servings: 4

Ingredients:

- 1 lb. beef chuck roast
- 1 fresh lime juice
- 1 garlic clove, crushed
- 1 teaspoon chili powder
- 2 cups lemon-lime soda
- 1/2 teaspoon salt

Directions:

1. Place beef chuck roast into a pot.
2. Season roast with garlic, chili powder, and salt.
3. Pour lemon-lime soda over the roast.
4. Cover the pot then cook on low flame for 3 hours. Shred the meat using fork.
5. Add lime juice over shredded roast and serve.

Nutrition:

Calories 355

Fat 16.8 g

Carbohydrates 14 g

Protein 35.5 g

Herb Pork Roast

Preparation Time: 10 Minutes

Cooking Time: 2 Hours

Servings: 8

Ingredients:

- 5 lbs. pork roast, boneless or bone-in
- 1 tablespoon dry herb mix
- 4 garlic cloves, cut into slivers
- 1 tablespoon salt

Directions:

1. By means of a sharp knife make small slices all over meat then insert garlic slivers into the cuts.
2. In a small bowl, mix together Italian herb mix and salt and rub all over pork roast.
3. Place the pork roast into a pot.
4. Cover then cook on low flame for 2 hours.
5. Uncover the pot and roast at high flame for 10 minutes.
6. Take away the meat from the pot and slice it.
7. Serve and enjoy.

Nutrition:

Calories 327

Fat 8 g

Carbohydrates 0.5 g

Protein 59 g

Seasoned Pork Chops

Preparation Time: 10 Minutes

Cooking Time: 4 Hours

Servings: 4

Ingredients:

- 4 pork chops
- 2 garlic cloves, minced
- 1 cup chicken broth
- 1 tablespoon poultry seasoning
- 1/4 cup olive oil
- Pepper and salt

Directions:

1. In a bowl, whisk together olive oil, poultry seasoning, garlic, broth, pepper, and salt.
2. Pour olive oil mixture into the slow cooker then place pork chops in the pot.
3. Cover and cook on low flame for about 3 hours.
4. Uncover the pot and roast at high flame for 10 minutes.
5. Dress the pork in the cooking sauce and serve along with vegetables.

Nutrition:

Calories 386

Fat 32.9 g

Carbohydrates 3 g

Protein 20 g

Greek Beef Roast

Preparation Time: 10 Minutes

Cooking Time: 2 Hours

Servings: 6

Ingredients:

- 2 lbs. lean top round beef roast
- 1 tablespoon Italian seasoning
- 6 garlic cloves, minced
- 1 onion, sliced
- 2 cups beef broth
- ½ cup red wine
- 1 teaspoon red pepper flakes
- Pepper
- Salt

Directions:

1. Season meat with pepper and salt and place into a pot.
2. Pour remaining ingredients over meat.
3. Cover then cook on low flame for 2 hours.
4. Slice the meat, dress with cooking sauce and serve.

Nutrition:

Calories 231

Fat 6 g

Carbohydrates 4 g

Protein 35 g

Tomato Pork Chops

Preparation Time: 10 Minutes

Cooking Time: 1 Hour 10 Minutes

Servings: 4

Ingredients:

- 4 pork chops, bone-in
- 1 tablespoon garlic, minced
- ½ small onion, chopped
- 6 oz can tomato paste
- 1 bell pepper, chopped
- ¼ teaspoon red pepper flakes
- 1 teaspoon Worcestershire sauce
- 1 tablespoon dried Italian seasoning
- 14.5 oz can tomato, diced

- 2 teaspoon olive oil
- ¼ teaspoon pepper
- 1 teaspoon kosher salt

Directions:

1. Warmth oil in a pan over medium-high heat.
2. Season pork chops with pepper and salt.
3. Sear pork chops in pan until brown from both the sides.
4. Transfer the pork chops into a pot.
5. Add the remaining ingredients to the pot.
6. Cover and cook on low flame for 1 hour.
7. Remove the lid and roast for about 10 minutes.
8. Serve and enjoy.

Nutrition:

Calories 325

Fat 23.4 g

Carbohydrates 10 g

Protein 20 g

Pork Roast

Preparation Time: 10 Minutes

Cooking Time: 1 Hour 35 Minutes

Servings: 6

Ingredients:

- 3 lbs. pork roast, boneless
- 1 cup water
- 1 onion, chopped
- 3 garlic cloves, chopped
- 1 tablespoon black pepper
- 1 rosemary sprig
- 2 fresh oregano sprigs
- 2 fresh thyme sprigs
- 1 tablespoon olive oil

- 1 tablespoon kosher salt

Directions:

1. Preheat the oven to 350 F.
2. Season pork roast with pepper and salt.
3. Heat olive oil in a stockpot and sear pork roast on each side, about 4 minutes.
4. Add onion and garlic. Pour in the water, oregano, and thyme and bring to boil for a minute.
5. Cover pot and roast in the preheated oven for 1 1/2 hours.
6. Serve and enjoy.

Nutrition:

Calories 502

Fat 23.8 g

Carbohydrates 3 g

Protein 65 g

Greek Pork Chops

Preparation Time: 10 Minutes

Cooking Time: 15 Minutes

Servings: 4

Ingredients:

- 8 pork chops, boneless
- 4 teaspoon dried oregano
- 2 tablespoon Worcestershire sauce
- 3 tablespoon fresh lemon juice
- ¼ cup olive oil
- 1 teaspoon ground mustard
- 2 teaspoon garlic powder
- 2 teaspoon onion powder
- Pepper
- Salt

Directions:

1. Whisk together oil, garlic powder, onion powder, oregano, Worcestershire sauce, lemon juice, mustard, pepper, and salt.
2. Place pork chops in a baking dish then pour marinade over pork chops and coat well. Place in refrigerator overnight.
3. Preheat the grill.
4. Place pork chops on hot grill and cook for 7-8 minutes on each side.
5. Serve and enjoy.

Nutrition:

Calories 324

Fat 26.5 g

Carbohydrates 2.5 g

Sugar 1.3 g

Protein 18 g

Cholesterol 69 mg

Pork Cacciatore

Preparation Time: 10 Minutes

Cooking Time: 2 Hours

Servings: 4

Ingredients:

- 1 ½ lbs. pork chops
- 1 teaspoon dried oregano
- 1 cup beef broth
- 3 tablespoon tomato paste
- 14 oz can tomato, diced
- 2 cups mushrooms, sliced
- 1 small onion, diced
- 1 garlic clove, minced
- 2 tablespoon olive oil
- ¼ teaspoon pepper
- ½ teaspoon salt

Directions:

1. Warmth oil in a pan over medium-high heat.
2. Add pork chops in pan and cook until brown on both the sides.
3. Transfer pork chops into a pot.
4. Pour remaining ingredients over the pork chops.
5. Cover then cook on low flame for 2 hours.
6. Serve and enjoy.

Nutrition:

Calories 440

Fat 33 g

Carbohydrates 6 g

Protein 28 g

Easy Beef Kofta

Preparation Time: 10 Minutes

Cooking Time: 10 Minutes

Servings: 6

Ingredients:

- 2 lbs. ground beef
- 4 garlic cloves, minced
- 1 onion, minced
- 2 teaspoon cumin
- 1 cup fresh parsley, chopped
- ¼ teaspoon pepper
- 1 teaspoon salt
- 1 tablespoon oil

Directions:

1. With a knife, chop the beef very well.
2. Add all the fixings excluding oil into the mixing bowl and mix until combined.
3. Roll meat mixture into mini-kabab shapes.
4. Add the oil to a pan then warm up at high flame.

5. Roast the meat in the hot pan for 4-6 minutes on each side or until cooked.
6. Serve with some vegetables and a sauce if you like.

Nutrition:

Calories 223

Fat 7.3 g

Carbohydrates 2.5 g

Protein 35 g

Pork with Tomato & Olives

Preparation Time: 10 Minutes

Cooking Time: 30 Minutes

Servings: 6

Ingredients:

- 6 pork chops, boneless and cut into thick slices
- 1/8 teaspoon ground cinnamon
- 1/2 cup olives, pitted and sliced
- 8 oz can tomato, crushed
- 1/4 cup beef broth
- 2 garlic cloves, chopped
- 1 large onion, sliced
- 1 tablespoon olive oil

Directions:

1. Warm up olive oil in a pan over medium heat.
2. Place pork chops in a pan and cook until lightly brown and set aside.
3. Cook garlic and onion in the same pan over medium heat, until onion is softened.
4. Add broth and bring to boil over high heat.
5. Return pork to pan and stir in crushed tomatoes and remaining ingredients.
6. Cover and simmer for 20 minutes.
7. Serve and enjoy.

Nutrition:

Calories 321

Fat 23 g

Carbohydrates 7 g

Protein 19 g

Jalapeno Lamb Patties

Preparation Time: 10 Minutes

Cooking Time: 8 Minutes

Servings: 4

Ingredients:

- 1 lb. ground lamb
- 1 jalapeno pepper, minced
- 5 basil leaves, minced
- 10 mint leaves, minced
- ¼ cup fresh parsley, chopped
- 1 cup feta cheese, crumbled
- 1 tablespoon garlic, minced
- 1 teaspoon dried oregano
- ¼ teaspoon pepper
- ½ teaspoon kosher salt

Directions:

1. Add all fixings into the mixing bowl and mix until well combined.
2. Preheat the grill to 450 F.
3. Spray grill with cooking spray.
4. Make four equal shape patties from meat mixture and place on hot grill and cook for 3 minutes. Turn patties to another side and cook for 4 minutes.
5. Serve and enjoy.

Nutrition:

Calories 317

Fat 16 g

Carbohydrates 3 g

Protein 37.5 g

Red Pepper Pork Tenderloin

Preparation Time: 10 Minutes

Cooking Time: 25 Minutes

Servings: 4

Ingredients:

- 1 lb. pork tenderloin
- 3/4 teaspoon red pepper
- 2 teaspoon dried oregano
- 1 tablespoon olive oil
- 3 tablespoon feta cheese, crumbled
- 3 tablespoon olive tapenades

Directions:

1. Add pork, oil, red pepper, and oregano in a zip-lock bag and rub well and place in a refrigerator for 2 hours.
2. Remove pork from zip-lock bag. Using sharp knife make lengthwise cut through the center of the tenderloin.
3. Spread olive tapenade on half tenderloin and sprinkle with feta cheese.
4. Fold another half of meat over to the original shape of tenderloin.
5. Tie close pork tenderloin with twine at 2-inch intervals.
6. Grill the pork tenderloin for 20 minutes.
7. Cut into slices and serve with some vegetables.

Nutrition:

Calories 215

Fat 9.1 g

Carbohydrates 1 g

Protein 30.8 g

Basil Parmesan Pork Roast

Preparation Time: 10 Minutes

Cooking Time: 2 Hours

Servings: 8

Ingredients:

- 2 lbs. lean pork roast, boneless
- 1 tablespoon parsley
- ½ cup parmesan cheese, grated
- 28 oz can tomato, diced
- 1 teaspoon dried oregano
- 1 teaspoon dried basil
- 1 teaspoon garlic powder
- Pepper
- Salt

Directions:

1. Add the meat into the crock pot.
2. Mix together tomatoes, oregano, basil, garlic powder, parsley, cheese, pepper, and salt and pour over meat.
3. Cook on low for 6 hours.
4. Serve and enjoy.

Nutrition:

Calories 294

Fat 11.6 g

Carbohydrates 5 g

Protein 38 g

Sun-dried Tomato Chuck Roast

Preparation Time: 10 Minutes

Cooking Time: 2 Hours

Servings: 6

Ingredients:

- 2 lbs. beef chuck roast
- ½ cup beef broth

- ¼ cup sun-dried tomatoes, chopped
- 25 garlic cloves, peeled
- ¼ cup olives, sliced
- 1 teaspoon dried Italian seasoning, crushed
- 2 tablespoon balsamic vinegar

Directions:

1. Place meat into a pot.
2. Pour remaining ingredients over meat.
3. Cover then cook on low flame for 2 hours.
4. Shred the meat using fork.
5. Serve and enjoy.

Nutrition:

Calories 582

Fat 43 g

Carbohydrates 5 g

Protein 40g

Lamb Stew

Preparation Time: 10 Minutes

Cooking Time: 3 Hours

Servings: 2

Ingredients:

- 1/2 lb. lamb, boneless
- 1/4 cup green olives, sliced
- 2 tablespoon lemon juice
- 1/2 onion, chopped
- 2 garlic cloves, minced
- 2 fresh thyme sprigs
- 1/4 teaspoon turmeric
- 1/2 teaspoon pepper
- 1/4 Teaspoon salt
- 1/2 teaspoon sesame seeds

Directions:

1. Slice the lamb into thin pieces.

2. Add every ingredient into a pot and stir.
3. Cover and cook on low flame for 3 hours.
4. Stir well, garnish with sesame seeds and serve.

Nutrition:

Calories 297

Fat 20.3 g

Carbohydrates 5.4 g

Protein 21 g

Lemon Lamb Leg

Preparation Time: 10 Minutes

Cooking Time: 2 Hours

Servings: 8

Ingredients:

- 4 lbs. lamb leg, boneless and slice of fat
- 1 tablespoon rosemary, crushed
- 1/4 cup water
- 1/4 cup lemon juice
- 1 teaspoon black pepper
- 1/4 teaspoon salt

Directions:

1. Place lamb into a pot.
2. Add remaining ingredients over the lamb, into the pot.
3. Cover then cook on low flame for 2 hours.
4. Remove lamb from the pot and slice it.
5. Serve and enjoy.

Nutrition:

Calories 275

Fat 10.2 g

Carbohydrates 0.4 g

Protein 42 g

Turkey and Cranberry Sauce

Preparation Time: 10 Minutes

Cooking Time: 50 Minutes

Servings: 4

Ingredients:

- 1 cup chicken stock
- 2 tablespoons avocado oil
- ½ cup cranberry sauce
- 1 big turkey breast, skinless, boneless and sliced
- 1 yellow onion, roughly chopped
- Salt and black pepper to the taste

Directions:

1. Heat up a pan with the avocado oil over medium-high heat, add the onion and sauté for 5 minutes.
2. Add the turkey and brown for 5 minutes more.
3. Add the rest of the ingredients, toss, introduce in the oven at 350 degrees F and cook for 40 minutes

Nutrition:

Calories:382,

Fat:12.6,

Fiber:9.6,

Carbs:26.6,

Protein:17.6

Sage Turkey Mix

Preparation Time: 10 Minutes

Cooking Time: 40 Minutes

Servings: 4

Ingredients:

- 1 big turkey breast, skinless, boneless and roughly cubed
- Juice of 1 lemon
- 2 tablespoons avocado oil
- 1 red onion, chopped
- 2 tablespoons sage, chopped
- 1 garlic clove, minced
- 1 cup chicken stock

Directions:

1. Heat up a pan with the avocado oil over medium-high heat, add the turkey and brown for 3 minutes on each side.
2. Add the rest of the fixings, let it simmer and cook over medium heat for 35 minutes.
3. Divide the mix between plates and serve with a side dish.

Nutrition:

Calories:382,

Fat:12.6,

Fiber:9.6,

Carbs:16.6,

Protein:33.2

Turkey and Asparagus Mix

Preparation Time: 10 Minutes

Cooking Time: 30 Minutes

Servings: 4

Ingredients:

- 1 bunch asparagus, trimmed and halved
- 1 big turkey breast, skinless, boneless and cut into strips
- 1 teaspoon basil, dried
- 2 tablespoons olive oil
- A pinch of salt and black pepper

- ½ cup tomato sauce
- 1 tablespoon chives, chopped

Directions:

1. Heat up a pan with the oil with medium heat, then put the turkey and brown for 4 minutes.
2. Add the asparagus and the rest of the ingredients except the chives, bring to a simmer and cook over medium heat for 25 minutes.
3. Add the chives, divide the mix between plates and serve.

Nutrition:

Calories:337,

Fat:21.2,

Fiber:10.2,

Carbs:21.4,

Protein:17.6

Herbed Almond Turkey

Preparation Time: 10 Minutes

Cooking Time: 40 Minutes

Servings: 4

Ingredients:

- 1 big turkey breast, skinless, boneless and cubed
- 1 tablespoon olive oil
- ½ cup chicken stock
- 1 tablespoon basil, chopped
- 1 tablespoon rosemary, chopped
- 1 tablespoon oregano, chopped
- 1 tablespoon parsley, chopped
- 3 garlic cloves, minced
- ½ cup almonds, toasted and chopped
- 3 cups tomatoes, chopped

Directions:

1. Warmth up a pan through the oil over medium-high heat, add the turkey and the garlic and brown for 5 minutes.
2. Add the stock in addition the rest of the fixings, bring to a simmer over medium heat and cook for 35 minutes.
3. Divide the mix between plates and serve.

Nutrition:

Calories:297,

Fat:11.2,

Fiber:9.2,

Carbs:19.4,

Protein:23.6

Thyme Chicken

Preparation Time: 10 Minutes

Cooking Time: 50 Minutes

Servings: 4

Ingredients:

- 1 tablespoon olive oil
- 4 garlic cloves, minced
- A pinch of salt and black pepper
- 2 teaspoons thyme, dried
- 12 small red potatoes, halved
- 2 pounds chicken breast, skinless, boneless and cubed
- 1 cup red onion, sliced
- ¾ cup chicken stock
- 2 tablespoons basil, chopped

Directions:

1. In a baking dish greased with the oil, add the potatoes, chicken and the rest of the ingredients, toss a bit, introduce in the oven and bake at 400 degrees F for 50 minutes.
2. Divide between plates and serve.

Nutrition:

Calories:281,

Fat:9.2,

Fiber:10.9,

Carbs:21.6,

Protein:13.6

Turkey, Artichokes and Asparagus

Preparation Time: 10 Minutes

Cooking Time: 30 Minutes

Servings: 4

Ingredients:

- 2 turkey breasts, boneless, skinless and halved
- 3 tablespoons olive oil
- 1 and ½ pounds asparagus, trimmed and halved
- 1 cup chicken stock
- A pinch of salt and black pepper
- 1 cup canned artichoke hearts, drained
- ¼ cup kalamata olives, pitted and sliced
- 1 shallot, chopped
- 3 garlic cloves, minced
- 3 tablespoons dill, chopped

Directions:

1. Warmth up a pan through the oil over medium-high heat, add the turkey and the garlic and brown for 4 minutes on each side.
2. Add the asparagus, the stock and the rest of the ingredients except the dill, bring to a simmer and cook over medium heat for 20 minutes.
3. Add the dill, divide the mix between plates and serve.

Nutrition:

Calories:291,

Fat:16,

Fiber:10.3,

Carbs:22.8,

Protein:34.5

Lemony Turkey and Pine Nuts

Preparation Time: 10 Minutes

Cooking Time: 30 Minutes

Servings: 4

Ingredients:

- 2 turkey breasts, boneless, skinless and halved
- A pinch of salt and black pepper
- 2 tablespoons avocado oil
- Juice of 2 lemons
- 1 tablespoon rosemary, chopped
- 3 garlic cloves, minced
- ¼ cup pine nuts, chopped
- 1 cup chicken stock

Directions:

1. Warmth up a pan through the oil over medium-high heat, add the garlic and the turkey and brown for 4 minutes on each side.
2. Add the rest of the fixings, let it simmer and cook over medium heat for 20 minutes.
3. Divide the mix between plates and serve with a side salad.

Nutrition:

Calories:293,

Fat:12.4,

Fiber:9.3,

Carbs:17.8,

Protein:24.5

Yogurt Chicken and Red Onion Mix

Preparation Time: 10 Minutes

Cooking Time: 30 Minutes

Servings: 4

Ingredients:

- 2 pounds chicken breast, skinless, boneless and sliced
- 3 tablespoons olive oil
- ¼ cup Greek yogurt
- 2 garlic cloves, minced
- ½ teaspoon onion powder
- A pinch of salt and black pepper
- 4 red onions, sliced

Directions:

1. In a roasting pan, combine the chicken with the oil, the yogurt and the other ingredients, introduce in the oven at 375 degrees F and bake for 30 minutes.
2. Divide chicken mix between plates and serve hot.

Nutrition:

Calories:278,

Fat:15,

Fiber:9.2,

Carbs:15.1,

Protein:23.3

Chicken and Mint Sauce

Preparation Time: 10 Minutes

Cooking Time: 30 Minutes

Servings: 4

Ingredients:

- 2 and ½ tablespoons olive oil
- 2 pounds chicken breasts, skinless, boneless and halved
- 3 tablespoons garlic, minced
- 2 tablespoons lemon juice
- 1 tablespoon red wine vinegar
- 1/3 cup Greek yogurt
- 2 tablespoons mint, chopped
- A pinch of salt and black pepper

Directions:

1. Blend the garlic plus lemon juice and the other ingredients except the oil and the chicken and pulse well.
2. Warmth up a pan through the oil over medium-high heat, add the chicken and brown for 3 minutes on each side.
3. Add the mint sauce, introduce in the oven and bake everything at 370 degrees F for 25 minutes.
4. Divide the mix between plates and serve.

Nutrition:

Calories:278,

Fat;12,

Fiber:11.2,

Carbs:18.1,

Protein:13.3

Oregano Turkey and Peppers

Preparation Time: 10 Minutes

Cooking Time: 1 Hour

Servings: 4

Ingredients:

- 2 red bell peppers, cut into strips
- 2 green bell peppers, cut into strips
- 1 red onion, chopped
- 4 garlic cloves, minced

- ½ cup black olives, pitted and sliced
- 2 cups chicken stock
- 1 big turkey breast, skinless, boneless and cut into strips
- 1 tablespoon oregano, chopped
- ½ cup cilantro, chopped

Directions:

1. In a baking pan, combine the peppers with the turkey and the rest of the ingredients, toss, introduce in the oven at 400 degrees F and roast for 1 hour.
2. Divide everything between plates and serve.

Nutrition:

Calories:229,

Fat:8.9,

Fiber:8.2,

Carbs:17.8,

Protein:33.6

Chicken and Mustard Sauce

Preparation Time: 10 Minutes

Cooking Time: 26 Minutes

Servings: 4

Ingredients:

- 1/3 cup mustard
- Salt and black pepper to the taste
- 1 red onion, chopped
- 1 tablespoon olive oil
- 1 and ½ cups chicken stock
- 4 chicken breasts, skinless, boneless, and halved
- ¼ teaspoon oregano, dried

Directions:

1. Heat up a pan with the stock over medium heat, add the mustard, onion, salt, pepper and the oregano, whisk, bring to a simmer and cook for 8 minutes.
2. Warmth up a pan through the oil over medium-high heat, add the chicken and brown for 3 minutes on each side.
3. Add chicken into the pan with the sauce, toss, simmer everything for 12 minutes more, divide between plates and serve.

Nutrition:

Calories:247,

Fat:15.1,

Fiber:9.1,

Carbs:16.6,

Protein:26.1

Chicken and Sausage Mix

Preparation Time: 10 Minutes

Cooking Time: 50 Minutes

Servings: 4

Ingredients:

- 2 zucchinis, cubed
- 1-pound Italian sausage, cubed
- 2 tablespoons olive oil
- 1 red bell pepper, chopped
- 1 red onion, sliced
- 2 tablespoons garlic, minced
- 2 chicken breasts, boneless, skinless and halved
- Salt and black pepper to the taste
- ½ cup chicken stock
- 1 tablespoon balsamic vinegar

Directions:

1. Heat up a pan with half of the oil over medium-high heat, add the sausages,

brown for 3 minutes on each side and transfer to a bowl.
2. Heat up the pan again with the rest of the oil over medium-high heat, add the chicken and brown for 4 minutes on each side.
3. Return the sausage, add the rest of the ingredients as well, bring to a simmer, introduce in the oven and bake at 400 degrees F for 30 minutes.
4. Divide everything between plates and serve.

Nutrition:

Calories:293,

Fat:13.1,

Fiber:8.1,

Carbs:16.6,

Protein:26.1

Coriander and Coconut Chicken

Preparation Time: 10 Minutes

Cooking Time: 30 Minutes

Servings: 4

Ingredients:

- 2 pounds chicken thighs, skinless, boneless and cubed
- 2 tablespoons olive oil
- Salt and black pepper to the taste
- 3 tablespoons coconut flesh, shredded
- 1 and ½ teaspoons orange extract
- 1 tablespoon ginger, grated
- ¼ cup orange juice
- 2 tablespoons coriander, chopped
- 1 cup chicken stock
- ¼ teaspoon red pepper flakes

Directions:

1. Warmth up a pan through the oil over medium-high heat, add the chicken and brown for 4 minutes on each side.
2. Add salt, pepper and the rest of the ingredients, bring to a simmer and cook over medium heat for 20 minutes.
3. Divide the mix between plates and serve hot.

Nutrition:

Calories:297,

Fat:14.4,

Fiber:9.6,

Carbs:22,

Protein:25

Saffron Chicken Thighs and Green Beans

Preparation Time: 10 Minutes

Cooking Time: 25 Minutes

Servings: 4

Ingredients:

- 2 pounds chicken thighs, boneless and skinless
- 2 teaspoons saffron powder
- 1-pound green beans, trimmed and halved
- ½ cup Greek yogurt
- Salt and black pepper to the taste
- 1 tablespoon lime juice
- 1 tablespoon dill, chopped

Directions:

1. In a roasting pan, combine the chicken with the saffron, green beans and the rest of the ingredients, toss a bit, introduce in the oven and bake at 400 degrees F for 25 minutes.

2. Divide everything between plates and serve.

Nutrition:

Calories:274,

Fat:12.3,

Fiber:5.3,

Carbs:20.4,

Protein:14.3

Chicken and Olives Salsa

Preparation Time: 10 Minutes

Cooking Time: 25 Minutes

Servings: 4

Ingredients:

- 2 tablespoon avocado oil
- 4 chicken breast halves, skinless and boneless
- Salt and black pepper to the taste
- 1 tablespoon sweet paprika
- 1 red onion, chopped
- 1 tablespoon balsamic vinegar
- 2 tablespoons parsley, chopped
- 1 avocado, peeled, pitted and cubed
- 2 tablespoons black olives, pitted and chopped

Directions:

1. Heat up your grill over medium-high heat, add the chicken brushed with half of the oil and seasoned with paprika, salt and pepper, cook for 7 minutes on each side and divide between plates.
2. Meanwhile, in a bowl, mix the onion with the rest of the ingredients and the remaining oil, toss, add on top of the chicken and serve.

Nutrition:

Calories:289,

Fat:12.4,

Fiber:9.1,

Carbs:23.8,

Protein:14.3

Carrots and Tomatoes Chicken

Preparation Time: 10 Minutes

Cooking Time: 1 Hour 10 Minutes

Servings: 4

Ingredients:

- 2 pounds chicken breasts, skinless, boneless and halved
- Salt and black pepper to the taste
- 3 garlic cloves, minced
- 3 tablespoons avocado oil
- 2 shallots, chopped
- 4 carrots, sliced
- 3 tomatoes, chopped
- ¼ cup chicken stock
- 1 tablespoon Italian seasoning
- 1 tablespoon parsley, chopped

Directions:

1. Warmth up a pan through the oil over medium-high heat, add the chicken, garlic, salt and pepper and brown for 3 minutes on each side.
2. Add the rest of the fixings excluding the parsley, bring to a simmer and cook over medium-low heat for 40 minutes.
3. Add the parsley, divide the mix between plates and serve.

Nutrition:

Calories:309,

Fat:12.4,

Fiber:11.1,

Carbs:23.8,

Protein:15.3

Smoked and Hot Turkey Mix

Preparation Time: 10 Minutes

Cooking Time: 40 Minutes

Servings: 4

Ingredients:

- 1 red onion, sliced
- 1 big turkey breast, skinless, boneless and roughly cubed
- 1 tablespoon smoked paprika
- 2 chili peppers, chopped
- Salt and black pepper to the taste
- 2 tablespoons olive oil
- ½ cup chicken stock
- 1 tablespoon parsley, chopped
- 1 tablespoon cilantro, chopped

Directions:

1. Grease a roasting pan through the oil, add the turkey, onion, paprika and the rest of the ingredients, toss, introduce in the oven and bake at 425 degrees F for 40 minutes.
2. Divide the mix between plates and serve right away.

Nutrition:

Calories:310,

Fat:18.4,

Fiber:10.4,

Carbs:22.3,

Protein:33.4

Spicy Cumin Chicken

Preparation Time: 10 Minutes

Cooking Time: 25 Minutes

Servings: 4

Ingredients:

- 2 teaspoons chili powder
- 2 and ½ tablespoons olive oil
- Salt and black pepper to the taste
- 1 and ½ teaspoons garlic powder
- 1 tablespoon smoked paprika
- ½ cup chicken stock
- 1-pound chicken breasts, skinless, boneless and halved
- 2 teaspoons sherry vinegar
- 2 teaspoons hot sauce
- 2 teaspoons cumin, ground
- ½ cup black olives, pitted and sliced

Directions:

1. Warm up a pan with the oil over medium-high heat, add the chicken and brown for 3 minutes on each side.
2. Add the chili powder, salt, pepper, garlic powder and paprika, toss and cook for 4 minutes more.
3. Add the rest of the ingredients, toss, bring to a simmer and cook over medium heat for 15 minutes more.
4. Divide the mix between plates and serve.

Nutrition:

Calories:230,

Fat:18.4,

Fiber:9.4,

Carbs:15.3,

Protein:13.4

Chicken with Artichokes and Beans

Preparation Time: 10 Minutes

Cooking Time: 40 Minutes

Servings: 4

Ingredients:

- 2 tablespoons olive oil
- 2 chicken breasts, skinless, boneless and halved
- Zest of 1 lemon, grated
- 3 garlic cloves, crushed
- Juice of 1 lemon
- Salt and black pepper to the taste
- 1 tablespoon thyme, chopped
- 6 ounces canned artichokes hearts, drained
- 1 cup canned fava beans, drained and rinsed
- 1 cup chicken stock
- A pinch of cayenne pepper
- Salt and black pepper to the taste

Directions:

1. Warmth up a pan with the oil on medium-high heat, add chicken and brown for 5 minutes.
2. Add lemon juice, lemon zest, salt, pepper and the rest of the ingredients, bring to a simmer and cook over medium heat for 35 minutes.
3. Divide the mix between plates and serve right away.

Nutrition:

Calories:291,

Fat:14.9,

Fiber:10.5,

Carbs:23.8,

Protein:24.2

Chicken and Olives Tapenade

Preparation Time: 10 Minutes

Cooking Time: 25 Minutes

Servings: 4

Ingredients:

- 2 chicken breasts, boneless, skinless and halved
- 1 cup black olives, pitted
- ½ cup olive oil
- Salt and black pepper to the taste
- ½ cup mixed parsley, chopped
- ½ cup rosemary, chopped
- Salt and black pepper to the taste
- 4 garlic cloves, minced
- Juice of ½ lime

Directions:

1. In a blender, combine the olives with half of the oil and the rest of the ingredients except the chicken and pulse well.
2. Heat up a pan with the rest of the oil over medium-high heat, add the chicken and brown for 4 minutes on each side.
3. Add the olives mix, and cook for 20 minutes more tossing often.

Nutrition:

Calories:291,

Fat:12.9,

Fiber:8.5,

Carbs:15.8,

Protein:34.2

Chapter 8: Sides Recipes

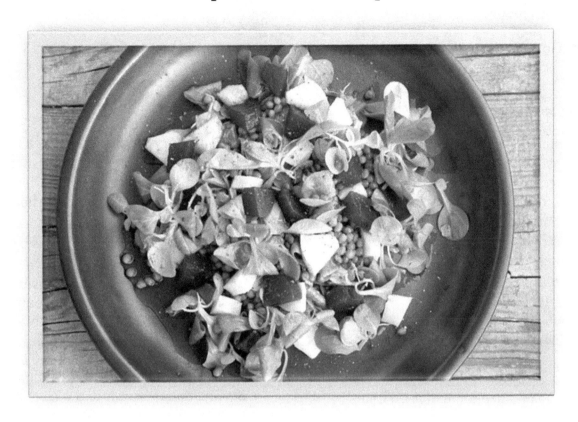

Nachos

Preparation Time: 5 Minutes

Cooking Time: 10 Minutes

Servings: 4

Ingredients:

- 4-ounce restaurant-style corn tortilla chips
- 1 medium green onion, thinly sliced (about 1 tbsp.)
- 1 (4 ounces) package finely crumbled feta cheese
- 1 finely chopped and drained plum tomato
- 2 tbsp Sun-dried tomatoes in oil, finely chopped
- 2 tbsp Kalamata olives

Directions:

1. Mix an onion, plum tomato, oil, sun-dried tomatoes, and olives in a small bowl.
2. Arrange the tortillas chips on a microwavable plate in a single layer topped evenly with cheese—microwave on high for one minute.
3. Rotate the plate half turn and continue microwaving until the cheese is bubbly. Spread the tomato mixture over the chips and cheese and enjoy.

Nutrition:

Calories: 140

Carbs: 19g

Fat: 7g

Protein: 2g

Stuffed Celery

Preparation Time: 15 Minutes

Cooking Time: 20 Minutes

Servings: 3

Ingredients:

- Olive oil
- 1 clove garlic, minced
- 2 tbsp Pine nuts
- 2 tbsp dry-roasted sunflower seeds
- ¼ cup Italian cheese blend, shredded
- 8 stalks celery leaves
- 1 (8-ounce) fat-free cream cheese
- Cooking spray

Directions:

1. Sauté garlic and pine nuts over a medium setting for the heat until the nuts are golden brown. Cut off the wide base and tops from celery.
2. Remove two thin strips from the round side of the celery to create a flat surface.
3. Mix Italian cheese and cream cheese in a bowl and spread into cut celery stalks.
4. Sprinkle half of the celery pieces with sunflower seeds and a half with the pine nut mixture. Cover mixture and let stand for at least 4 hours before eating.

Nutrition:

Calories: 64

Carbs: 2g

Fat: 6g

Protein: 1g

Butternut Squash Fries

Preparation Time: 5 Minutes

Cooking Time: 10 Minutes

Servings: 2

Ingredients:

- 1 Butternut squash
- 1 tbsp Extra virgin olive oil
- ½ tbsp Grapeseed oil
- 1/8 tsp Sea salt

Directions:

1. Remove seeds from the squash and cut into thin slices. Coat with extra virgin olive oil and grapeseed oil. Add a sprinkle of salt and toss to coat well.
2. Arrange the squash slices onto three baking sheets and bake for 10 minutes until crispy.

Nutrition:

Calories: 40

Carbs: 10g

Fat: 0g

Protein: 1g

Dried Fig Tapenade

Preparation Time: 5 Minutes

Cooking Time: 0 Minutes

Servings: 1

Ingredients:

- 1 cup Dried figs
- 1 cup Kalamata olives
- ½ cup Water
- 1 tbsp Chopped fresh thyme
- 1 tbsp extra virgin olive oil
- ½ tsp Balsamic vinegar

Directions:

1. Prepare figs in a food processor until well chopped, add water, and continue processing to form a paste.
2. Add olives and pulse until well blended. Add thyme, vinegar, and extra virgin olive oil and pulse until very smooth.

Best served with crackers of your choice.

Nutrition:

Calories: 249

Carbs: 64g

Fat: 1g

Protein: 3g

Speedy Sweet Potato Chips

Preparation Time: 15 Minutes

Cooking Time: 0 Minutes

Servings: 4

Ingredients:

- 1 large Sweet potato
- 1 tbsp Extra virgin olive oil
- Salt

Directions:

1. 300°F preheated oven. Slice your potato into nice, thin slices that resemble fries.
2. Toss the potato slices with salt and extra virgin olive oil in a bowl. Bake for about one hour, flipping every 15 minutes until crispy and browned.

Nutrition:

Calories: 150

Carbs: 16g

Fat: 9g

Protein: 1g

Nachos with Hummus (Mediterranean Inspired)

Preparation Time: 15 Minutes

Cooking Time: 20 Minutes

Servings: 4

Ingredients:

- 4 cups salted pita chips
- 1 (8 oz.) red pepper (roasted)
- Hummus
- 1 tsp Finely shredded lemon peel
- ¼ cup Chopped pitted Kalamata olives
- ¼ cup crumbled feta cheese
- 1 plum (Roma) tomato, seeded, chopped
- ½ cup chopped cucumber
- 1 tsp Chopped fresh oregano leaves

Directions:

1. 400°F preheated oven. Arrange the pita chips on a heatproof platter and drizzle with hummus.
2. Top with olives, tomato, cucumber, and cheese and bake until warmed through. Sprinkle lemon zest and oregano and enjoy while it's hot.

Nutrition:

Calories: 130

Carbs: 18g

Fat: 5g

Protein: 4g

Hummus and Olive Pita Bread

Preparation Time: 5 Minutes

Cooking Time: 0 Minutes

Servings: 3

Ingredients:

- 7 pita bread cut into 6 wedges each
- 1 (7 ounces) container plain hummus
- 1 tbsp Greek vinaigrette
- ½ cup Chopped pitted Kalamata olives

Directions:

1. Spread the hummus on a serving plate—Mix vinaigrette and olives in a bowl and spoon over the hummus. Enjoy with wedges of pita bread.

Nutrition:

Calories: 225

Carbs: 40g

Fat: 5g

Protein: 9g

Roast Asparagus

Preparation Time: 15 Minutes

Cooking Time: 5 Minutes

Servings: 4

Ingredients:

- 1 tbsp Extra virgin olive oil (1 tablespoon)
- 1 medium lemon
- ½ tsp Freshly grated nutmeg
- ½ tsp black pepper
- ½ tsp Kosher salt

Directions:

2. Warm the oven to 500°F. Put the asparagus on an aluminum foil and drizzle with extra virgin olive oil, and toss until well coated.
3. Roast the asparagus in the oven for about five minutes; toss and continue roasting until browned. Sprinkle the roasted asparagus with nutmeg, salt, zest, and pepper.

Nutrition:

Calories: 123

Carbs: 5g

Fat: 11g

Protein: 3g

Chicken Kale Wraps

Preparation Time: 10 Minutes

Cooking Time: 10 Minutes

Servings: 4

Ingredients:

- 4 kale leaves
- 4 oz chicken fillet
- ½ apple
- 1 tablespoon butter
- ¼ teaspoon chili pepper
- ¾ teaspoon salt
- 1 tablespoon lemon juice
- ¾ teaspoon dried thyme

Directions:

1. Chop the chicken fillet into small cubes. Then mix up the chicken with chili pepper and salt.
2. Heat butter in the skillet. Add chicken cubes. Roast them for 4 minutes.
3. Meanwhile, chop the apple into small cubes and add to the chicken. Mix up well.
4. Sprinkle the ingredients with lemon juice and dried thyme. Cook them for 5 minutes over medium-high heat.
5. Fill the kale leaves with the hot chicken mixture and wrap.

Nutrition:

Calories 106

Fat 5.1

Fiber 1.1

Carbs 6.3

Protein 9

Tomato Triangles

Preparation Time: 10 Minutes

Cooking Time: 0 Minutes

Servings: 6

Ingredients:

- 6 corn tortillas
- 1 tablespoon cream cheese
- 1 tablespoon ricotta cheese
- ½ teaspoon minced garlic
- 1 tablespoon fresh dill, chopped
- 2 tomatoes, sliced

Directions:

1. Cut every tortilla into 2 triangles. Then mix up cream cheese, ricotta cheese, minced garlic, and dill.
2. Spread 6 triangles with cream cheese mixture.
3. Then place the sliced tomato on them and cover with remaining tortilla triangles. Serve.

Nutrition:

Calories 71

Fat 1.6

Fiber 2.1

Carbs 12.8

Protein 2.3

Zaatar Fries

Preparation Time: 10 Minutes

Cooking Time: 35 Minutes

Servings: 5

Ingredients:

- 1 teaspoon Zaatar spices

- 3 sweet potatoes
- 1 tablespoon dried dill
- 1 teaspoon salt
- 3 teaspoons sunflower oil
- ½ teaspoon paprika

Directions:

1. Pour water into the crockpot. Cut the sweet potatoes into fries.
2. Line the baking tray with parchment. Place the layer of the sweet potato in the tray.
3. Sprinkle the vegetables with dried dill, salt, and paprika. Then sprinkle sweet potatoes with Za'atar and mix up well with the help of the fingertips.
4. Sprinkle the sweet potato fries with sunflower oil—Preheat the oven to 375F.
5. Bake the sweet potato fries within 35 minutes. Stir the fries every 10 minutes.

Nutrition:

Calories 28

Fat 2.9

Fiber 0.2

Carbs 0.6

Protein 0.2

Summertime Vegetable Chicken Wraps

Preparation Time: 15 Minutes

Cooking Time: 0 Minutes

Servings: 4

Ingredients:

- 2 cups cooked chicken, chopped
- ½ English cucumbers, diced
- ½ red bell pepper, diced
- ½ cup carrot, shredded

- 1 scallion, white and green parts, chopped
- ¼ cup plain Greek yogurt
- 1 tablespoon freshly squeezed lemon juice
- ½ teaspoon fresh thyme, chopped
- Pinch of salt
- Pinch of ground black pepper
- 4 multigrain tortillas

Directions:

1. Take a medium bowl and mix in chicken, red bell pepper, cucumber, carrot, yogurt, scallion, lemon juice, thyme, sea salt and pepper.
2. Mix well.
3. Spoon one quarter of chicken mix into the middle of the tortilla and fold the opposite ends of the tortilla over the filling.
4. Roll the tortilla from the side to create a snug pocket.
5. Repeat with the remaining ingredients and serve.
6. Enjoy!

Nutrition:

Calories: 278

Fat: 4g

Carbohydrates: 28g

Protein: 27g

Premium Roasted Baby Potatoes

Preparation Time: 10 Minutes

Cooking Time: 35 Minutes

Servings: 4

Ingredients:

- 2 pounds new yellow potatoes, scrubbed and cut into wedges

- 2 tablespoons extra virgin olive oil
- 2 teaspoons fresh rosemary, chopped
- 1 teaspoon garlic powder
- 1 teaspoon sweet paprika
- ½ teaspoon sea salt
- ½ teaspoon freshly ground black pepper

Directions:

1. Pre-heat your oven to 400 degrees Fahrenheit.
2. Take a large bowl and add potatoes, olive oil, garlic, rosemary, paprika, sea salt and pepper.
3. Spread potatoes in single layer on baking sheet and bake for 35 minutes.
4. Serve and enjoy!

Nutrition:

Calories: 225

Fat: 7g

Carbohydrates: 37g

Protein: 5g

Tomato and Cherry Linguine

Preparation Time: 10 Minutes

Cooking Time: 15 Minutes

Servings: 4

Ingredients:

- 2 pounds cherry tomatoes
- 3 tablespoons extra virgin olive oil
- 2 tablespoons balsamic vinegar
- 2 teaspoons garlic, minced
- Pinch of fresh ground black pepper
- ¾ pound whole-wheat linguine pasta
- 1 tablespoon fresh oregano, chopped
- ¼ cup feta cheese, crumbled

Directions:

1. Pre-heat your oven to 350 degrees Fahrenheit.
2. Take a large bowl and add cherry tomatoes, 2 tablespoons olive oil, balsamic vinegar, garlic, pepper and toss.
3. Spread tomatoes evenly on baking sheet and roast for 15 minutes.
4. While the tomatoes are roasting, cook the pasta according to the package instructions and drain the paste into a large bowl.
5. Toss pasta with 1 tablespoon olive oil.
6. Add roasted tomatoes (with juice) and toss.
7. Serve with topping of oregano and feta cheese.
8. Enjoy!

Nutrition:

Calories: 397

Fat: 15g

Carbohydrates: 55g

Protein: 13g

Mediterranean Zucchini Mushroom Pasta

Preparation Time: 10 Minutes

Cooking Time: 10 Minutes

Servings: 4

Ingredients:

- ½ pound pasta
- 2 tablespoons olive oil
- 6 garlic cloves, crushed
- 1 teaspoon red chili
- 2 spring onions, sliced
- 3 teaspoons rosemary
- 1 large zucchini, cut in half
- 5 large portabella mushrooms
- 1 can tomatoes

- 4 tablespoons Parmesan cheese
- Fresh ground black pepper

Directions:

1. Cook the pasta.
2. Take a large-sized frying pan and place it over medium heat.
3. Add oil and allow the oil to heat up.
4. Add garlic, onion and chili and sauté for a few minutes until golden.
5. Add zucchini, rosemary and mushroom and sauté for a few minutes.
6. Increase the heat to medium-high and add tinned tomatoes to the sauce until thick.
7. Drain your boiled pasta and transfer to serving platter.
8. Pour the tomato mix on top and mix using tongs.
9. Garnish with Parmesan and freshly ground black pepper.
10. Enjoy!

Nutrition:

Calories: 361

Fat: 12g

Carbohydrates: 47g

Protein: 14g

Lemon and Garlic Fettucine

Preparation Time: 5 Minutes

Cooking Time: 15 Minutes

Servings: 5

Ingredients:

- 8 ounces of whole wheat fettuccine
- 4 tablespoons of extra virgin olive oil
- 4 cloves of minced garlic
- 1 cup of fresh breadcrumbs
- ¼ cup of lemon juice
- 1 teaspoon of freshly ground pepper

- ½ teaspoon of salt
- 2 cans of 4 ounce boneless and skinless sardines (dipped in tomato sauce)
- ½ cup of chopped up fresh parsley
- ¼ cup of finely shredded Parmesan cheese

Directions:

1. Take a large-sized pot and bring water to a boil.
2. Cook pasta for 10 minutes until Al Dente.
3. Take a small-sized skillet and place it over medium heat.
4. Add 2 tablespoons of oil and allow it to heat up.
5. Add garlic and cook for 20 seconds.
6. Transfer the garlic to a medium-sized bowl
7. Add breadcrumbs to the hot skillet and cook for 5-6 minutes until golden
8. Whisk in lemon juice, pepper and salt into the garlic bowl
9. Add pasta to the bowl (with garlic) and sardines, parsley and Parmesan
10. Stir well and sprinkle bread crumbs
11. Enjoy!

Nutrition:

Calories: 480

Fat: 21g

Carbohydrates: 53g

Protein: 23g

Roasted Broccoli with Parmesan

Preparation Time: 10 Minutes

Cooking Time: 10 Minutes

Servings: 4

Ingredients:

- 2 head broccolis, cut into florets

- 2 tablespoons extra-virgin olive oil
- 2 teaspoons garlic, minced
- Zest of 1 lemon
- Pinch of salt
- ½ cup Parmesan cheese, grated

Directions:

1. Pre-heat your oven to 400 degrees Fahrenheit.
2. Take a large bowl and add broccoli with 2 tablespoons olive oil, lemon zest, garlic, lemon juice and salt.
3. Spread mix on the baking sheet in single layer and sprinkle with Parmesan cheese.
4. Bake for 10 minutes until tender.
5. Transfer broccoli to serving the dish.
6. Serve and enjoy!

Nutrition:

Calories: 154

Fat: 11g

Carbohydrates: 10g

Protein: 9g

Spinach and Feta Bread

Preparation Time: 10 Minutes

Cooking Time: 12 Minutes

Servings: 6

Ingredients:

- 6 ounces of sun-dried tomato pesto
- 6 pieces of 6-inch whole wheat pita bread
- 2 chopped up Roma plum tomatoes
- 1 bunch of rinsed and chopped spinach
- 4 sliced fresh mushrooms
- ½ cup of crumbled feta cheese
- 2 tablespoons of grated Parmesan cheese

- 3 tablespoons of olive oil
- Ground black pepper as needed

Directions:

1. Pre-heat your oven to 350 degrees Fahrenheit.
2. Spread your tomato pesto onto one side of your pita bread and place on your baking sheet (with the pesto side up).
3. Top up the pitas with spinach, tomatoes, feta cheese, mushrooms and Parmesan cheese.
4. Drizzle with some olive oil and season nicely with pepper.
5. Bake in your oven for around 12 minutes until the breads are crispy.
6. Cut up the pita into quarters and serve!

Nutrition:

Calories: 350

Fat: 17g

Carbohydrates: 41g

Protein:11g

Quick Zucchini Bowl

Preparation Time: 10 Minutes

Cooking Time: 10 Minutes

Servings: 4

Ingredients:

- ½ pound of pasta
- 2 tablespoons of olive oil
- 6 crushed garlic cloves
- 1 teaspoon of red chili
- 2 finely sliced spring onions
- 3 teaspoons of chopped rosemary
- 1 large zucchini cut up in half, lengthways and sliced
- 5 large portabella mushrooms
- 1 can of tomatoes

- 4 tablespoons of Parmesan cheese
- Fresh ground black pepper

Directions:

1. Cook the pasta.
2. Take a large-sized frying pan and place over medium heat.
3. Add oil and allow the oil to heat up.
4. Add garlic, onion and chili and sauté for a few minutes until golden.
5. Add zucchini, rosemary and mushroom and sauté for a few minutes.
6. Increase the heat to medium-high and add tinned tomatoes to the sauce until thick.
7. Drain your boiled pasta and transfer to a serving platter.
8. Pour the tomato mix on top and mix using tongs.
9. Garnish with Parmesan cheese and freshly ground black pepper.
10. Enjoy!

Nutrition:

Calories: 361

Fat: 12g

Carbohydrates: 47g

Protein: 14g

Healthy Basil Platter

Preparation Time: 25 Minutes

Cooking Time: 15 Minutes

Servings: 4

Ingredients:

- 2 pieces of red pepper seeded and cut up into chunks
- 2 pieces of red onion cut up into wedges
- 2 mild red chilies, diced and seeded
- 3 coarsely chopped garlic cloves
- 1 teaspoon of golden caster sugar

- 2 tablespoons of olive oil (plus additional for serving)
- 2 pounds of small ripe tomatoes quartered up
- 12 ounces of dried pasta
- Just a handful of basil leaves
- 2 tablespoons of grated Parmesan

Directions:

1. Pre-heat the oven to 392 degrees Fahrenheit.
2. Take a large-sized roasting tin and scatter pepper, red onion, garlic and chilies.
3. Sprinkle sugar on top.
4. Drizzle olive oil then season with pepper and salt.
5. Roast the veggies in your oven for 15 minutes.
6. Take a large-sized pan and cook the pasta in boiling, salted water until Al Dente.
7. Drain them.
8. Remove the veggies from the oven and tip in the pasta into the veggies.
9. Toss well and tear basil leaves on top.
10. Sprinkle Parmesan and enjoy!

Nutrition:

Calories: 452

Fat: 8g

Carbohydrates: 88g

Protein: 14g

Spiced Vegetable Couscous

Preparation Time: 10 minutes

Cooking Time: 20 minutes

Servings: 2

Ingredients

- Cauliflower – 1 head, cut into 1 –inch florets
- Extra-virgin olive oil – 6 tbsp. plus extra for serving
- Salt and pepper
- Couscous – 1 ½ cups
- Zucchini – 1, cut into ½ inch pieces
- Red bell pepper – 1, stemmed, seeded, and cut into ½ inch pieces
- Garlic – 4 cloves, minced
- Ras el hanout – 2 tsp.
- Grated lemon zest -1 tsp. plus lemon wedges for serving
- Chicken broth – 1 ¾ cups
- Minced fresh marjoram – 1 tbsp.

Directions

1. In a skillet, heat 2 tbsp. oil over medium heat.
2. Add cauliflowers, ¾ tsp. salt, and ½ tsp. pepper. Mix.
3. Cover and cook for 5 minutes, or until the florets start to brown and the edges are just translucent.
4. Remove the lid and cook, stirring for 10 minutes, or until the florets turn golden brown. Transfer to a bowl and clean the skillet.
5. Heat 2 tbsp. oil in the skillet.
6. Add the couscous. Cook and stir for 3 to 5 minutes, or until grains are just beginning to brown. Transfer to a bowl and clean the skillet.
7. Heat the remaining 3 tbsp. oil in the skillet and add bell pepper, zucchini, and ½ tsp. salt. Cook for 6 to 8 minutes, or until tender.
8. Stir in lemon zest, ras el hanout, and garlic. Cook until fragrant (about 30 seconds).
9. Stir in the broth and bring to a simmer.
10. Stir in the couscous. Cover, remove from the heat, and set aside until tender (about 7 minutes).
11. Add marjoram and cauliflower; then gently fluff with a fork to combine.
12. Drizzle with extra oil and season with salt and pepper.
13. Serve with lemon wedges.

Nutrition

Calories: 787

Fat: 18.3g

Carb: 129.6g

Protein: 24.5g

Pasta e Fagioli with Orange and Fennel

Preparation Time: 10 minutes

Cooking Time: 30 minutes

Servings: 5

Ingredients

- Extra-virgin olive oil – 1 tbsp. plus extra for serving
- Pancetta – 2 ounces, chopped fine
- Onion – 1, chopped fine
- Fennel – 1 bulb, stalks discarded, bulb halved, cored, and chopped fine
- Celery – 1 rib, minced
- Garlic – 2 cloves, minced
- Anchovy fillets – 3, rinsed and minced
- Minced fresh oregano – 1 tbsp.
- Grated orange zest – 2 tsp.
- Fennel seeds – ½ tsp.
- Red pepper flakes – ¼ tsp.
- Diced tomatoes – 1 (28-ounce) can
- Parmesan cheese – 1 rind, plus more for serving
- Cannellini beans – 1 (7-ounce) cans, rinsed
- Chicken broth – 2 ½ cups
- Water – 2 ½ cups
- Salt and pepper
- Orzo – 1 cup

- Minced fresh parsley – ¼ cup

Directions

1. Heat oil in a Dutch oven over medium heat. Add pancetta.
2. Stir-fry for 3 to 5 minutes or until beginning to brown.
3. Stir in celery, fennel, and onion and stir-fry until softened (about 5 to 7 minutes).
4. Stir in pepper flakes, fennel seeds, orange zest, oregano, anchovies, and garlic. Cook for 1 minute.
5. Stir in tomatoes and their juice. Stir in Parmesan rind and beans.
6. Bring to a simmer and cook for 10 minutes.
7. Stir in water, broth, and 1 tsp. salt.
8. Increase heat to high and bring to a boil.
9. Stir in pasta and cook for 10 minutes, or until al dente.
10. Remove from heat and discard parmesan rind.
11. Stir in parsley and season with salt and pepper to taste.
12. Drizzle with olive oil and sprinkle with grated Parmesan.
13. Serve.

Nutrition

Calories: 502

Fat: 8.8g

Carb: 72.2g

Protein: 34.9g

Spaghetti al Limone

Preparation Time: 10 minutes

Cooking Time: 15 minutes

Servings: 2

Ingredients

- Extra-virgin olive oil – ½ cup
- Grated lemon zest – 2 tsp.
- Lemon juice – 1/3 cup
- Garlic – 1 clove, minced to pate
- Salt and pepper
- Parmesan cheese – 2 ounces, grated
- Spaghetti – 1 pound
- Shredded fresh basil – 6 tbsp.

Directions

1. In a bowl, whisk garlic, oil, lemon zest, juice, ½ tsp. salt and ¼ tsp. pepper. Stir in the Parmesan and mix until creamy.
2. Meanwhile, cook the pasta according to package directions. Drain and reserve ½ cup cooking water.
3. Add the oil mixture and basil to the pasta and toss to combine.
4. Season with salt and pepper to taste and add the cooking water as needed.
5. Serve.

Nutrition:

Calories: 398

Fat: 20.7g

Carb: 42.5g

Protein: 11.9g

Spiced Baked Rice with Fennel

Preparation Time: 10 minutes

Cooking Time: 45 minutes

Servings: 2

Ingredients
- Sweet potatoes – 1 ½ pounds, peeled and cut into 1-inch pieces
- Extra-virgin olive oil – ¼ cup
- Salt and pepper
- Fennel – 1 bulb, chopped fine
- Small onion – 1, chopped fine
- Long-grain white rice – 1 ½ cups, rinsed
- Garlic – 4 cloves, minced

- Ras el hanout – 2 tsp.
- Chicken broth – 2 ¾ cups
- Large pitted brine-cured green olives – ¾ cup, halved
- Minced fresh cilantro – 2 tbsp.
- Lime wedges

Directions

1. Adjust the oven rack to the middle position and heat the oven to 400F. Toss the potatoes with ½ tsp. salt and 2 tbsp. oil.
2. Arrange the potatoes in a single layer in a rimmed baking sheet and roast for 25 to 30 minutes, or until tender. Stir the potatoes halfway through roasting.
3. Remove the potatoes from the oven and lower the oven temperature to 350F.
4. In a Dutch oven, heat the remaining 2 tbsp. oil over medium heat.
5. Add onion and fennel; next, cook for 5 to 7 minutes, or until softened. Stir in ras el hanout, garlic, and rice. Stir-fry for 3 minutes.
6. Stir in the olives and broth and let sit for 10 minutes. Add the potatoes to the rice and fluff gently with a fork to combine.
7. Season with salt and pepper to taste.
8. Sprinkle with cilantro and serve with lime wedges.

Nutrition

Calories: 207

Fat: 8.9g

Carb: 29.4g

Protein: 3.9g

Moroccan-Style Couscous with Chickpeas

Preparation Time: 5 minutes

Cooking Time: 18 minutes

Servings: 2

Ingredients

- Extra-virgin olive oil – ¼ cup, extra for serving
- Couscous – 1 ½ cups
- Peeled and chopped fine carrots – 2
- Chopped fine onion – 1
- Salt and pepper
- Garlic – 3 cloves, minced
- Ground coriander – 1 tsp.
- Ground ginger - tsp.
- Ground anise seed – ¼ tsp.
- Chicken broth – 1 ¾ cups
- Chickpeas - 1 (15-ounce) can, rinsed
- Frozen peas – 1 ½ cups
- Chopped fresh parsley or cilantro – ½ cup
- Lemon wedges

Directions

1. Heat 2 tbsp. oil in a skillet over medium heat.
2. Add the couscous and cook for 3 to 5 minutes, or until just beginning to brown.
3. Transfer to a bowl and clean the skillet.
4. Heat remaining 2 tbsp. oil in the skillet and add the onion, carrots, and 1 tsp. salt.
5. Cook for 5 to 7 minutes, or until softened.
6. Stir in anise, ginger, coriander, and garlic. Cook until fragrant (about 30 seconds).
7. Stir in the chickpeas and broth and bring to simmer.
8. Stir in the couscous and peas. Cover and remove from the heat. Set aside for 7 minutes, or until the couscous is tender.
9. Add the parsley to the couscous and fluff with a fork to combine.
10. Drizzle with extra oil and season with salt and pepper.

11. Serve with lemon wedges.

Nutrition

Calories: 649

Fat: 14.2g

Carb: 102.8g

Protein: 30.1g

Vegetarian Paella with Green Beans and Chickpeas

Preparation Time: 10 minutes

Cooking Time: 35 minutes

Servings: 2

Ingredients

- Pinch of saffron
- Vegetable broth – 3 cups
- Olive oil – 1 tbsp.
- Yellow onion – 1 large, diced
- Garlic – 4 cloves, sliced
- Red bell pepper – 1, diced
- Crushed tomatoes – ¾ cup, fresh or canned
- Tomato paste – 2 tbsp.
- Hot paprika – 1 ½ tsp.
- Salt – 1 tsp.
- Freshly ground black pepper – ½ tsp.
- Green beans – 1 ½ cups, trimmed and halved
- Chickpeas – 1 (15-ounce) can, drained and rinsed
- Short-grain white rice – 1 cup
- Lemon – 1, cut into wedges

Directions

1. Mix the saffron threads with 3 tbsp. warm water in a small bowl.

2. In a saucepan, bring the water to a simmer over medium heat. Lower the heat to low and let the broth simmer.
3. Heat the oil in a skillet over medium heat. Add the onion and stir-fry for 5 minutes.
4. Add the bell pepper and garlic and stir-fry for 7 minutes or until pepper is softened.
5. Stir in the saffron-water mixture, salt, pepper, paprika, tomato paste, and tomatoes.
6. Add the rice, chickpeas, and green beans. Add the warm broth and bring to a boil.
7. Lower the heat and simmer uncovered for 20 minutes.
8. Serve hot, garnished with lemon wedges.

Nutrition

Calories: 709

Fat: 12g

Carb: 121g

Protein: 33g

Garlic Prawns with Tomatoes and Basil

Preparation Time: 10 minutes

Cooking Time: 10 minutes

Servings: 2

Ingredients
- Olive oil – 2 tbsp.
- Prawns – 1 ¼ pounds, peeled and deveined
- Garlic – 3 cloves, minced
- Crushed red pepper flakes – 1/8 tsp.
- Dry white wine – ¾ cup
- Grape tomatoes – 1 ½ cups
- Finely chopped fresh basil – ¼ cup, plus more for garnish

- Salt – ¾ tsp.
- Ground black pepper – ½ tsp.

Directions

1. In a skillet, heat oil over medium-high heat. Add the prawns and cook for 1 minute, or until just cooked through. Transfer to a plate.
2. Add the red pepper flakes, and garlic to the oil in the pan and cook, stirring, for 30 seconds. Stir in the wine and cook until it's reduced by about half.
3. Add the tomatoes and stir-fry until tomatoes begin to break down (about 3 to 4 minutes). Stir in the reserved shrimp, salt, pepper, and basil. Cook for 1 to 2 minutes more.
4. Serve garnished with the remaining basil.

Nutrition

Calories: 282

Fat: 10g

Carb: 7g

Protein: 33g

Stuffed Calamari in Tomato Sauce

Preparation Time: 10 minutes

Cooking Time: 25 minutes

Servings: 2

Ingredients

- Olive oil – ½ cup, plus 3 tbsp. divided
- Large onions - 2, finely chopped
- Garlic – 4 cloves, finely chopped
- Grated Pecorino Romano – 1 cup, plus ¼ cup, divided
- Chopped flat-leaf parsley – ½ cup, plus ¼ cup, divided

- Breadcrumbs – 6 cups
- Raisins – 1 cup
- Large squid tubes – 12, cleaned
- Toothpicks – 12
- For the tomato sauce
- Olive oil – 2 tbsp.
- Garlic – 4 cloves, chopped
- Crushed tomatoes – 2 (28-ounce) cans
- Finely chopped basil – ½ cup
- Salt – 1 tsp.
- Pepper – 1 tsp.

Directions

1. Combine the saffron threads with 2 tbsp. of warm water.
2. In a Dutch oven, heat ½ cup of olive oil. Add the onions and ½ tsp. of salt and stir-fry for 5 minutes. Add the tomato paste and cook for 1 minute more.
3. Add the wine and bring to a boil. Add the fish broth and soaked saffron and bring back to a boil. Lower the heat to low and simmer, uncovered, for 10 minutes.
4. Meanwhile, in a food processor, combine the bread and garlic, and process until ground.
5. Add the remaining ¼ cup olive oil and ½ tsp. salt and pulse just to mix.
6. Add the fish to the pot, cover, and cook until the fish is just cooked through, about 6 minutes. Stir in the sauce. Taste and adjust the seasoning.
7. Ladle the stew into the serving bowls.
8. Serve garnished with parsley.

Nutrition

Calories: 779

Fat: 41g

Carb: 31g

Protein: 67g

Provencal Braised Hake

Preparation Time: 10 minutes

Cooking Time: 20 minutes

Servings: 2

Ingredients

- Extra-virgin olive oil – 2 tbsp. plus extra for serving
- Onion – 1, halved and sliced thin
- Fennel bulb – 1, stalks discarded, bulb halved, cored and sliced thin
- Salt and black pepper
- Garlic clove – 4, minced
- Minced fresh thyme – 1 tsp.
- Diced tomatoes – 1 (14.5 ounce) can, drained
- Dry white wine – ½ cup
- Skinless hake fillets – 4 (4 to 6 ounce) 1 to 1 ½ inches thick
- Minced fresh parsley – 2 Tbsp.

Directions

1. Heat the oil in a skillet over medium heat. Add fennel, onion, and ½ tsp. salt and cook for 5 minutes. Stir in thyme and garlic and cook for 30 seconds.
2. Stir in the wine and tomatoes and then bring to a simmer.
3. Pat the hake dry with paper towels and season with salt and pepper. Place the hake into the skillet (skin side down). Spoon some sauce over the top and bring to a simmer.
4. Lower the heat to medium-low, cover, and cook for 10 to 12 minutes, or until the hake flakes apart when prodded with a knife.
5. Serve the hake into individual bowls. Stir parsley into the sauce and season with salt and pepper to taste.

Spoon the sauce over the hake and drizzle with extra oil.
6. Serve.

Nutrition

Calories: 292

Fat: 11.1g

Carb: 11g

Protein: 33g

Pan-Roasted Sea Bass

Preparation Time: 5 minutes

Cooking Time: 10 minutes

Servings: 2

Ingredients

- Skinless sea bass fillets – 4 (4 to 6 ounces) 1 to 1 ½ inches thick
- Salt and pepper
- Sugar – ½ tsp.
- Extra-virgin olive oil – 1 tbsp.
- Lemon wedges

Directions

1. Place the oven rack in the middle and preheat the oven to 425F. Pat the sea bass dry with paper towels and season with salt and pepper. On one side of each fillet, sprinkle the sugar evenly.
2. In a skillet, heat the oil over medium-high. Place the sea bass sugared side down in the skillet and cook for 2 minutes, or until browned.
3. Then flip and transfer the skillet to the oven and roast for 7 to 10 minutes, or until the fish registers 140F.
4. Serve with lemon wedges.

Nutrition

Calories: 225

Fat: 4.3g

Carb: 1g

Protein: 45.5g

Delicious Quinoa & Dried

Preparation Time: 10 minutes

Cooking Time: 17 minutes

Servings: 2

Ingredients:

- 3 c. water
- ¼ c. cashew nut
- 8 dried apricots
- 4 dried figs
- 1 tsp. cinnamon

Directions:

1. In a pot, mix water and quinoa and
2. Let simmer for 15 minutes, until the water evaporates.
3. Chop dried fruit.
4. When quinoa is cooked, stir in all other ingredients.
5. Serve cold. Add milk, if desired.

Nutrition:

44g Carbs,

7g Fat,

13g Protein,

285 Calories 65

Classic Apple Oats

Preparation Time: 10 minutes

Cooking Time: 15 minutes

Servings: 2

Ingredients:

- ½ tsp. cinnamon
- ¼ tsp. ginger
- 2 apples make half-inch chunks
- ½ c. oats, steel cut
- 1½ c. water
- Maple syrup
- ¼ tsp. salt
- Clove
- ¼ tsp. nutmeg

Directions:

1. Take Instant Pot and careful y arrange it over a clean, dry kitchen platform.
2. Turn on the appliance.
3. In the cooking pot area, add the water, oats, cinnamon, ginger, clove, nutmeg, apple, and salt. Stir the ingredients gently.
4. Close the pot lid and seal the valve to avoid any leakage. Find and press the "Manual" cooking setting and set cooking time to 5 minutes.
5. Allow the recipe ingredients to cook for the set time, and after that, the timer reads "zero."
6. Press "Cancel" and press "NPR" setting for natural pressure release. It takes 8-10 times for all inside pressure to release.
7. Open the pot and arrange the cooked recipe in serving plates.
8. Sweeten as needed with maple or agave syrup and serve immediately.
9. Top with some chopped nuts, optional.

Nutrition:

Calories: 232,

Fat: 5.7 g,

Carbs: 48.1 g,

Protein: 5.2 g 66

Peach & Chia Seed

Preparation Time: 10 minutes

Cooking Time: 10 minutes

Servings: 2

Ingredients:

- ½ oz. chia seeds
- 1 tbsp. pure maple syrup
- 1 c. coconut milk
- 1 tsp. ground cinnamon
- 3 diced peaches
- 2/3 c. granola

Directions:

1. Find a small bowl and add the chia seeds, maple syrup, and coconut milk.
2. Stir well, then cover and pop into the fridge for at least one hour.
3. Find another bowl, add the peaches and sprinkle with the cinnamon. Pop to one side
4. When it's time to serve, take two glasses, and pour the chia mixture between the two.
5. Sprinkle the granola over the top, keeping a tiny amount to one side to use to decorate later.
6. Top with the peaches and top with the reserved granola and serve.

Nutrition:

Calories: 415,

Protein: 13.9g,

Carbs: 54.4g,

Fat: 16.9g 68

Avocado Spread

Preparation Time: 10 minutes

Cooking Time: 1 minutes

Servings: 2

Ingredients:

- 2 peeled and pitted avocados
- 1 tbsp. olive oil
- 1 tbsp. minced shallots
- 1 tbsp. lime juice
- 1 tbsp. heavy coconut cream
- Salt
- Black pepper
- 1 tbsp. chopped chives

Directions:

1. In a blender, combine the avocado flesh with the oil, shallots, and the other ingredients except for the chopped chives.
2. Pulse well, divide into bowls, sprinkle the chives on top, and serve as a morning spread.

Nutrition:

Calories: 79,

Fat: 0.4 g,

Carbs: 15 g,

Protein: 1.3 g 71

Almond Butter and Blueberry Smoothie

Preparation Time: 10 minutes

Cooking Time: 1 minutes

Servings: 2

Ingredients:

- 1 c. almond milk
- 1 c. blueberries
- 4 ice cubes
- 1 scoop vanilla protein powder
- 1 tbsp. almond butter
- 1 tbsp. chia seeds

Directions:

1. Use a blender to mix the almond butter, vanilla protein powder, chia seeds, almond milk, ice cubes and blueberries together until the consistency is smooth.

Nutrition:

Calories: 230,

Carbs: 20 g,

Fat: 8.1 g,

Protein: 21.6 g 72

Salmon and Egg Muffins

Preparation Time: 10 minutes

Cooking Time: 15 minutes

Servings: 2

Ingredients:

- 4 eggs
- 1/3 c. milk
- Salt and pepper
- 1½ oz. smoked salmon
- 1 tbsp. chopped chives
- Green onions, optional

Directions:

2. Preheat the oven to 356 degrees Fahrenheit and grease 6 muffin tin holes with a small amount of olive oil.

3. Place the eggs, milk, and a pinch of salt and pepper into a small bowl and lightly beat to combine.
4. Divide the egg mixture between the 6 muffin holes, then divide the salmon between the muffins and place into each hole, gently pressing down to submerge in the egg mixture, chopped
5. Sprinkle each muffin with chopped chives and place in the oven for about 8-10 minutes or until just set.
6. Leave to cool for about 5 minutes before turning out and storing in an airtight container in the fridge.

Nutrition:

Calories: 93,

Fat: 6g,

Protein: 8g,

Carbs: 1g 74

Nachos

Preparation Time: 5 Minutes

Cooking Time: 10 Minutes

Servings: 4

Ingredients:

- 4-ounce restaurant-style corn tortilla chips
- 1 medium green onion, thinly sliced (about 1 tbsp.)
- 1 (4 ounces) package finely crumbled feta cheese
- 1 finely chopped and drained plum tomato
- 2 tbsp Sun-dried tomatoes in oil, finely chopped
- 2 tbsp Kalamata olives

Directions:

1. Mix an onion, plum tomato, oil, sun-dried tomatoes, and olives in a small bowl.
2. Arrange the tortillas chips on a microwavable plate in a single layer topped evenly with cheese—microwave on high for one minute.
3. Rotate the plate half turn and continue microwaving until the cheese is bubbly. Spread the tomato mixture over the chips and cheese and enjoy.

Nutrition:

Calories: 140

Carbs: 19g

Fat: 7g

Protein: 2g

Stuffed Celery

Preparation Time: 15 Minutes

Cooking Time: 20 Minutes

Servings: 3

Ingredients:

- Olive oil
- 1 clove garlic, minced
- 2 tbsp Pine nuts
- 2 tbsp dry-roasted sunflower seeds
- ¼ cup Italian cheese blend, shredded
- 8 stalks celery leaves
- 1 (8-ounce) fat-free cream cheese
- Cooking spray

Directions:

1. Sauté garlic and pine nuts over a medium setting for the heat until the nuts are golden brown. Cut off the wide base and tops from celery.
2. Remove two thin strips from the round side of the celery to create a flat surface.

3. Mix Italian cheese and cream cheese in a bowl and spread into cut celery stalks.
4. Sprinkle half of the celery pieces with sunflower seeds and a half with the pine nut mixture. Cover mixture and let stand for at least 4 hours before eating.

Nutrition:

Calories: 64

Carbs: 2g

Fat: 6g

Protein: 1g

Butternut Squash Fries

Preparation Time: 5 Minutes

Cooking Time: 10 Minutes

Servings: 2

Ingredients:

- 1 Butternut squash
- 1 tbsp Extra virgin olive oil
- ½ tbsp Grapeseed oil
- 1/8 tsp Sea salt

Directions:

1. Remove seeds from the squash and cut into thin slices. Coat with extra virgin olive oil and grapeseed oil. Add a sprinkle of salt and toss to coat well.
2. Arrange the squash slices onto three baking sheets and bake for 10 minutes until crispy.

Nutrition:

Calories: 40

Carbs: 10g

Fat: 0g

Protein: 1g

Dried Fig Tapenade

Preparation Time: 5 Minutes

Cooking Time: 0 Minutes

Servings: 1

Ingredients:

- 1 cup Dried figs
- 1 cup Kalamata olives
- ½ cup Water
- 1 tbsp Chopped fresh thyme
- 1 tbsp extra virgin olive oil
- ½ tsp Balsamic vinegar

Directions:

1. Prepare figs in a food processor until well chopped, add water, and continue processing to form a paste.
2. Add olives and pulse until well blended. Add thyme, vinegar, and extra virgin olive oil and pulse until very smooth. Best served with crackers of your choice.

Nutrition:

Calories: 249

Carbs: 64g

Fat: 1g

Protein: 3g

Speedy Sweet Potato Chips

Preparation Time: 15 Minutes

Cooking Time: 0 Minutes

Servings: 4

Ingredients:

- 1 large Sweet potato
- 1 tbsp Extra virgin olive oil
- Salt

Directions:

1. 300°F preheated oven. Slice your potato into nice, thin slices that resemble fries.
2. Toss the potato slices with salt and extra virgin olive oil in a bowl. Bake for about one hour, flipping every 15 minutes until crispy and browned.

Nutrition:

Calories: 150

Carbs: 16g

Fat: 9g

Protein: 1g

Nachos with Hummus (Mediterranean Inspired)

Preparation Time: 15 Minutes

Cooking Time: 20 Minutes

Servings: 4

Ingredients:

- 4 cups salted pita chips
- 1 (8 oz.) red pepper (roasted)

Hummus

- 1 tsp Finely shredded lemon peel
- ¼ cup Chopped pitted Kalamata olives
- ¼ cup crumbled feta cheese
- 1 plum (Roma) tomato, seeded, chopped
- ½ cup chopped cucumber
- 1 tsp Chopped fresh oregano leaves

Directions:

1. 400°F preheated oven. Arrange the pita chips on a heatproof platter and drizzle with hummus.
2. Top with olives, tomato, cucumber, and cheese and bake until warmed through.

Sprinkle lemon zest and oregano and enjoy while it's hot.

Nutrition:

Calories: 130

Carbs: 18g

Fat: 5g

Protein: 4g

Hummus and Olive Pita Bread

Preparation Time: 5 Minutes

Cooking Time: 0 Minutes

Servings: 3

Ingredients:

- 7 pita bread cut into 6 wedges each
- 1 (7 ounces) container plain hummus
- 1 tbsp Greek vinaigrette
- ½ cup Chopped pitted Kalamata olives

Directions:

1. Spread the hummus on a serving plate—Mix vinaigrette and olives in a bowl and spoon over the hummus. Enjoy with wedges of pita bread.

Nutrition:

Calories: 225

Carbs: 40g

Fat: 5g

Protein: 9g

Roast Asparagus

Preparation Time: 15 Minutes

Cooking Time: 5 Minutes

Servings: 4

Ingredients:

- 1 tbsp Extra virgin olive oil (1 tablespoon)
- 1 medium lemon
- ½ tsp Freshly grated nutmeg
- ½ tsp black pepper
- ½ tsp Kosher salt

Directions:

1. Warm the oven to 500°F. Put the asparagus on an aluminum foil and drizzle with extra virgin olive oil, and toss until well coated.
2. Roast the asparagus in the oven for about five minutes; toss and continue roasting until browned. Sprinkle the roasted asparagus with nutmeg, salt, zest, and pepper.

Nutrition:

Calories: 123

Carbs: 5g

Fat: 11g

Protein: 3g

Chicken Kale Wraps

Preparation Time: 10 Minutes

Cooking Time: 10 Minutes

Servings: 4

Ingredients:

- 4 kale leaves
- 4 oz chicken fillet
- ½ apple
- 1 tablespoon butter
- ¼ teaspoon chili pepper
- ¾ teaspoon salt
- 1 tablespoon lemon juice
- ¾ teaspoon dried thyme

Directions:

1. Chop the chicken fillet into small cubes. Then mix up the chicken with chili pepper and salt.
2. Heat butter in the skillet. Add chicken cubes. Roast them for 4 minutes.
3. Meanwhile, chop the apple into small cubes and add to the chicken. Mix up well.
4. Sprinkle the ingredients with lemon juice and dried thyme. Cook them for 5 minutes over medium-high heat.
5. Fill the kale leaves with the hot chicken mixture and wrap.

Nutrition:

Calories 106

Fat 5.1

Fiber 1.1

Carbs 6.3

Protein 9

Tomato Triangles

Preparation Time: 10 Minutes

Cooking Time: 0 Minutes

Servings: 6

Ingredients:

- 6 corn tortillas
- 1 tablespoon cream cheese
- 1 tablespoon ricotta cheese
- ½ teaspoon minced garlic
- 1 tablespoon fresh dill, chopped
- 2 tomatoes, sliced

Directions:

1. Cut every tortilla into 2 triangles. Then mix up cream cheese, ricotta cheese, minced garlic, and dill.
2. Spread 6 triangles with cream cheese mixture.
3. Then place the sliced tomato on them and cover with remaining tortilla triangles. Serve.

Nutrition:

Calories 71

Fat 1.6

Fiber 2.1

Carbs 12.8

Protein 2.3

Zaatar Fries

Preparation Time: 10 Minutes

Cooking Time: 35 Minutes

Servings: 5

Ingredients:

- 1 teaspoon Zaatar spices
- 3 sweet potatoes
- 1 tablespoon dried dill
- 1 teaspoon salt
- 3 teaspoons sunflower oil
- ½ teaspoon paprika

Directions:

1. Pour water into the crockpot. Cut the sweet potatoes into fries.
2. Line the baking tray with parchment. Place the layer of the sweet potato in the tray.
3. Sprinkle the vegetables with dried dill, salt, and paprika. Then sprinkle sweet potatoes with Za'atar and mix up well with the help of the fingertips.
4. Sprinkle the sweet potato fries with sunflower oil—Preheat the oven to 375F.

5. Bake the sweet potato fries within 35 minutes. Stir the fries every 10 minutes.

Nutrition:

Calories 28

Fat 2.9

Fiber 0.2

Carbs 0.6

Protein 0.2

Summertime Vegetable Chicken Wraps

Preparation Time: 15 Minutes

Cooking Time: 0 Minutes

Servings: 4

Ingredients:

- 2 cups cooked chicken, chopped
- ½ English cucumbers, diced
- ½ red bell pepper, diced
- ½ cup carrot, shredded
- 1 scallion, white and green parts, chopped
- ¼ cup plain Greek yogurt
- 1 tablespoon freshly squeezed lemon juice
- ½ teaspoon fresh thyme, chopped
- Pinch of salt
- Pinch of ground black pepper
- 4 multigrain tortillas

Directions:

1. Take a medium bowl and mix in chicken, red bell pepper, cucumber, carrot, yogurt, scallion, lemon juice, thyme, sea salt and pepper.
2. Mix well.
3. Spoon one quarter of chicken mix into the middle of the tortilla and fold the opposite ends of the tortilla over the filling.
4. Roll the tortilla from the side to create a snug pocket.
5. Repeat with the remaining ingredients and serve.
6. Enjoy!

Nutrition:

Calories: 278

Fat: 4g

Carbohydrates: 28g

Protein: 27g

Premium Roasted Baby Potatoes

Preparation Time: 10 Minutes

Cooking Time: 35 Minutes

Servings: 4

Ingredients:

- 2 pounds new yellow potatoes, scrubbed and cut into wedges
- 2 tablespoons extra virgin olive oil
- 2 teaspoons fresh rosemary, chopped
- 1 teaspoon garlic powder
- 1 teaspoon sweet paprika
- ½ teaspoon sea salt
- ½ teaspoon freshly ground black pepper

Directions:

1. Pre-heat your oven to 400 degrees Fahrenheit.
2. Take a large bowl and add potatoes, olive oil, garlic, rosemary, paprika, sea salt and pepper.
3. Spread potatoes in single layer on baking sheet and bake for 35 minutes.
4. Serve and enjoy!

Nutrition:

Calories: 225

Fat: 7g

Carbohydrates: 37g

Protein: 5g

Tomato and Cherry Linguine

Preparation Time: 10 Minutes

Cooking Time: 15 Minutes

Servings: 4

Ingredients:

- 2 pounds cherry tomatoes
- 3 tablespoons extra virgin olive oil
- 2 tablespoons balsamic vinegar
- 2 teaspoons garlic, minced
- Pinch of fresh ground black pepper
- ¾ pound whole-wheat linguine pasta
- 1 tablespoon fresh oregano, chopped
- ¼ cup feta cheese, crumbled

Directions:

1. Pre-heat your oven to 350 degrees Fahrenheit.
2. Take a large bowl and add cherry tomatoes, 2 tablespoons olive oil, balsamic vinegar, garlic, pepper and toss.
3. Spread tomatoes evenly on baking sheet and roast for 15 minutes.
4. While the tomatoes are roasting, cook the pasta according to the package instructions and drain the paste into a large bowl.
5. Toss pasta with 1 tablespoon olive oil.
6. Add roasted tomatoes (with juice) and toss.
7. Serve with topping of oregano and feta cheese.
8. Enjoy!

Nutrition:

Calories: 397

Fat: 15g

Carbohydrates: 55g

Protein: 13g

Mediterranean Zucchini Mushroom Pasta

Preparation Time: 10 Minutes

Cooking Time: 10 Minutes

Servings: 4

Ingredients:

- ½ pound pasta
- 2 tablespoons olive oil
- 6 garlic cloves, crushed
- 1 teaspoon red chili
- 2 spring onions, sliced
- 3 teaspoons rosemary
- 1 large zucchini, cut in half
- 5 large portabella mushrooms
- 1 can tomatoes
- 4 tablespoons Parmesan cheese
- Fresh ground black pepper

Directions:

1. Cook the pasta.
2. Take a large-sized frying pan and place it over medium heat.
3. Add oil and allow the oil to heat up.
4. Add garlic, onion and chili and sauté for a few minutes until golden.
5. Add zucchini, rosemary and mushroom and sauté for a few minutes.
6. Increase the heat to medium-high and add tinned tomatoes to the sauce until thick.
7. Drain your boiled pasta and transfer to serving platter.
8. Pour the tomato mix on top and mix using tongs.

9. Garnish with Parmesan and freshly ground black pepper.
10. Enjoy!

Nutrition:

Calories: 361

Fat: 12g

Carbohydrates: 47g

Protein: 14g

Lemon and Garlic Fettucine

Preparation Time: 5 Minutes

Cooking Time: 15 Minutes

Servings: 5

Ingredients:

- 8 ounces of whole wheat fettuccine
- 4 tablespoons of extra virgin olive oil
- 4 cloves of minced garlic
- 1 cup of fresh breadcrumbs
- ¼ cup of lemon juice
- 1 teaspoon of freshly ground pepper
- ½ teaspoon of salt
- 2 cans of 4 ounce boneless and skinless sardines (dipped in tomato sauce)
- ½ cup of chopped up fresh parsley
- ¼ cup of finely shredded Parmesan cheese

Directions:

1. Take a large-sized pot and bring water to a boil.
2. Cook pasta for 10 minutes until Al Dente.
3. Take a small-sized skillet and place it over medium heat.
4. Add 2 tablespoons of oil and allow it to heat up.
5. Add garlic and cook for 20 seconds.

6. Transfer the garlic to a medium-sized bowl
7. Add breadcrumbs to the hot skillet and cook for 5-6 minutes until golden
8. Whisk in lemon juice, pepper and salt into the garlic bowl
9. Add pasta to the bowl (with garlic) and sardines, parsley and Parmesan
10. Stir well and sprinkle bread crumbs
11. Enjoy!

Nutrition:

Calories: 480

Fat: 21g

Carbohydrates: 53g

Protein: 23g

Roasted Broccoli with Parmesan

Preparation Time: 10 Minutes

Cooking Time: 10 Minutes

Servings: 4

Ingredients:

- 2 head broccolis, cut into florets
- 2 tablespoons extra-virgin olive oil
- 2 teaspoons garlic, minced
- Zest of 1 lemon
- Pinch of salt
- ½ cup Parmesan cheese, grated

Directions:

1. Pre-heat your oven to 400 degrees Fahrenheit.
2. Take a large bowl and add broccoli with 2 tablespoons olive oil, lemon zest, garlic, lemon juice and salt.
3. Spread mix on the baking sheet in single layer and sprinkle with Parmesan cheese.
4. Bake for 10 minutes until tender.
5. Transfer broccoli to serving the dish.

6. Serve and enjoy!

Nutrition:

Calories: 154

Fat: 11g

Carbohydrates: 10g

Protein: 9g

Spinach and Feta Bread

Preparation Time: 10 Minutes

Cooking Time: 12 Minutes

Servings: 6

Ingredients:

- 6 ounces of sun-dried tomato pesto
- 6 pieces of 6-inch whole wheat pita bread
- 2 chopped up Roma plum tomatoes
- 1 bunch of rinsed and chopped spinach
- 4 sliced fresh mushrooms
- ½ cup of crumbled feta cheese
- 2 tablespoons of grated Parmesan cheese
- 3 tablespoons of olive oil
- Ground black pepper as needed

Directions:

1. Pre-heat your oven to 350 degrees Fahrenheit.
2. Spread your tomato pesto onto one side of your pita bread and place on your baking sheet (with the pesto side up).
3. Top up the pitas with spinach, tomatoes, feta cheese, mushrooms and Parmesan cheese.
4. Drizzle with some olive oil and season nicely with pepper.
5. Bake in your oven for around 12 minutes until the breads are crispy.
6. Cut up the pita into quarters and serve!

Nutrition:

Calories: 350

Fat: 17g

Carbohydrates: 41g

Protein:11g

Quick Zucchini Bowl

Preparation Time: 10 Minutes

Cooking Time: 10 Minutes

Servings: 4

Ingredients:

- ½ pound of pasta
- 2 tablespoons of olive oil
- 6 crushed garlic cloves
- 1 teaspoon of red chili
- 2 finely sliced spring onions
- 3 teaspoons of chopped rosemary
- 1 large zucchini cut up in half, lengthways and sliced
- 5 large portabella mushrooms
- 1 can of tomatoes
- 4 tablespoons of Parmesan cheese
- Fresh ground black pepper

Directions:

1. Cook the pasta.
2. Take a large-sized frying pan and place over medium heat.
3. Add oil and allow the oil to heat up.
4. Add garlic, onion and chili and sauté for a few minutes until golden.
5. Add zucchini, rosemary and mushroom and sauté for a few minutes.
6. Increase the heat to medium-high and add tinned tomatoes to the sauce until thick.
7. Drain your boiled pasta and transfer to a serving platter.

8. Pour the tomato mix on top and mix using tongs.
9. Garnish with Parmesan cheese and freshly ground black pepper.
10. Enjoy!

Nutrition:

Calories: 361

Fat: 12g

Carbohydrates: 47g

Protein: 14g

Healthy Basil Platter

Preparation Time: 25 Minutes

Cooking Time: 15 Minutes

Servings: 4

Ingredients:

- 2 pieces of red pepper seeded and cut up into chunks
- 2 pieces of red onion cut up into wedges
- 2 mild red chilies, diced and seeded
- 3 coarsely chopped garlic cloves
- 1 teaspoon of golden caster sugar
- 2 tablespoons of olive oil (plus additional for serving)
- 2 pounds of small ripe tomatoes quartered up
- 12 ounces of dried pasta
- Just a handful of basil leaves
- 2 tablespoons of grated Parmesan

Directions:

1. Pre-heat the oven to 392 degrees Fahrenheit.
2. Take a large-sized roasting tin and scatter pepper, red onion, garlic and chilies.
3. Sprinkle sugar on top.

4. Drizzle olive oil then season with pepper and salt.
5. Roast the veggies in your oven for 15 minutes.
6. Take a large-sized pan and cook the pasta in boiling, salted water until Al Dente.
7. Drain them.
8. Remove the veggies from the oven and tip in the pasta into the veggies.
9. Toss well and tear basil leaves on top.
10. Sprinkle Parmesan and enjoy!

Nutrition:

Calories: 452

Fat: 8g

Carbohydrates: 88g

Protein: 14g

Tomato Bruschetta

Preparation Time: 10 Minutes

Cooking Time: 10 Minutes

Servings: 6

Ingredients:

- 1 baguette, sliced
- 1/3 cup basil, chopped
- 6 tomatoes, cubed
- 2 garlic cloves, minced
- A pinch of salt and black pepper
- 1 teaspoon olive oil
- 1 tablespoon balsamic vinegar
- ½ teaspoon garlic powder
- Cooking spray

Directions:

1. Arrange the baguette slices in the baking sheet lined with parchment paper, grease them with cooking spray

and bake at 400 degrees F for 10 minutes.
2. In a bowl, mix the tomatoes with the basil and the remaining ingredients, toss well and leave aside for 10 minutes.
3. Divide the tomato mix on each baguette slice, arrange them all on a platter and serve.

Nutrition:

Calories: 162,

Fat: 4,

Fiber: 7,

Carbs: 29,

Protein: 4

Artichoke Flatbread

Preparation Time: 10 Minutes

Cooking Time: 15 Minutes

Servings: 4

Ingredients:

- 5 tablespoons olive oil
- 2 garlic cloves, minced
- 2 tablespoons parsley, chopped
- 2 round whole wheat flatbreads
- 4 tablespoons parmesan, grated
- ½ cup mozzarella cheese, grated
- 14 ounces canned artichokes, drained and quartered
- 1 cup baby spinach, chopped
- ½ cup cherry tomatoes, halved
- ½ teaspoon basil, dried
- Salt and black pepper to the taste

Directions:

1. In a bowl, mix the parsley with the garlic and 4 tablespoons oil, whisk well and spread this over the flatbreads.

2. Sprinkle the mozzarella and half of the parmesan.
3. In a bowl, mix the artichokes with the spinach, tomatoes, basil, salt, pepper and the rest of the oil, toss and divide over the flatbreads as well.
4. Sprinkle the remaining of the parmesan on top, arrange the flatbreads on a baking sheet lined with parchment paper and bake at 425 degrees F for 15 minutes.
5. Serve.

Nutrition:

Calories: 223,

Fat: 11.2,

Fiber: 5.34,

Carbs: 15.5,

Protein: 7.4

Red Pepper Tapenade

Preparation Time: 10 Minutes

Cooking Time: 0 Minutes

Servings: 4

Ingredients:

- 7 ounces roasted red peppers, chopped
- ½ cup parmesan, grated
- 1/3 cup parsley, chopped
- 14 ounces canned artichokes, drained and chopped
- 3 tablespoons olive oil
- ¼ cup capers, drained
- 1 and ½ tablespoons lemon juice
- 2 garlic cloves, minced

Directions:

1. In your blender, combine the red peppers with the parmesan and the rest of the ingredients and pulse well.

2. Divide into cups and serve.

Nutrition:

Calories: 200,

Fat: 5.6,

Fiber: 4.5,

Carbs: 12.4,

Protein: 4.6

Coriander Falafel

Preparation Time: 10 Minutes

Cooking Time: 10 Minutes

Servings: 8

Ingredients:

- 1 cup canned garbanzo beans, drained and rinsed
- 1 bunch parsley leaves
- 1 yellow onion, chopped
- 5 garlic cloves, minced
- 1 teaspoon coriander, ground
- A pinch of salt and black pepper
- ¼ teaspoon cayenne pepper
- ¼ teaspoon baking soda
- ¼ teaspoon cumin powder
- 1 teaspoon lemon juice
- 3 tablespoons tapioca flour
- Olive oil for frying

Directions:

1. In your food processor, combine the beans with the parsley, onion and the rest the ingredients except the oil and the flour and pulse well.
2. Transfer the mix to a bowl, add the flour, stir well, shape 16 balls out of this mix and flatten them a bit.
3. Heat up a pan with some oil over medium-high heat, add the falafels, cook them for 5 minutes on each side, transfer to paper towels, drain excess grease, arrange them on a platter and serve as an appetizer.

Nutrition:

Calories: 112,

Fat: 6.2,

Fiber: 2,

Carbs: 12.3,

Protein: 3.1

Chapter 9: Snacks Recipes

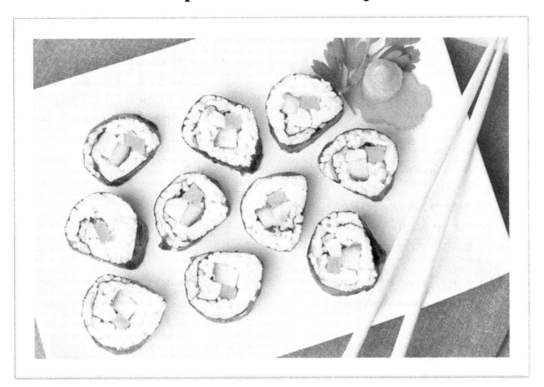

Cinnamon and Hemp Seed Coffee Shake

Preparation Time: 5 Minutes

Cooking Time: 0 Minutes

Servings: 1

Ingredients:

- 1 ½ frozen bananas, sliced into coins
- 1/8 teaspoon ground cinnamon
- 2 tablespoons hemp seeds
- 1 tablespoon maple syrup
- ¼ teaspoon vanilla extract, unsweetened
- 1 cup regular coffee, cooled
- ¼ cup almond milk, unsweetened
- ½ cup of ice cubes

Directions:

1. Pour milk into a blender, add vanilla, cinnamon, and hemp seeds and then pulse until smooth.
2. Add banana, pour in the coffee, and then pulse until smooth.
3. Add ice, blend until well combined, blend in maple syrup and then serve.

Nutrition:

Calories: 410 Cal;

Fat: 19.5 g;

Protein: 4.9 g;

Carbs: 60.8 g;

Fiber: 6.8 g

Green Smoothie

Preparation Time: 5 Minutes

Cooking Time: 0 Minutes

Servings: 1

Ingredients:

- ½ cup strawberries, frozen
- 4 leaves of kale
- ¼ of a medium banana
- 2 Medjool dates, pitted
- 1 tablespoon flax seed
- ¼ cup pumpkin seeds, hulled
- 1 cup of water

Directions:

1. Place all the ingredients in the jar of a food processor or blender and then cover it with the lid.
2. Pulse until smooth and then serve.

Nutrition:

Calories: 204 Cal;

Fat: 1.1 g;

Protein: 6.5 g;

Carbs: 48 g;

Fiber: 8.3 g

Strawberry and Banana Smoothie

Preparation Time: 5 Minutes

Cooking Time: 0 Minutes

Servings: 1

Ingredients:

- 1 cup sliced banana, frozen
- 2 tablespoons chia seeds
- 2 cups strawberries, frozen
- 2 teaspoons honey
- ¼ teaspoon vanilla extract, unsweetened
- 6 ounces coconut yogurt
- 1 cup almond milk, unsweetened

Directions:

1. Place all the ingredients in the jar of a food processor or blender and then cover it with the lid.
2. Pulse until smooth and then serve.

Nutrition:

Calories: 114 Cal;

Fat: 2.1 g;

Protein: 3.7 g;

Carbs: 22.3 g;

Fiber: 3.8 g

Orange Smoothie

Preparation Time: 5 Minutes

Cooking Time: 0 Minutes

Servings: 1

Ingredients:

- 1 cup slices of oranges
- ½ teaspoon grated ginger
- 1 cup of mango pieces
- 1 cup of coconut water
- 1 cup chopped strawberries
- 1 cup crushed ice

Directions:

1. Place all the ingredients in the jar of a food processor or blender and then cover it with the lid.
2. Pulse until smooth and then serve.

Nutrition:

Calories: 198.7 Cal;

Fat: 1.2 g;

Protein: 6.1 g;

Carbs: 34.3 g;

Fiber: 0 g

Pumpkin Chai Smoothie

Preparation Time: 5 Minutes

Cooking Time: 0 Minutes

Servings: 1

Ingredients:

- 1 cup cooked pumpkin
- ¼ cup pecans
- 1 frozen banana
- ¼ teaspoon ground cinnamon
- ¼ teaspoon cardamom
- ¼ teaspoon ground nutmeg
- 2 teaspoons maple syrup
- 1 cup of water, cold
- ½ cup of ice cubes

Directions:

1. Place pecans in a small bowl, cover with water, and then let them soak for 10 minutes.
2. Drain the pecans, add them into a blender, and then add the remaining ingredients.
3. Pulse for 1 minute until smooth, and then serve.

Nutrition:

Calories: 157.5 Cal;

Fat: 3.8 g;

Protein: 3 g;

Carbs: 32.3 g;

Fiber: 4.5 g

Banana Shake

Preparation Time: 5 Minutes

Cooking Time: 0 Minutes

Servings: 1

Ingredients:

- 3 medium frozen bananas
- 1 tablespoon cocoa powder, unsweetened
- 1 teaspoon shredded coconut
- 1 tablespoon maple syrup
- 1 tablespoon peanut butter
- 1 teaspoon vanilla extract, unsweetened
- 2 cups of coconut water
- 1 cup of ice cubes

Directions:

1. Add banana in a food processor, add maple syrup and vanilla, pour in water and then add ice.
2. Pulse until smooth and then pour half of the smoothie into a glass.
3. Add butter and cocoa powder into the blender, pulse until smooth, and then add to the smoothie glass.
4. Sprinkle coconut over the smoothie and then serve.

Nutrition:

Calories: 301 Cal;

Fat: 9.3 g;

Protein: 6.8 g;

Carbs: 49 g;

Fiber: 1.9 g

Green Honeydew Smoothie

Preparation Time: 5 Minutes

Cooking Time: 15 Minutes

Servings: 4

Ingredients:

- 1 large banana
- 6 large leaves of basil
- ½ cup frozen pineapple
- 1 teaspoon lime juice
- 1 cup pieces of honeydew melon
- 1 teaspoon green tea matcha powder
- ¼ cup almond milk, unsweetened

Directions:

1. Place all the ingredients in the jar of a food processor or blender and then cover it with the lid.
2. Pulse until smooth and then serve.

Nutrition:

Calories: 223.5 Cal;

Fat: 2.7 g;

Protein: 20.1 g;

Carbs: 32.7 g;

Fiber: 5.2 g

Summer Salsa

Preparation Time: 5 Minutes

Cooking Time: 15 Minutes

Servings: 8

Ingredients:

- 1 cup cherry tomatoes, chopped
- ¼ cup chopped cilantro
- 2 tablespoons chopped red onion
- 1 teaspoon minced garlic
- 1 small jalapeno, deseeded, chopped
- ½ of a lime, juiced
- 1/8 teaspoon salt
- 1 tablespoon olive oil

Directions:

1. Place all the ingredients in the jar of a food processor or blender except for cilantro and then cover with its lid.
2. Pulse until smooth and then pulse in cilantro until evenly mixed.

3. Tip the salsa into a bowl and then serve with vegetable sticks.

Nutrition:

Calories: 51 Cal;

Fat: 0.1 g;

Protein: 1.7 g;

Carbs: 11.4 g;

Fiber: 3.1 g

Red Salsa

Preparation Time: 35 Minutes

Cooking Time: 15 Minutes

Servings: 8

Ingredients:

- 4 Roma tomatoes, halved
- ¼ cup chopped cilantro
- 1 jalapeno pepper, deseeded, halved
- ½ of a medium white onion, peeled, cut into quarters
- 3 cloves of garlic, peeled
- ½ teaspoon salt
- 1 tablespoon brown sugar
- 1 teaspoon apple cider vinegar

Directions:

1. Switch on the oven, then set it to 425 degrees F and let it preheat.
2. Meanwhile, take a baking sheet, line it with foil, and then spread tomato, jalapeno pepper, onion, and garlic.
3. Bake the vegetables for 15 minutes until vegetables have cooked and begin to brown and then let the vegetables cool for 3 minutes.
4. Transfer the roasted vegetables into a blender, add remaining ingredients and then pulse until smooth.

5. Tip the salsa into a medium bowl and then chill it for 30 minutes before serving with vegetable sticks.

Nutrition:

Calories: 240 Cal;

Fat: 0 g;

Protein: 0 g;

Carbs: 48 g;

Fiber: 16 g

Pinto Bean Dip

Preparation Time: 5 Minutes

Cooking Time: 0 Minutes

Servings: 4

Ingredients:

- 15 ounces canned pinto beans
- 1 jalapeno pepper
- 2 teaspoons ground cumin
- 3 tablespoons nutritional yeast
- 1/3 cup basil salsa

Directions:

1. Place all the ingredients in a food processor, cover with the lid, and then pulse until smooth.
2. Tip the dip in a bowl and then serve with vegetable slices.

Nutrition:

Calories: 360 Cal;

Fat: 0 g;

Protein: 24 g;

Carbs: 72 g;

Fiber: 24 g

Smoky Red Pepper Hummus

Preparation Time: 5 Minutes

Cooking Time: 0 Minutes

Servings: 4

Ingredients:

- ¼ cup roasted red peppers
- 1 cup cooked chickpeas
- 1/8 teaspoon garlic powder
- ½ teaspoon salt
- 1/8 teaspoon ground black pepper
- ¼ teaspoon ground cumin
- ¼ teaspoon red chili powder
- 1 tablespoon Tahini
- 2 tablespoons water

Directions:

1. Place all the ingredients in the jar of the food processor and then pulse until smooth.
2. Tip the hummus in a bowl and then serve with vegetable slices.

Nutrition:

Calories: 489 Cal;

Fat: 30 g;

Protein: 9 g;

Carbs: 15 g;

Fiber: 6 g

Spinach Dip

Preparation Time: 20 Minutes

Cooking Time: 5 Minutes

Servings: 8

Ingredients:

- ¾ cup cashews
- 3.5 ounces soft tofu
- 6 ounces of spinach leaves
- 1 medium white onion, peeled, diced
- 2 teaspoons minced garlic
- ½ teaspoon salt
- 3 tablespoons olive oil

Directions:

1. Place cashews in a bowl, cover with hot water, and then let them soak for 15 minutes.
2. After 15 minutes, drain the cashews and then set aside until required.
3. Take a medium skillet pan, add oil to it and then place the pan over medium heat.
4. Add onion, cook for 3 to 5 minutes until tender, stir in garlic and then continue cooking for 30 seconds until fragrant.
5. Spoon the onion mixture into a blender, add remaining ingredients and then pulse until smooth.
6. Tip the dip into a bowl and then serve with chips.

Nutrition:

Calories: 134.6 Cal;

Fat: 8.6 g;

Protein: 10 g;

Carbs: 6.3 g;

Fiber: 1.4 g

Tomatillo Salsa

Preparation Time: 5 Minutes

Cooking Time: 20 Minutes

Servings: 8

Ingredients:

- 5 medium tomatillos, chopped
- 3 cloves of garlic, peeled, chopped

- 3 Roma tomatoes, chopped
- 1 jalapeno, chopped
- ½ of a medium red onion, peeled, chopped
- 1 Anaheim chili
- 2 teaspoons salt
- 1 teaspoon ground cumin
- 1 lime, juiced
- ¼ cup cilantro leaves
- ¾ cup of water

Directions:

1. Take a medium pot, place it over medium heat, pour in water, and then add onion, tomatoes, tomatillo, jalapeno, and Anaheim chili.
2. Sauté the vegetables for 15 minutes, remove the pot from heat, add cilantro and lime juice and then stir in salt.
3. Remove pot from heat and then pulse by using an immersion blender until smooth.
4. Serve the salsa with chips.

Nutrition:

Calories: 317.4 Cal;

Fat: 0 g;

Protein: 16 g;

Carbs: 64 g;

Fiber: 16 g

Arugula Pesto Couscous

Preparation Time: 10 Minutes

Cooking Time: 20 Minutes

Servings: 4

Ingredients:

- 8 ounces Israeli couscous
- 3 large tomatoes, chopped
- 3 cups arugula leaves
- ½ cup parsley leaves
- 6 cloves of garlic, peeled
- ½ cup walnuts
- ¾ teaspoon salt
- 1 cup and 1 tablespoon olive oil
- 2 cups vegetable broth

Directions:

1. Take a medium saucepan, place it over medium-high heat, add 1 tablespoon oil and then let it heat.
2. Add couscous, stir until mixed, and then cook for 4 minutes until fragrant and toasted.
3. Pour in the broth, stir until mixed, bring it to a boil, switch heat to medium level and then simmer for 12 minutes until the couscous has absorbed all the liquid and turn tender.
4. When done, remove the pan from heat, fluff it with a fork, and then set aside until required.
5. While couscous cooks, prepare the pesto, and for this, place walnuts in a blender, add garlic, and then pulse until nuts have broken.
6. Add arugula, parsley, and salt, pulse until well combined, and then blend in oil until smooth.
7. Transfer couscous to a salad bowl, add tomatoes and prepared pesto, and then toss until mixed.
8. Serve straight away.

Nutrition:

Calories: 73 Cal;

Fat: 4 g;

Protein: 2 g;

Carbs: 8 g;

Fiber: 2 g

Oatmeal and Raisin Balls

Preparation Time: 40 Minutes

Cooking Time: 0 Minutes

Servings: 4

Ingredients:

- 1 cup rolled oats
- ¼ cup raisins
- ½ cup peanut butter

Directions:

1. Place oats in a large bowl, add raisins and peanut butter, and then stir until well combined.
2. Shape the mixture into twelve balls, 1 tablespoon of mixture per ball, and then arrange the balls on a baking sheet.
3. Place the baking sheet into the freezer for 30 minutes until firm and then serve.

Nutrition:

Calories: 135 Cal;

Fat: 6 g;

Protein: 8 g;

Carbs: 13 g;

Fiber: 4 g

Nacho Cheese

Preparation Time: 10 Minutes

Cooking Time: 15 Minutes

Servings: 4

Ingredients:

- 1 cup chopped carrots
- ½ teaspoon onion powder
- 2 cups peeled and chopped potatoes

- ½ teaspoon garlic powder
- 1 teaspoon salt
- ½ cup nutritional yeast
- 1 tablespoon lemon juice
- ¼ cup of salsa
- ½ cup of water

Directions:

1. Take a medium pot, place carrots and potato in it, cover with water and then place the pot over medium-high heat.
2. Boil the vegetables for 10 minutes, drain them, and then transfer into a blender.
3. Add remaining ingredients and then pulse until smooth.
4. Tip the cheese into a bowl and then serve with vegetable slices.

Nutrition:

Calories: 611.7 Cal;

Fat: 17.2 g;

Protein: 32.1 g;

Carbs: 62.1 g;

Fiber: 12.1 g

Pico de Gallo

Preparation Time: 5 Minutes

Cooking Time: 0 Minutes

Servings: 6

Ingredients:

- ½ of a medium red onion, peeled, chopped
- 2 cups diced tomato
- ½ cup chopped cilantro
- 1 jalapeno pepper, minced
- 1/8 teaspoon salt
- ¼ teaspoon ground black pepper
- ½ of a lime, juiced

- 1 teaspoon olive oil

Directions:

1. Take a large bowl, place all the ingredients in it and then stir until well mixed.
2. Serve the Pico de Gallo with chips.

Nutrition:

Calories: 790 Cal;

Fat: 6.4 g;

Protein: 25.6 g;

Carbs: 195.2 g;

Fiber: 35.2 g

Beet Balls

Preparation Time: 10 Minutes

Cooking Time: 0 Minutes

Servings: 6

Ingredients:

- ½ cup oats
- 1 medium beet, cooked
- ½ cup almond flour
- 1/3 cup shredded coconut and more for coating
- ¾ cup Medjool dates, pitted
- 1 tablespoon cocoa powder
- ½ cup peanuts
- ¼ cup chocolate chips, unsweetened

Directions:

1. Place cooked beets in a blender and then pulse until chopped into very small pieces.
2. Add remaining ingredients and then pulse until the dough comes together.

3. Shape the dough into eighteen balls, coat them in some more coconut and then serve.

Nutrition:

Calories: 114.2 Cal;

Fat: 2.4 g;

Protein: 5 g;

Carbs: 19.6 g;

Fiber: 4.9 g

Cheesy Crackers

Preparation Time: 10 Minutes

Cooking Time: 20 Minutes

Servings: 3

Ingredients:

- 1 ¾ cup almond meal
- 3 tablespoons nutritional yeast
- ½ teaspoon of sea salt
- 2 tablespoons lemon juice
- 1 tablespoon melted coconut oil
- 1 tablespoon ground flaxseed
- 2 ½ tablespoons water

Directions:

1. Switch on the oven, then set it to 350 degrees F and let it preheat.
2. Meanwhile, take a medium bowl, place flaxseed in it, stir in water, and then let the mixture rest for 5 minutes until thickened.
3. Place almond meal in a medium bowl, add salt and yeast and then stir until mixed.
4. Add lemon juice and oil into the flaxseed mixture and then whisk until mixed.
5. Pour the flaxseed mixture into the almond meal mixture and then stir until dough comes together.

6. Place a piece of a wax paper on a clean working space, place the dough on it, cover with another piece of wax paper, and then roll dough into a 1/8-inch-thick crust.
7. Cut the dough into a square shape, sprinkle salt over the top and then bake for 15 to 20 minutes until done.
8. Serve straight away.

Nutrition:

Calories: 30 Cal;

Fat: 1 g;

Protein: 1 g;

Carbs: 5 g;

Fiber: 0 g

Tomato Soup

Preparation Time: 10 Minutes

Cooking Time: 10 Minutes

Servings: 2

Ingredients:

- 56 ounces stewed tomatoes
- ¼ teaspoon salt
- ¼ teaspoon ground black pepper
- 1 medium red bell pepper, cored, diced
- ¼ teaspoon dried thyme
- 6 leaves of basil, chopped
- ¼ teaspoon dried oregano
- 1 teaspoon olive oil

Directions:

1. Take a medium pot, place it over medium heat, add oil, and when hot, add bell pepper and then cook for 4 minutes.
2. Add remaining ingredients into the pot, stir until mixed, switch heat to medium-high heat, and bring the mixture to simmer.

3. Remove pot from the heat and then puree the soup until smooth.
4. Taste to adjust seasoning, ladle soup into bowls and then serve.

Nutrition:

Calories: 170 Cal;

Fat: 1.1 g;

Protein: 3.5 g;

Carbs: 36 g;

Fiber: 2.6 g

Meatballs Platter

Preparation Time: 10 Minutes

Cooking Time: 15 Minutes

Servings: 4

Ingredients:

- 1-pound beef meat, ground
- ¼ cup panko breadcrumbs
- A pinch of salt and black pepper
- 3 tablespoons red onion, grated
- ¼ cup parsley, chopped
- 2 garlic cloves, minced
- 2 tablespoons lemon juice
- Zest of 1 lemon, grated
- 1 egg
- ½ teaspoon cumin, ground
- ½ teaspoon coriander, ground
- ¼ teaspoon cinnamon powder
- 2 ounces feta cheese, crumbled
- Cooking spray

Directions:

1. In a bowl, blend the beef with the breadcrumbs, salt, pepper and the rest of the ingredients except the cooking spray, stir well and shape medium balls out of this mix.

2. Arrange the meatballs on a baking sheet lined with parchment paper, grease them with cooking spray and bake at 450 degrees F for 15 minutes.
3. Position the meatballs on a platter and serve as a snack.

Nutrition:

Calories: 300,

Fat: 15.4,

Fiber: 6.4,

Carbs: 22.4,

Protein: 35

Yogurt Dip

Preparation Time: 10 Minutes

Cooking Time: 0 Minutes

Servings: 6

Ingredients:

- 2 cups Greek yogurt
- 2 tablespoons pistachios, toasted and chopped
- A pinch of salt and white pepper
- 2 tablespoons mint, chopped
- 1 tablespoon kalamata olives, pitted and chopped
- ¼ cup za'atar spice
- ¼ cup pomegranate seeds
- 1/3 cup olive oil

Directions:

1. In a bowl, blend the yogurt with the pistachios and the rest of the ingredients, whisk well.
2. Divide into small cups and serve with pita chips on the side.

Nutrition:

Calories: 294,

Fat: 18,

Fiber: 1,

Carbs: 21,

Protein: 10

Tomato Bruschetta

Preparation Time: 10 Minutes

Cooking Time: 10 Minutes

Servings: 6

Ingredients:

- 1 baguette, sliced
- 1/3 cup basil, chopped
- 6 tomatoes, cubed
- 2 garlic cloves, minced
- A pinch of salt and black pepper
- 1 teaspoon olive oil
- 1 tablespoon balsamic vinegar
- ½ teaspoon garlic powder
- Cooking spray

Directions:

1. Arrange the baguette slices in the baking sheet lined with parchment paper, grease them with cooking spray and bake at 400 degrees F for 10 minutes.
2. In a bowl, mix the tomatoes with the basil and the remaining ingredients, toss well and leave aside for 10 minutes.
3. Divide the tomato mix on each baguette slice, arrange them all on a platter and serve.

Nutrition:

Calories: 162,

Fat: 4,

Fiber: 7,

Carbs: 29,

Protein: 4

Artichoke Flatbread

Preparation Time: 10 Minutes

Cooking Time: 15 Minutes

Servings: 4

Ingredients:

- 5 tablespoons olive oil
- 2 garlic cloves, minced
- 2 tablespoons parsley, chopped
- 2 round whole wheat flatbreads
- 4 tablespoons parmesan, grated
- ½ cup mozzarella cheese, grated
- 14 ounces canned artichokes, drained and quartered
- 1 cup baby spinach, chopped
- ½ cup cherry tomatoes, halved
- ½ teaspoon basil, dried
- Salt and black pepper to the taste

Directions:

1. In a bowl, mix the parsley with the garlic and 4 tablespoons oil, whisk well and spread this over the flatbreads.
2. Sprinkle the mozzarella and half of the parmesan.
3. In a bowl, mix the artichokes with the spinach, tomatoes, basil, salt, pepper and the rest of the oil, toss and divide over the flatbreads as well.
4. Sprinkle the remaining of the parmesan on top, arrange the flatbreads on a baking sheet lined with parchment paper and bake at 425 degrees F for 15 minutes.
5. Serve a snack.

Nutrition:

Calories: 223,

Fat: 11.2,

Fiber: 5.34,

Carbs: 15.5,

Protein: 7.4

Red Pepper Tapenade

Preparation Time: 10 Minutes

Cooking Time: 0 Minutes

Servings: 4

Ingredients:

- 7 ounces roasted red peppers, chopped
- ½ cup parmesan, grated
- 1/3 cup parsley, chopped
- 14 ounces canned artichokes, drained and chopped
- 3 tablespoons olive oil
- ¼ cup capers, drained
- 1 and ½ tablespoons lemon juice
- 2 garlic cloves, minced

Directions:

1. In your blender, combine the red peppers with the parmesan and the rest of the ingredients and pulse well.
2. Divide into cups and serve as a snack.

Nutrition:

Calories: 200,

Fat: 5.6,

Fiber: 4.5,

Carbs: 12.4,

Protein: 4.6

Coriander Falafel

Preparation Time: 10 Minutes

Cooking Time: 10 Minutes

Servings: 8

Ingredients:

- 1 cup canned garbanzo beans, drained and rinsed
- 1 bunch parsley leaves
- 1 yellow onion, chopped
- 5 garlic cloves, minced
- 1 teaspoon coriander, ground
- A pinch of salt and black pepper
- ¼ teaspoon cayenne pepper
- ¼ teaspoon baking soda
- ¼ teaspoon cumin powder
- 1 teaspoon lemon juice
- 3 tablespoons tapioca flour
- Olive oil for frying

Directions:

1. In your food processor, combine the beans with the parsley, onion and the rest the ingredients except the oil and the flour and pulse well.
2. Transfer the mix to a bowl, add the flour, stir well, shape 16 balls out of this mix and flatten them a bit.
3. Heat up a pan with some oil over medium-high heat, add the falafels, cook them for 5 minutes on each side, transfer to paper towels, drain excess grease, arrange them on a platter and serve as an appetizer.

Nutrition:

Calories: 112,

Fat: 6.2,

Fiber: 2,

Carbs: 12.3,

Protein: 3.1

Red Pepper Hummus

Preparation Time: 10 Minutes

Cooking Time: 0 Minutes

Servings: 6

Ingredients:

- 6 ounces roasted red peppers, peeled and chopped
- 16 ounces canned chickpeas, drained and rinsed
- ¼ cup Greek yogurt
- 3 tablespoons tahini paste
- Juice of 1 lemon
- 3 garlic cloves, minced
- 1 tablespoon olive oil
- A pinch of salt and black pepper
- 1 tablespoon parsley, chopped

Directions:

1. In your food processor, combine the red peppers with the rest of the ingredients except the oil and the parsley and pulse well.
2. Add the oil, pulse again, divide into cups, sprinkle the parsley on top and serve as a party spread.

Nutrition:

Calories: 255,

Fat: 11.4,

Fiber: 4.5,

Carbs: 17.4,

Protein: 6.5

White Bean Dip

Preparation Time: 10 Minutes

Cooking Time: 0 Minutes

Servings: 4

Ingredients:

- 15 ounces canned white beans

- 6 ounces canned artichoke hearts, drained and quartered
- 4 garlic cloves, minced
- 1 tablespoon basil, chopped
- 2 tablespoons olive oil
- Juice of ½ lemon
- Zest of ½ lemon, grated
- Salt and black pepper to the taste

Directions:

1. In your food processor, combine the beans with the artichokes and the rest of the ingredients except the oil and pulse well.
2. Add the oil gradually, pulse the mix again, divide into cups and serve as a party dip.

Nutrition:

Calories: 274,

Fat: 11.7,

Fiber: 6.5,

Carbs: 18.5,

Protein: 16.5

Hummus with Ground Lamb

Preparation Time: 10 Minutes

Cooking Time: 15 Minutes

Servings: 8

Ingredients:

- 10 ounces hummus
- 12 ounces lamb meat, ground
- ½ cup pomegranate seeds
- ¼ cup parsley, chopped
- 1 tablespoon olive oil
- Pita chips for serving

Directions:

1. Heat up a pan with the oil over medium-high heat, add the meat, and brown for 15 minutes stirring often.
2. Spread the hummus on a platter, spread the ground lamb all over, also spread the pomegranate seeds and the parsley and serve with pita chips as a snack.

Nutrition:

Calories: 133,

Fat: 9.7,

Fiber: 1.7,

Carbs: 6.4,

Protein: 5.4

Bulgur Lamb Meatballs

Preparation Time: 10 Minutes

Cooking Time: 15 Minutes

Servings: 6

Ingredients:

- 1 and ½ cups Greek yogurt
- ½ teaspoon cumin, ground
- 1 cup cucumber, shredded
- ½ teaspoon garlic, minced
- A pinch of salt and black pepper
- 1 cup bulgur
- 2 cups water
- 1-pound lamb, ground
- ¼ cup parsley, chopped
- ¼ cup shallots, chopped
- ½ teaspoon allspice, ground
- ½ teaspoon cinnamon powder
- 1 tablespoon olive oil

Directions:

1. In a bowl, blend the bulgur with the water, cover the bowl, leave aside for 10 minutes, drain and transfer to a bowl.

2. Add the meat, the yogurt and the rest of the ingredients except the oil, stir well and shape medium meatballs out of this mix.
3. Heat up a pan with the oil over medium-high heat, add the meatballs, cook them for 7 minutes on each side, arrange them all on a platter and serve as a snack.

Nutrition:

Calories: 300,

Fat: 9.6,

Fiber: 4.6,

Carbs: 22.6,

Protein: 6.6

Eggplant Dip

Preparation Time: 10 Minutes

Cooking Time: 40 Minutes

Servings: 4

Ingredients:

- 1 eggplant, poked with a fork
- 2 tablespoons tahini paste
- 2 tablespoons lemon juice
- 2 garlic cloves, minced
- 1 tablespoon olive oil
- Salt and black pepper to the taste
- 1 tablespoon parsley, chopped

Directions:

1. Put the eggplant in a roasting pan, bake at 400 degrees F for 40 minutes, cool down, peel and transfer to your food processor.
2. Add the rest of the fixings excluding the parsley, pulse well, divide into small bowls and serve as a snack with the parsley sprinkled on top.

Nutrition:

Calories: 121,

Fat: 4.3,

Fiber: 1,

Carbs: 1.4,

Protein: 4.3

Veggie Fritters

Preparation Time: 10 Minutes

Cooking Time: 10 Minutes

Servings: 8

Ingredients:

- 2 garlic cloves, minced
- 2 yellow onions, chopped
- 4 scallions, chopped
- 2 carrots, grated
- 2 teaspoons cumin, ground
- ½ teaspoon turmeric powder
- Salt and black pepper to the taste
- ¼ teaspoon coriander, ground
- 2 tablespoons parsley, chopped
- ¼ teaspoon lemon juice
- ½ cup almond flour
- 2 beets, peeled and grated
- 2 eggs, whisked
- ¼ cup tapioca flour
- 3 tablespoons olive oil

Directions:

1. In a bowl, combine the garlic with the onions, scallions and the rest of the ingredients except the oil, stir well and shape medium fritters out of this mix.
2. Heat up a pan with the oil on medium-high heat, add the fritters, cook for 5 minutes on each side, arrange on a platter and serve.

Nutrition:

Calories: 209,

Fat: 11.2,

Fiber: 3,

Carbs: 4.4,

Protein: 4.8

Cucumber Bites

Preparation Time: 10 Minutes

Cooking Time: 0 Minutes

Servings: 12

Ingredients:

- 1 English cucumber, sliced into 32 rounds
- 10 ounces hummus
- 16 cherry tomatoes, halved
- 1 tablespoon parsley, chopped
- 1-ounce feta cheese, crumbled

Directions:

1. Spread the hummus on each cucumber round, divide the tomato halves on each, sprinkle the cheese and parsley on to and serve as a snack.

Nutrition:

Calories: 162,

Fat: 3.4,

Fiber: 2,

Carbs: 6.4,

Protein: 2.4

Stuffed Avocado

Preparation Time: 10 Minutes

Cooking Time: 0 Minutes

Servings: 2

Ingredients:

- 1 avocado, halved and pitted
- 10 ounces canned tuna, drained
- 2 tablespoons sun-dried tomatoes, chopped
- 1 and ½ tablespoon basil pesto
- 2 tablespoons black olives, pitted and chopped
- Salt and black pepper to the taste
- 2 teaspoons pine nuts, toasted and chopped
- 1 tablespoon basil, chopped

Directions:

1. In a bowl, blend the tuna with the sun-dried tomatoes and the rest of the ingredients except the avocado and stir.
2. Stuff the avocado halves with the tuna mix and serve as a snack.

Nutrition:

Calories: 233,

Fat: 9,

Fiber: 3.5,

Carbs: 11.4,

Protein: 5.6

Wrapped Plums

Preparation Time: 5 Minutes

Cooking Time: 0 Minutes

Servings: 8

Ingredients:

- 2 ounces prosciutto, cut into 16 pieces
- 4 plums, quartered

- 1 tablespoon chives, chopped
- A pinch of red pepper flakes, crushed

Directions:

1. Wrap each plum quarter in a prosciutto slice, arrange them all on a platter, sprinkle the chives and pepper flakes all over and serve.

Nutrition:

Calories: 30,

Fat: 1,

Fiber: 0,

Carbs: 4,

Protein: 2

Cucumber Sandwich Bites

Preparation Time: 5 Minutes

Cooking Time: 0 Minutes

Servings: 12

Ingredients:

- 1 cucumber, sliced
- 8 slices whole wheat bread
- 2 tablespoons cream cheese, soft
- 1 tablespoon chives, chopped
- ¼ cup avocado, peeled, pitted and mashed
- 1 teaspoon mustard
- Salt and black pepper to the taste

Directions:

1. Spread the mashed avocado on each bread slice, also spread the rest of the ingredients except the cucumber slices.
2. Divide the cucumber slices on the bread slices, cut each slice in thirds,

arrange on a platter and serve as a snack.

Nutrition:

Calories: 187,

Fat: 12.4,

Fiber: 2.1,

Carbs: 4.5,

Protein: 8.2

Cucumber Rolls

Preparation Time: 5 Minutes

Cooking Time: 0 Minutes

Servings: 6

Ingredients:

- 1 big cucumber, sliced lengthwise
- 1 tablespoon parsley, chopped
- 8 ounces canned tuna, drained and mashed
- Salt and black pepper to the taste
- 1 teaspoon lime juice

Directions:

1. Arrange cucumber slices on a working surface, divide the rest of the ingredients, and roll.
2. Arrange all the rolls on a platter and serve as a snack.

Nutrition:

Calories: 200,

Fat: 6,

Fiber: 3.4,

Carbs: 7.6,

Protein: 3.5

Olives and Cheese Stuffed Tomatoes

Preparation Time: 10 Minutes

Cooking Time: 0 Minutes

Servings: 24

Ingredients:

- 24 cherry tomatoes, top cut off and insides scooped out
- 2 tablespoons olive oil
- ¼ teaspoon red pepper flakes
- ½ cup feta cheese, crumbled
- 2 tablespoons black olive paste
- ¼ cup mint, torn

Directions:

2. In a bowl, mix the olives paste with the rest of the ingredients except the cherry tomatoes and whisk well.
3. Stuff the cherry tomatoes with this mix, arrange them all on a platter and serve as a snack.

Nutrition:

Calories: 136,

Fat: 8.6,

Fiber: 4.8,

Carbs: 5.6,

Protein: 5.1

Vinegar Beet Bites

Preparation Time: 10 Minutes

Cooking Time: 30 Minutes

Servings: 4

Ingredients:

- 2 beets, sliced
- Sea salt and black pepper

- 1/3 cup balsamic vinegar
- 1 cup olive oil

Directions:

1. Spread the beet slices on a baking sheet lined with parchment paper, add the rest of the ingredients, toss and bake at 350 degrees F for 30 minutes.
2. Serve the beet bites cold as a snack.

Nutrition:

Calories: 199,

Fat: 5.4,

Fiber: 3.5,

Carbs: 8.5,

Protein: 3.5

Lentils Stuffed Potato Skins

Preparation Time: 10 Minutes

Cooking Time: 30 Minutes

Servings: 8

Ingredients:

- 16 red baby potatoes
- ¾ cup red lentils, cooked and drained
- 2 tablespoons olive oil
- 2 garlic cloves, minced
- 1 tablespoon chives, chopped
- ½ teaspoon hot chili sauce
- Salt and black pepper to the taste

Directions:

1. Put potatoes in a pot, add water to cover them, bring to a boil over medium low heat, cook for 15 minutes, drain, cool them down, cut in halves, remove the pulp, transfer it to a blender and pulse it a bit.

2. Add the rest of the ingredients to the blender, pulse again well and stuff the potato skins with this mix.
3. Arrange the stuffed potatoes on a baking sheet lined with parchment paper, introduce them in the oven at 375 degrees F and bake for 15 minutes.
4. Arrange on a platter and serve as an appetizer.

Nutrition:

Calories: 300,

Fat: 9.3,

Fiber: 14.5,

Carbs: 22.5,

Protein: 8.5

Fresh Black Bean Dip

Preparation time: 5 minutes

Cooking time: 30 minutes

Servings: 5

Ingredients:

- 1 small yellow onion, peeled and chopped
- 2 jalapeño peppers
- 1 clove garlic, peeled and chopped
- 1/4 cup red bell pepper
- 2 (15-ounce) cans black beans, drained
- 3 tablespoons water
- 1 teaspoon ground cumin
- 2 teaspoons cocoa powder
- 3 tablespoons fresh lime juice
- 2 tablespoons fresh chopped cilantro

- 4 cherry tomatoes, sliced

Directions:

1. Add onion, jalapeño, garlic, bell pepper, black beans, and water to a food processor bowl. Pulse three times, pushing down contents that go up sides of bowl. Add cumin and cocoa powder and pulse again until smooth.

2. Pour into a medium microwave-safe container and cook 60 seconds. Stir and repeat. Remove from microwave and let cool 1 minute.

3. Stir in lime juice and cilantro. Cover and refrigerate up to 5 days or freeze up to 2 months. To serve, cook in microwave in 30-second intervals until heated through, then garnish with sliced cherry tomatoes.

Nutrition:

Calories: 88

Fat: 0.3 g

Protein: 5.5 g

Sodium: 191 mg

Fiber: 6.5 g

Carbohydrates: 18.9 g

Sugar: 1.4 g

Easy Vegan Quest Dip

Preparation time: 5 minutes

Cooking time: 15minutes

Servings: 6

Ingredients:

- 1 (8-ounce) package vegan cream cheese

- 1 (10-ounce) can mild green chili enchilada sauce
- 3 tablespoons nutritional yeast flakes
- 1 teaspoon garlic powder
- 1/2 teaspoon salt
- 1/4 teaspoon black pepper

Directions:

1. Scoop vegan cream cheese into a small microwave-safe bowl and microwave about 20 seconds. Remove, stir, and repeat until sauce is smooth and stirs easily.

2. Pour green chili enchilada sauce over cream cheese. Stir to combine. Stir in nutritional yeast flakes, garlic powder, salt, and pepper. Let cool about 5 minutes before covering and refrigerating up to 7 days.

3. To serve, remove from refrigerator and cook in microwave in 30-second intervals until heated through.

Nutrition:

Calories: 78

Fat: 0.3 g

Protein: 2.5 g

Sodium: 191 mg

Fiber: 5.5 g

Carbohydrates: 19.9 g

Sugar: 1.4 g

Vegan Seven-Layer Dip

Preparation time: 5 minutes

Cooking time: 15minutes

Servings: 10

Ingredients:

- 1 (12-ounce) package vegan meat crumbles
- 1 tablespoon olive oil
- 3 tablespoons taco seasoning
- 1 can black beans
- 1.1/2 cups mild chunky salsa, divided
- 2 cups vegan Cheddar shreds
- 1 cup vegan sour cream
- 1 cup guacamole
- 1 (2.25-ounce) can black olives, chopped
- 1/2 cup chopped tomatoes
- 1/2 cup chopped green onion

Directions:

1. In a large skillet, brown vegan meat crumbles in olive oil over medium heat about 5 minutes. Add taco seasoning. Set aside to cool to room temperature, about 5 minutes.

2. Place beans in a blender or food processor with 1/2 cup salsa. Blend about 20 seconds until beans are consistency of refried beans.

3. Spread beans into bottom of a large serving tray that is about 11/2" deep. Sprinkle shredded cheese on top of beans. Sprinkle vegan meat crumbles on top of cheese. Carefully spread sour cream on top of vegan crumbles, and then spread guacamole on top of sour cream. Pour remaining salsa over guacamole and spread evenly. Sprinkle with olives. Garnish with tomatoes and green onions. Cover and refrigerate up to 3 days.

Nutrition:

Calories: 58

Fat: 3.3 g

Protein: 2.5 g

Sodium: 191 mg

Fiber: 5.5 g

Carbohydrates: 19.9 g

Sugar: 1.4 g

Chocolate Chip Peanut Butter Dip

Preparation time: 5 minutes

Cooking time: 10minutes

Servings: 10

Ingredients:

- 1 (15-ounce) can chickpeas, rinsed and drained
- 3/4 cup creamy peanut butter
- 1/2 cup agave nectar
- 1 teaspoon vanilla extract
- 3 tablespoons filtered water
- 1 cup dairy-free chocolate chips

Directions:

1. Pour all ingredients except chocolate chips into bowl of a food processor.

2. Pulse 3 seconds. Use a spatula to push down ingredients from sides of bowl. Pulse an additional 40 seconds.

3. Transfer to a small lidded container and stir in chocolate chips. Store in refrigerator up to 5 days.

Nutrition:

Calories: 79

Fat: 7.3 g

Protein: 4.5 g

Sodium: 191 mg

Fiber: 8.5 g

Carbohydrates: 20.9 g

Sugar: 1.4 g

Air-Fried Tofu

Preparation time: 5 minutes

Cooking time: 15minutes

Servings: 4

Ingredients:

- 1 (15-ounce) package extra-firm tofu, pressed and cut into 1/2" cubes
- 2 teaspoons olive oil
- 1/4 teaspoon salt

Directions:

1. Preheat air fryer to 375°F and set timer for 18 minutes. Allow air fryer to heat up 30 seconds. Remove fryer basket and spray with vegetable cooking spray. Add tofu cubes and olive oil. Toss to coat, then place basket back in air fryer.

2. Every 5 minutes, remove basket and stir tofu by shaking basket carefully. Cook until timer goes off and tofu is crispy. Remove from basket and sprinkle with salt.

3. Let cool 10 minutes, then transfer tofu to a large sealed container and refrigerate up to 5 days.

4. To serve, reheat tofu in the air fryer heated at 350°F for 5 minutes.

Nutrition:

Calories: 49

Fat: 8.3 g

Protein: 4.5 g

Sodium: 191 mg

Fiber: 8.5 g

Carbohydrates: 20.9 g

Sugar: 1.4 g

Green Chili Hummus with Salsa

Preparation time: 5 minutes

Cooking time: 15minutes

Servings: 12

Ingredients:

- 1 (15-ounce) can chickpeas, rinsed and drained
- 2 tablespoons tahini
- 2 tablespoons nutritional yeast flakes
- 2 teaspoons garlic powder
- 1 (4-ounce) can green chilies
- 1/2 cup fresh spinach
- 1 (8-ounce) jar mild chunky salsa

Directions:

1. Combine chickpeas, tahini, nutritional yeast flakes, garlic powder, green chilies, and spinach in a food processor. Pulse 3 seconds until coarse and crumbly.

2. Set a colander and pour salsa into colander to strain liquid.

3. Add liquid 1 tablespoon at a time to food processor and pulse until a spreadable consistency is reached.

4. Spoon hummus into a small serving dish and top with strained salsa.

5. Cover and keep refrigerated until ready to serve (up to 4 days). Alternatively, it can be frozen up to 1 month.

6. Serve and enjoy.

Nutrition:

Calories: 69

Fat: 8.3 g

Protein: 4.5 g

Sodium: 121 mg

Fiber: 6.5 g

Carbohydrates: 20.9 g

Sugar: 1.4 g

Crostini with Pecan Basil Pesto

Preparation time: 5 minutes

Cooking time: 15minutes

Servings: 8

Ingredients:

- 1/3 cup pecans
- 1 cup fresh spinach
- 1/3 cup olive oil
- 2 teaspoons vegan Parmesan
- 1 teaspoon garlic powder
- 5 fresh basil leaves
- 1 baguette, sliced into 24 (1/2"-thick) slices

Directions:

1. Set oven and place pecans on an ungreased baking sheet and toast in oven about 5 minutes. Remove and cool about 2 minutes.

2. Place cooled pecans, spinach, olive oil, vegan Parmesan, garlic powder, and basil leaves in a food processor. Pulse 3 seconds to combine.

3. Set bread slices in one layer on a large ungreased baking sheet. Place in oven and toast about 5 minutes. Remove from oven and cool about 5 minutes, then transfer to a medium sealed container and refrigerate up to 3 days.

4. To serve, wrap toast with foil and heat in toaster oven at 350°F for 5 minutes, until heated through. Top with Pecan Basil Pesto.

Nutrition:

Calories: 65

Fat: 2.3 g

Protein: 9.5 g

Sodium: 121 mg

Fiber: 6.5 g

Carbohydrates: 14.9 g

Sugar: 1.4 g

Black-Eyed Pea Dip

Preparation time: 5 minutes

Cooking time: 35minutes

Servings: 6

Ingredients:

- 1 (15-ounce) can black eye peas, drained

- 3 tablespoons finely chopped peeled yellow onion
- 1/4 cup vegan sour cream
- 1/2 (8-ounce) jar mild chunky salsa
- 1 cup vegan Cheddar shred.

Directions:

1. Place black eye peas in an ungreased 8" × 8" casserole dish and use a fork to mash up most of beans.

2. Add in onions, sour cream, salsa, and 1/2 vegan Cheddar shreds. Stir to combine. Top mixture with remaining vegan Cheddar shreds.

3. Bake 25 minutes until top cheese layer melts. Remove from oven and allow to cool 15 minutes.

4. Transfer dip to a large sealable container and refrigerate up to 5 days. To serve, cook in microwave in 30-second intervals until heated through.

Nutrition:

Calories: 55

Fat: 2.3 g

Protein: 9.5 g

Sodium: 111 mg

Fiber: 6.5 g

Carbohydrates: 18.9 g

Sugar: 1.4 g

Caramelized Onion Hummus

Preparation time: 5 minutes

Cooking time: 35minutes

Servings: 10

Ingredients:

- 1 small yellow onion
- 3 tablespoons olive oil, divided
- 1 teaspoon agave nectar
- 1 (15-ounce) can chickpeas, rinsed and drained
- 1/4 cup pine nuts
- 3 tablespoons lime juice
- 1/2 teaspoon dried basil
- 1 tablespoon nutritional yeast flakes
- 1 clove garlic, peeled

Directions:

1. Set a skillet on a low heat and add onions. Drizzle with 1 tablespoon olive oil. Cook until tender, about 5 minutes. Then add agave nectar and continue cooking about 10 minutes, until caramelized. Remove from heat and set aside.

2. Add chickpeas into a food processor with pine nuts and pulse 5 seconds. Add remaining tablespoons olive oil, lime juice, basil, nutritional yeast flakes, garlic, and 1/2 caramelized onions. Pulse 3 seconds until smooth. Top with remaining caramelized onions. Transfer to a medium lidded container and refrigerate up to 5 days.

Nutrition:

Calories: 79

Fat: 8.3 g

Protein: 17.5 g

Sodium: 231 mg

Fiber: 6.5 g

Carbohydrates: 18.9 g

Sugar: 1.4 g

Spicy Roasted Chickpeas

Preparation time: 5 minutes

Cooking time: 35minutes

Servings: 4

Ingredients:

- 1 can chickpeas
- 11/2 teaspoons olive oil
- 1 tablespoon Southwest Chipotle seasoning
- 1/2 teaspoon salt
- 1/8 teaspoon ground black pepper

Directions:

1. Preheat oven to 400°F.

2. Add chickpeas and olive oil to a medium bowl and stir until each chickpea is coated with oil. Place chickpeas on prepared pan.

3. Bake 25 minutes until chickpeas are crispy on outside.

4. Remove from oven and sprinkle seasoning over top. Stir until thoroughly coated. Sprinkle with salt and pepper, then transfer to a small sealed container and refrigerate up to 5 days.

Nutrition:

Calories: 56

Fat: 8.3 g

Protein: 15.5 g

Sodium: 121 mg

Fiber: 6.5 g

Carbohydrates: 18.9 g

Sugar: 1.4 g

Southwestern Hummus

Preparation time: 5 minutes

Cooking time: minutes

Servings: 10

Ingredients:

- 1 (15-ounce) can chickpeas, rinsed and drained
- 1/4 cup tahini
- 1/4 cup lime juice
- 1 cup mild chunky salsa
- 1 tablespoon Southwest Chipotle seasoning

Directions:

1. Pour all ingredients in bowl of food processor and pulse 3 seconds. Use a spatula to scrape down any ingredients on side of bowl. Pulse again until consistency is smooth.
2. Transfer to a small sealed container and refrigerate up to 5 days.

Nutrition:

Calories: 56

Fat: 8.3 g

Protein: 15.5 g

Sodium: 121 mg

Fiber: 6.5 g

Carbohydrates: 18.9 g

Sugar: 1.4 g

Vegan Bacon Ricotta Crostini

Preparation time: 5 minutes

Cooking time: 10 minutes

Servings: 10

Ingredients:

- 1 baguette, cut into 24 slices
- 1 tablespoon olive oil
- 1 clove garlic, peeled and chopped
- 8 slices vegan bacon
- 1 cup cashews
- 1/2 cup unsweetened almond milk
- 1 tablespoon nutritional yeast flakes
- 1 teaspoon dried basil
- 1 tablespoon mild miso paste
- 1/4 cup maple syrup

Directions:

1. Preheat oven to 375°F. Set a baking sheet.
2. Set slices on prepared baking sheet and bake 10 minutes until toasted. Transfer to a large sealable bag and refrigerate up to 5 days.
3. Place a medium skillet over medium heat. Add olive oil and garlic. Set aside.
4. In same skillet, cook vegan bacon 3 minutes per side. Take off from skillet and set aside to cool about 5 minutes, and then break into pieces.
5. Add soaked cashews, almond milk, nutritional yeast flakes, basil, and miso paste to bowl of food processor. Pulse 3

seconds. Repeat process until mixture is smooth and leaves no large pieces of cashews.

6. Transfer to a medium sealable container and refrigerate up to 5 days. To serve, top each piece of toasted crostini with one dollop cashew ricotta, followed by divided-out vegan bacon pieces and maple syrup. Toast in toaster oven at 300°F for 5 minutes until crispy.

Nutrition:

Calories: 56

Fat: 8.3 g

Protein: 15.5 g

Sodium: 121 mg

Fiber: 6.5 g

Carbohydrates: 18.9 g

Sugar: 1.4 g

Vegan Beer Brats in a Blanket

Preparation time: 5 minutes

Cooking time: 20minutes

Servings: 10

Ingredients:

- 1/4 cup yellow mustard
- 1 tablespoon agave nectar
- 1 (12-ounce) bottle pale lager beer
- 4 vegan brats
- 8 dairy-free crescent rolls
- 1 cup dill and garlic sauerkraut
- 1 cup vegan mozzarella cheese
- 4 slices vegan bacon, halved

Directions:

1. Preheat oven to 350F.

2. Combine mustard and agave nectar in a small lidded bowl. Cover and refrigerate up to 7 days.

3. Pour beer into a medium saucepan and bring to a boil over medium heat. Add brats and cook. Once processed, cut each brat in half. Set aside.

4. Arrange dough pieces on prepared baking sheet, adding sauerkraut and vegan cheese evenly over each.

5. Wrap each brat piece in 1/2 slice vegan bacon. Place on piece of dough. Wrap dough tightly around each brat and pinch to seal dough. Bake 15 minutes.

6. Let rolls cool 10 minutes, then transfer to a large lidded container and refrigerate up to 5 days. To serve, remove from refrigerator and heat in microwave in 30-second intervals until heated through. Pour mustard sauce over each roll.

Nutrition:

Calories: 56

Fat: 8.3 g

Protein: 15 g

Sodium: 12 mg

Fiber: 6 g

Carbohydrates: 18.g

Sugar: 1.4 g

Baked Jalapeño Poppers

Preparation time: 5 minutes

Cooking time: 20minutes

Servings: 10

Ingredients:

- 1/2 (8-ounce) container dairy-free cream cheese, softened

- 1/2 (14.2-ounce) container Diana Jalapeño Garlic Havarti Style Wedge, shredded

- 3/4 cup + 1 tablespoon plain soy milk, divided

- 1/8 teaspoon garlic powder

- 1/2 teaspoon salt

- 10 jalapeños, halved and seeded

- 2 tablespoons ground flaxseed

- 1/2 cup all-purpose flour

- 1/2 cup bread crumbs

Directions:

1. Preheat oven to 350°F.

2. Place vegan cream cheese, shredded vegan cheese, 1 tablespoon soy milk, garlic powder, and salt in a medium bowl and stir until well combined. Stuff each halved jalapeño with an even amount cream cheese mixture.

3. In a separate medium bowl combine flaxseed and remaining soy milk. Set aside.

4. Pour flour into a small dish and bread crumbs into another. Set aside.

5. Roll a stuffed jalapeño in flour, and then dip in flaxseed mixture, followed by a final dip in bread crumbs. Place breaded popper on prepared pan and repeat dipping process with remaining stuffed jalapeños.

6. Take out from oven and let cool. Transfer to a large sealed container and refrigerate up to 5 days. To serve, heat in a toaster oven at 350°F for about 5 minutes.

Nutrition:

Calories: 12

Fat: 873 g

Protein: 12 g

Sodium: 12 mg

Fiber: 6 g

Carbohydrates: 18.g

Sugar: 1.4 g

Vegan Spinach Cheese Pinwheels

Preparation time: 15 minutes

Cooking time: 0minutes

Servings: 10

Ingredients:

- 1/2 cup shredded vegan jack cheese

- 1/4 cup vegan Parmesan cheese

- 2 tablespoons chopped green onion

- 1/4 teaspoon garlic powder

- 1/2 teaspoon salt

- 1/4 cup all-purpose flour

- 1 Pepperidge Farm Puff Pastry Sheet

- 1 tablespoon vegan butter, melted

- 1 tablespoon plain soy milk

- 1 package frozen chopped spinach

Directions:

1. In a medium bowl stir together vegan cheeses, green onions, garlic powder, and salt.

2. Prepare a work area by sprinkling with flour. Lay out pastry sheet on floured surface. Stir together melted vegan butter and soy milk in a small bowl and brush over top of pastry sheet, reserving remaining mixture.

3. Spread cheese mixture over buttered pastry sheet, and then spread drained spinach over cheese mixture.

4. Begin with side closest to you and roll pastry sheet, wrapping ingredients in as you roll. Wrap pastry roll in aluminum foil and freeze about 30 minutes.

5. Preheat oven to 400°F. Grease a baking sheet with vegetable cooking spray.

6. Use a serrated knife to cut pastry roll into 1/2" slices. Place slices on prepared pan and brush with reserved butter mixture.

7. Bake 20 minutes until pinwheels are a golden color.

8. Remove from oven and let cool about 5 minutes before transferring to a large sealed container. Refrigerate up to 5 days. To serve, cook in a toaster oven at 350°F until heated through, about 5 minutes.

Nutrition:

Calories: 10

Fat: 873 g

Protein: 121g

Sodium: 16 mg

Fiber: 6 g

Carbohydrates: 18.g

Sugar: 1.4 g

Cocktail Lentil Meatballs

Preparation time: 15 minutes

Cooking time: 25minutes

Servings: 9

Ingredients:

- 1 cup chopped peeled yellow onion
- 1 cup dried brown lentils
- 3 cups water
- 1 cup extra-firm tofu, pressed
- 2 tablespoons ground flaxseed, divided
- 11/4 cups rolled oats, divided
- 1 tablespoon cashews
- 2 teaspoons Better than Bouillon Seasoned Vegetable Base
- 1 tablespoon nutritional yeast flakes
- 1 teaspoon rubbed sage
- 1/4 teaspoon ground turmeric
- 1 teaspoon paprika
- 3/4 cup grape jelly
- 11/2 cups ketchup
- 1 teaspoon sriracha

Directions:

1. Add onions, lentils, and water to a small saucepan. Bring to a boil over high heat, then reduce heat to low, cover, and cook 25 minutes. Strain excess liquid and set aside.

2. In a food processor add tofu, 1 tablespoon flaxseed, and 1/2 cup rolled oats, cashews, better than Bouillon,

nutritional yeast flakes, sage, turmeric, and paprika. Pulse until combined.

3. Add 2 cups strained lentil mixture to tofu mixture. Pulse to combine. Add remaining lentil mixture and use a spatula to stir. Add remaining flaxseed and oats and stir to combine. Set aside about 5 minutes to allow mixture to thicken.

4. Preheat oven to 375°F. Line two baking sheets with parchment paper.

5. Use a cookie dough scoop to measure consistent portions from mixture. Form into balls.

6. Place lentil meatballs on prepared pans, allowing some space between them.

7. Bake 25 minutes, turning over once, halfway through bake. When lentil meatballs are done, remove from oven and let cool about 10 minutes.

8. To prepare sauce, combine grape jelly, ketchup, and sriracha in a large microwave-safe bowl. Heat in microwave 30 seconds then stir. Repeat heating until jelly has melted and a sauce form. Add meatballs to sauce, stirring gently to coat.

9. Transfer meatballs to a large lidded container and refrigerate up to 5 days, or freeze up to 2 months.

Nutrition:

Calories: 10

Fat: 30 g

Protein: 121g

Sodium: 16 mg

Fiber: 6 g

Carbohydrates: 18.g

Sugar: 1.4 g

Carrot Hummus

Preparation time: 15 minutes

Cooking time: 0minutes

Servings: 9

Ingredients:

- 1 (15-ounce) can chickpeas, rinsed and drained
- 1 cup roughly chopped peeled carrots
- 1 tablespoon balsamic vinegar
- 2 teaspoons garlic powder
- 1/2 teaspoon ground cumin
- 1/2 teaspoon ground turmeric
- 1 teaspoon dried basil
- 1 tablespoon tamari
- 2 tablespoons all-natural peanut butter
- 4 tablespoons water
- 2 tablespoons olive oil

Directions:

1. Place all ingredients except water and olive oil in a food processor and pulse until combined. Remove lid and stir ingredients, adding water 1 tablespoon at a time until desired consistency is reached.

2. Transfer to a medium lidded container and refrigerate up to 7 days. To serve, drizzle olive oil on top of hummus.

Nutrition:

Calories: 9

Fat: 20 g

Protein: 11g

Sodium: 16 mg

Fiber: 6 g

Carbohydrates: 18.g

Sugar: 1.4 g

Vegan Cheesy Popcorn

Preparation time: 5 minutes

Cooking time: 5minutes

Servings: 2

Ingredients:

- 1/3 cup popcorn kernels
- 2 teaspoons nutritional yeast flakes
- 1 teaspoon paprika
- 1/2 teaspoon ground turmeric
- 1/8 teaspoon salt

Directions:

1. Place popcorn kernels in a microwave popcorn popper. Place lid on container and microwave about 3minutes.

2. Place nutritional yeast flakes, paprika, and turmeric in a small bowl. Stir to combine.

3. Use oven mitts to remove popcorn popper from microwave, then carefully remove lid.

4. Pour popcorn into a large sealable container, removing unpeopled kernels. Spray popcorn generously with vegetable cooking spray. Sprinkle nutritional yeast mixture and salt over top and use your hands or a spoon to distribute seasonings evenly throughout popcorn.

Nutrition:

Calories: 9

Fat: 19 g

Protein: 11g

Sodium: 15 mg

Fiber: 6 g

Carbohydrates: 18.g

Sugar: 1.4 g

Easy Vegan Rangoon Dip

Preparation time: 5 minutes

Cooking time: 15minutes

Servings: 10

Ingredients:

- 1 cup Frank's Red-hot Sweet Chili Sauce
- 1 (15-ounce) container extra-firm tofu, pressed and cut into 1/2" cubes
- 1 (8-ounce) container vegan cream cheese, divided
- 1 green onion, chopped
- About 10 tortilla chips, crushed

Directions:

1. Preheat oven to 350°F.

2. Pour sauce in a medium skillet over medium heat. Add tofu and allow simmering in sauce 3 minutes. Be sure to stir tofu well while cooking. Use a spatula to break up tofu more.

3. Add 2 tablespoons cream cheese to tofu mixture and stir to incorporate. Remove from heat and set aside.

4. Spread remaining cream cheese in bottom of a 1.5-quart casserole dish. Top with green onions. Pour tofu and sauce over cream cheese and top with crushed tortilla chip pieces.

5. Bake 25 minutes, then remove from oven and let cool about 10 minutes.

6. Cover and refrigerate up to 7 days. To serve, let sit until room temperature or heat in microwave in 30-second intervals until heated through.

Nutrition:

Calories: 9

Fat: 17 g

Protein: 17g

Sodium: 10 mg

Fiber: 6 g

Carbohydrates: 18.g

Sugar: 1.4 g

Tapas Made of Swan and Hummus

Preparation time: 5 minutes

Cooking time: 15minutes

Servings: 6

Ingredients:

- 2/3 cup quinoa
- 1 cup vegetable cups
- 1/2 tsp. paprika
- 1/2 teaspoon chili powder with fries
- 1-teaspoon garlic powder
- 1 tsp. onion
- 1-cup cornstarch and one ear

- 1 cooked chickpea with a cup
- Divide 1 cup cherry tomatoes into wedges
- 2 tablespoons of lime juice
- 1/2 kosher or a teaspoon of salt to taste
- 1 tablespoon
- Spinach leaves
- 6 milk cakes (giant burrito)

Directions:

1. Always cook quinoa before cooking. Place the winch in a bowl with enough water to cover about an inch. Rub the quinoa seriously into your hands. The water becomes cloudy with sapiens; the layer of protective seeds disappears bitterly. Repeat three times, then rinse under running water. I use eye compression.

2. Combine quinoa, broth, paprika, pepper, garlic, and onion in a small saucepan over medium heat. Heat for 20 minutes, envelope, reduce heat and cool. You know the grain is ready in the package.

3. Pour quinoa into a large bowl and mix with corn, beans, tomatoes, and lemon juice. Salt to taste.

4. Spread the hummus on all types of mulch, gently cover the spinach leaves, and add about 1/3 of the casino quinoa mix in the center. Turn the other side of the turkey onto a crannog and wrap it tightly. Close the toothbrush.

Nutrition:

Calories: 9

Fat: 19 g

Protein: 17g

Sodium: 101mg

Fiber: 6 g

Carbohydrates: 187g

Sugar: 1.4 g

Keto Coconut Flake Balls

Preparation Time: 15 Minutes

Cooking Time: 0 Minutes

Servings: 2

Ingredients:

- 1 Vanilla shortbread collagen protein bar
- 1 tablespoon lemon
- ¼ teaspoon ground ginger
- ½ cup unsweetened coconut flakes,
- ¼ teaspoon ground turmeric

Directions:

1. Process protein bar, ginger, turmeric, and ¾ of the total flakes into a food processor.
2. Remove and add a spoon of water and roll till dough forms.
3. Roll into balls, and sprinkle the rest of the flakes on it. Serve.

Nutrition:

Calories: 204 kcal

Total Fat: 11g

Total Carbs: 4.2g

Protein: 1.5g

Tofu Nuggets with Cilantro Dip

Preparation Time: 10 Minutes

Cooking Time: 15 Minutes

Servings: 4

Ingredients:

- 1 lime, ½ juiced and ½ cut into wedges
- 1½ cups olive oil
- 28 oz tofu, pressed and cubed
- 1 egg, lightly beaten
- 1 cup golden flaxseed meal
- 1 ripe avocado, chopped
- ½ tablespoon chopped cilantro
- Salt and black pepper to taste
- ½ tablespoon olive oil

Directions:

1. Heat olive oil in a deep skillet. Coat tofu cubes in the egg and then in the flaxseed meal. Fry until golden brown. Transfer to a plate.
2. Place avocado, cilantro, salt, pepper, and lime juice in a blender; puree until smooth. Spoon into a bowl, add tofu nuggets, and lime wedges to serve.

Nutrition:

Calories: 665

Net Carbs: 6.2g

Fat: 54g

Protein: 32g

Keto Chocolate Greek Yoghurt Cookies

Preparation Time: 15 Minutes

Cooking Time: 30 Minutes

Servings: 3

Ingredients:

- 3 eggs
- 1/8 teaspoon tartar
- 5 tablespoons softened Greek yogurt

Directions:

1. Beat the egg whites, the tartar, and mix.
2. In the yolk, put in the Greek yogurt, and mix.
3. Combine both egg whites and yolk batter into a bowl.
4. Bake for 25-30 minutes, serve.

Nutrition:

Calories: 287 kcal

Total Fat: 19g

Total Carbs: 6.5g

Protein: 6.8g

Bacon-Wrapped Sausage Skewers

Preparation Time: 10 Minutes

Cooking Time: 8 Minutes

Servings: 4

Ingredients:

- 5 Italian chicken sausages
- 10 slices bacon

Directions:

1. Preheat the deep fryer to 370°F/190°C
2. Cut the sausage into four pieces.
3. Slice the bacon in half.
4. Wrap the bacon over the sausage.
5. Skewer the sausage.
6. Fry for 4-5 minutes until browned.
7. Remove from the fryer and serve hot.

Nutrition:

Calories: 331 kcal

Protein: 11.84 g

Fat: 30.92 g

Carbohydrates: 1.06g

Bacon-Wrapped Mozzarella Sticks

Preparation Time: 5 Minutes

Cooking Time: 5 Minutes

Servings: 2

Ingredients:

- 2 slices thick bacon
- 2 Frigo® Cheese Heads String Cheese sticks
- Coconut oil – for frying
- For Dipping: Low-sugar pizza sauce

Directions:

1. Warm the oil to 350º Fahrenheit in a deep fryer.
2. Slice the cheese stick in half. Wrap it with the bacon and close it using the toothpick.
3. Cook the sticks in the hot fryer for two to three minutes
4. Drain on a towel and cool. Serve with sauce.

Nutrition:

Calorie Count: 103

Protein: 7 g

Fat: 9 g

Carbohydrates: 1 g

Broiled Bacon Wraps with Dates

Preparation Time: 10 Minutes

Cooking Time: 20 Minutes

Servings: 6

Ingredients:

- 1 lb. sliced bacon
- 8 oz. pitted dates

Directions:

1. Heat the oven to reach 425° Fahrenheit.
2. Use a ½ slice of bacon and wrap each of the dates. Close with a toothpick.
3. Put the wraps on a baking tray and bake them for 15-20 minutes. Serve hot.

Nutrition:

Calorie: 203

Protein: 19 g

Fats: 10 g

Carbohydrates: 5 g

Caramelized Bacon Knots

Preparation Time: 10 Minutes

Cooking Time: 15 Minutes

Servings: 4

Ingredients:

- 8 sliced bacon
- 1 tablespoon black pepper
- 1 tablespoon Low-carb sweetener - your preference

Directions:

1. Mix the pepper blend and sweetener in a small bowl. Set aside.
2. Slice each bacon slice in half. Tie each half into a knot.
3. Press the bacon knots into the pepper mixture, turning them over to coat as much as possible. Place the dipped knots onto a wire rack placed on a baking tin.
4. Place the bacon knots under a hot broiler and cook until they're to your liking (5-7 min. per side).
5. Cool on a layer of paper towels to remove excess grease as needed.
6. Serve as soon as they're ready.

Nutrition:

Calorie Count: 187

Protein: 5 g

Fat: 17 g

Carbohydrates: 1 g

Chocolate Dipped Candied Bacon

Preparation Time: 20 Minutes

Cooking Time: 1 Hour 15 Minutes

Servings: 6

Ingredients:

- ½ teaspoon Cinnamon
- 2 tablespoon brown sugar alternative – ex. Surkin Gold
- 16 thin-cut slices of bacon
- ½ oz. cacao butter or coconut oil
- 3 oz. 85% dark chocolate
- 1 teaspoon Sugar-free maple extract

Directions:

1. Whisk the Surkin Gold and cinnamon together.
2. Arrange the bacon strips on a parchment paper-lined tray and sprinkle using half of the mixture. Do the other side with the rest of the seasoning mixture.
3. Set the oven to reach 275° Fahrenheit. Bake until caramelized and crispy (approximately 1 hour and 15 minutes).
4. Heat a skillet to melt the cocoa butter and chocolate. Pour the maple syrup into the mixture and stir well. Set aside until it's room temperature.
5. Arrange the bacon on a platter to cool thoroughly before dipping it into the chocolate.
6. Dip half of each strip of the bacon into the chocolate.

7. Arrange on a tray for the chocolate to solidify. Either place it in the refrigerator or on the countertop.

Nutrition:

Calorie Count: 54

Protein: 3 g

Fat: 4.1 g

Carbohydrates: 1.1 g

Tropical Coconut Balls

Preparation Time: 15 Minutes

Cooking Time: 20 Minutes

Servings: 2

Ingredients:

- 1 cup shredded coconut (unsweetened)
- 6 tablespoons coconut milk (full-fat)
- 2 tablespoons melted coconut oil
- 1/4 cup almond flour
- 2 tablespoons lemon juice
- 2 tablespoons ground chia seeds
- Zest of 1 lemon
- 10 drops stevia (alcohol-free)
- 1/8 teaspoons sea salt

Directions:

1. Preheat the oven to 250 degrees Fahrenheit
2. Place the shredded coconut in a large bowl and pour the coconut milk into it.
3. Add the almond flour, ground chia, sea salt, coconut oil, and lemon zest, and lemon juice to the bowl.
4. Mix everything until well combined.
5. Take 1 tablespoon of the mixture and form a ball out of it. Repeat with the remaining mixture.
6. Line a baking tray using parchment paper and place the small balls on it.

7. If you find the mixture too dry while making the balls, add one tablespoon (extra) of coconut oil to the mixture
8. Bake the coconut balls for 30 minutes and remove them from the oven.
9. Let it cool completely at room temperature.
10. Transfer the balls into another container carefully and refrigerate it for 30 minutes.
11. Serve chilled and enjoy!

Nutrition:

Calories 134 Kcal

Fat: 13.1 g

Protein: 2.2 g

Net carb: 1.1 g

Jicama Fries

Preparation Time: 5 Minutes

Cooking Time: 10 Minutes

Servings: 2

Ingredients:

- 1 Jicama (sliced into thin strips)
- 1/2 teaspoon onion powder
- 2 tablespoons avocado oil
- Cayenne pepper (pinch)
- 1 teaspoon paprika
- Sea salt, to taste

Directions:

1. Dry roast the jicama strips in a non-stick frying pan (or you can also grease the pan with a bit of avocado oil)
2. Place the roasted jicama fries into a large bowl and add the onion powder, cayenne pepper, paprika, and sea salt.
3. Drizzle over the avocado oil and toss the contents until the flavors are incorporated well.

4. Serve immediately and enjoy!

Nutrition:

Calories 92 Kcal

Fat: 7 g

Protein: 1 g

Net carb: 2 g

Ham 'n' Cheese Puffs

Preparation Time: 15 Minutes

Cooking Time: 30 Minutes

Servings: 8

Ingredients:

- 6 large eggs
- 10 oz. sliced deli ham, diced
- 1 ½ cup shredded cheddar cheese
- ¾ cup mayonnaise
- 1/3 cup coconut flour
- 1/3 cup coconut oil
- 1/3 teaspoon baking powder
- 1/3 teaspoon baking soda
- Nonstick cooking spray

Directions:

1. Set the oven to 350°F. Lightly coat rimmed baking sheet using nonstick cooking spray and set aside.
2. In a bowl, put together the eggs, coconut oil, and mayonnaise. Mix and set aside.
3. In a separate bowl, combine the baking soda, baking powder, and coconut flour. Add the dry ingredients to the wet ingredients and mix well until smooth.
4. Fold the ham and cheddar cheese into the mixture and set aside.
5. Cut the dough into 18 small pieces then arrange on the prepared baking sheet.
6. Bake for 30 minutes, or until the puffs are golden brown and set.

7. Arrange the puffs on a cooling rack and allow to cool slightly.
8. Store it in a sealed container for up to 5 days. If desired, reheat in the microwave before serving.

Nutrition:

Calories: 249

Fat: 20g

Carbs: 3g

Protein: 15g

Curry Spiced Almonds

Preparation Time: 5 Minutes

Cooking Time: 25 Minutes

Servings: 4

Ingredients:

- 1 cup whole almonds
- 2 teaspoons olive oil
- 1 teaspoon curry powder
- ¼ teaspoon salt
- ¼ teaspoon ground turmeric
- Pinch cayenne

Directions:

1. Preheat the oven to 300$\underline{o}$ F
2. In a mixing bowl, whisk the spices and olive oil.
3. Toss in the almonds then spread on the baking sheet.
4. Bake for 25 minutes until toasted, then cool and store in an airtight container.

Nutrition:

Calories: 155

Fat: 14g

Protein: 5g

Chia Peanut Butter Bites

Preparation Time: 10 Minutes

Cooking Time: 10 Minutes

Servings: 6

Ingredients:

- ½ ounce of raw almonds
- 1 tablespoon powdered erythritol
- 4 teaspoons coconut oil
- 2 tablespoons canned coconut milk
- ½ teaspoon vanilla extract
- 2 tablespoons chia seeds, ground to powder
- ¼ cup coconut cream

Directions:

1. Put the almonds in a skillet over medium-low heat, and cook until toasted. Takes about 5 minutes.
2. Transfer the almonds to a food processor with the erythritol and 1 teaspoon coconut oil.
3. Blend until it forms a smooth almond butter.
4. Heat the rest of the coconut oil in a skillet over medium heat.
5. Add the coconut milk and vanilla and bring to a simmer.
6. Stir in the ground chia seeds, coconut cream, and almond butter.
7. Cook for 2 minutes, then spread in a foil-lined square dish.
8. Chill until the mixture is firm, then cut into squares to serve.

Nutrition:

Calories: 110

Fat: 8g

Protein: 2g

Cheesy Sausage Dip

Preparation Time: 10 Minutes

Cooking Time: 120 Minutes

Servings: 12

Ingredients:

- ½ pound ground Italian sausage
- ½ cup diced tomatoes
- Two green onions, sliced thin
- 4 ounces cream cheese, cubed
- 4 ounces pepper jack cheese, cubed
- 1 cup sour cream

Directions:

1. Brown the sausage in a skillet, wait for it to cook completely, then stir in the tomatoes.
2. Cook for 2 minutes, stirring often, thereafter, add in the green onions.
3. Line the bottom of a slow cooker with the cheeses, then spoon the sausage mixture on top.
4. Spoon the sour cream over the sausage, then cover and cook on high heat for 2 hours, stirring once halfway through.
5. Serve with celery sticks or pork rinds for dipping.

Nutrition:

Calories: 170

Fat: 15g

Protein: 7g

Net Carbs: 2g

Salted Kale Chips

Preparation Time: 10 Minutes

Cooking Time: 12 Minutes

Servings: 2

Ingredients:

- ½ bunch fresh kale
- 1 tablespoon olive oil
- Salt and pepper to taste

Directions:

1. Preheat the oven to 350$\underline{o}$ F and line a baking sheet with foil.
2. Pick the thick stems from the kale and then tear the leaves into pieces.
3. Toss the kale with olive oil and spread it on the baking sheet.
4. Bake for 10 to 12 minutes until crisp, then sprinkle with salt and pepper.

Nutrition:

Calories: 75

Fat: 7g

Protein: 1g

Net Carbs: 3g

Bacon Jalapeno Quick Bread

Preparation Time: 20 Minutes

Cooking Time: 45 Minutes

Servings: 10

Ingredients:

- Four slices of thick-cut bacon
- Three jalapeno peppers
- ½ cup coconut flour sifted
- ½ teaspoon baking soda
- ½ teaspoon salt
- Six large eggs, beaten
- ½ cup coconut oil, melted
- ¼ cup of water

Directions:

1. Preheat the oven to 400$\underline{o}$ F

2. Grease a loaf pan with cooking spray.
3. Spread the bacon and jalapenos on a baking sheet and roast for 10 minutes, stirring halfway through.
4. Crumble the bacon and cut the jalapenos in half to remove the seeds.
5. Combine the bacon and jalapeno in a food processor and pulse until well chopped.
6. Beat together the coconut flour, baking soda, and salt in a bowl.
7. Add the eggs, coconut oil, and water, then stir in the bacon and jalapenos.
8. Spread in the loaf pan, then bake for 40 to 45 minutes, until a knife inserted in the center comes out clean.

Nutrition:

Calories: 225

Fat: 19g

Protein: 8g

Net Carbs: 3g

Toasted Pumpkin Seeds

Preparation Time: 5 Minutes

Cooking Time: 5 Minutes

Servings: 2

Ingredients:

- ½ cup hulled pumpkin seeds
- 2 teaspoons coconut oil
- 2 teaspoons chili powder
- ½ teaspoon salt

Directions:

1. Heat a cast-iron skillet over medium heat.
2. Add the pumpkin seeds and let them cook until toasted, about 3 to 5 minutes, stirring often.

3. Remove from heat and stir in the coconut oil, chili powder, and salt.
4. Let the seeds cool, then store in an airtight container.

Nutrition:

Calories: 100

Fat: 8.5g

Protein: 5.5g

Net Carbs: 0.5g

Bacon-Wrapped Burger Bites

Preparation Time: 5 Minutes

Cooking Time: 60 Minutes

Servings: 6

Ingredients:

- 6 ounces ground beef (80% lean)
- ¼ teaspoon onion powder
- ¼ teaspoon garlic powder
- ¼ teaspoon ground cumin
- Salt and pepper to taste
- Six slices bacon, uncooked

Directions:

1. Preheat the oven to 350o F
2. Combine the onion powder, garlic powder, cumin, salt, and pepper in a bowl.
3. Add the beef and stir until well combined.
4. Divide the ground beef mixture into six even portions and roll them into balls.
5. Wrap each ball with a slice of bacon and place it on the baking sheet.
6. Bake for 60 minutes until the bacon is crisp and the beef is cooked through.

Nutrition:

Calories: 150

Fat: 10g

Protein: 16g

Net Carbs: 0.5g

Almond Sesame Crackers

Preparation Time: 10 Minutes

Cooking Time: 15 Minutes

Servings: 6

Ingredients:

- 1 ½ cups almond flour
- ½ cup sesame seeds
- 1 teaspoon dried oregano
- ½ teaspoon salt
- 1 large egg, whisked
- 1 tablespoon coconut oil, melted

Directions:

1. Preheat the oven to 350o F
2. Whisk together the almond flour, sesame seeds, oregano, and salt in a bowl.
3. Add the eggs and coconut oil, stirring into a soft dough.
4. Sandwich the dough between two sheets of parchment and roll to 1/8" thickness.
5. Cut into squares and arrange them on the baking sheet.
6. Bake for 10 to 12 minutes or wait until browned around the edges.

Nutrition:

Calories: 145

Fat: 12.5g

Protein: 5g

Net Carbs: 2g

Cauliflower Cheese Dip

Preparation Time: 5 Minutes

Cooking Time: 15 Minutes

Servings: 6

Ingredients:

- One small head cauliflower, chopped
- ¾ cup chicken broth
- ¼ teaspoon ground cumin
- ¼ teaspoon chili powder
- ¼ teaspoon garlic powder
- Salt and pepper to taste
- 1/3 cup cream cheese, chopped
- Two tablespoons canned coconut milk

Directions:

1. Combine the cauliflower and chicken broth in a saucepan and simmer until the cauliflower is tender.
2. Add the cumin, chili powder, and garlic powder, then season with salt and pepper.
3. Stir in the cream cheese until melted, then blend everything with an immersion blender.
4. Whisk in the coconut milk, then spoon into a serving bowl.
5. Serve with sliced celery sticks.

Nutrition:

Calories: 75

Fat: 6g

Protein: 2.5g

Net Carbs: 2g

Chapter 10: Dessert Recipes

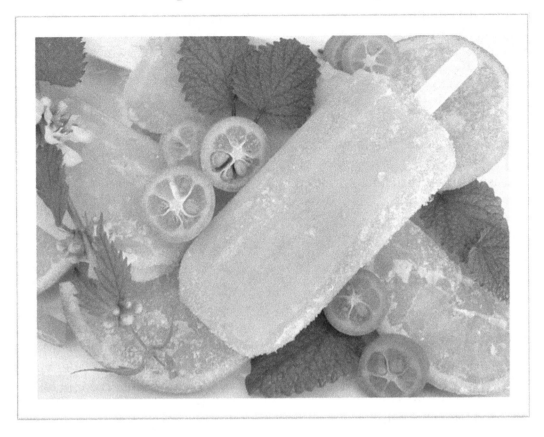

Raspberry Muffins

Preparation Time: 10 Minutes

Cooking Time: 25 Minutes

Servings: 12

Ingredients:

- ½ cup and 2 tablespoons whole-wheat flour
- 1 ½ cup raspberries, fresh and more for decorating
- 1 cup white whole-wheat flour
- 1/8 teaspoon salt
- ¾ cup of coconut sugar
- 2 teaspoons baking powder
- 1 teaspoon apple cider vinegar
- 1 ¼ cups water
- ½ cup olive oil

Directions:

1. Switch on the oven, then set it to 400 degrees F and let it preheat.
2. Meanwhile, take a large bowl, place both flours in it, add salt and baking powder and then stir until combined.
3. Take a medium bowl, add oil to it, and then whisk in the sugar until dissolved.
4. Whisk in vinegar and water until blended, slowly stir in flour mixture until smooth batter comes together, and then fold in berries.
5. Take a 12-cups muffin pan, grease it with oil, fill evenly with the prepared mixture and then put a raspberry on top of each muffin.
6. Bake the muffins for 25 minutes until the top golden brown, and then serve.

Nutrition:

Calories: 109 Cal;

Fat: 3.4 g;

Protein: 2.1 g;

Carbs: 17.6 g;

Fiber: 1 g

Chocolate Chip Cake

Preparation Time: 10 Minutes

Cooking Time: 50 Minutes

Servings: 10

Ingredients:

- 2 cups white whole-wheat flour
- ¼ teaspoon baking soda
- 1/3 cup coconut sugar
- 2 teaspoons baking powder
- ½ teaspoon salt
- ½ cup chocolate chips, vegan
- 1 teaspoon vanilla extract, unsweetened
- 1 tablespoon applesauce
- 1 teaspoon apple cider vinegar
- ¼ cup melted coconut oil
- ½ teaspoon almond extract, unsweetened
- 1 cup almond milk, unsweetened

Directions:

1. Switch on the oven, then set it to 360 degrees F and let it preheat.
2. Meanwhile, take a 9-by-5 inches loaf pan, grease it with oil, and then set aside until required.
3. Take a large bowl, add sugar to it, pour in oil, vanilla and almond extract, vinegar, apple sauce, and milk, and then whisk until well combined.
4. Take a large bowl, place flour in it, add salt, baking powder, and soda, and then stir until mixed.
5. Stir the flour mixture into the milk mixture until smooth batter comes together, and then fold in 1/3 cup of chocolate chips.

6. Spoon the batter into the loaf pan, scatter remaining chocolate chips on top and then bake for 50 minutes.
7. When done, let the bread cool for 10 minutes and then cut it into slices.
8. Serve straight away.

Nutrition:

Calories: 218 Cal;

Fat: 8 g;

Protein: 3.4 g;

Carbs: 32 g;

Fiber: 2 g

Coffee Cake

Preparation Time: 10 Minutes

Cooking Time: 45 Minutes

Servings: 9

Ingredients:

For the Cake:
- 1/3 cup coconut sugar
- 1 teaspoon vanilla extract, unsweetened
- ¼ cup olive oil
- 1/8 teaspoon almond extract, unsweetened
- 1 ¾ cup white whole-wheat flour
- 2 teaspoons baking powder
- ½ teaspoon salt
- ¼ teaspoon baking soda
- 1 teaspoon apple cider vinegar
- 1 tablespoon applesauce
- 1 cup almond milk, unsweetened
  For the Streusel:
- ½ cup white whole-wheat flour
- 2 teaspoons cinnamon
- 1/3 cup coconut sugar
- ½ teaspoon salt
- 2 tablespoons olive oil
- 1 tablespoon coconut butter

Directions:

1. Switch on the oven, then set it to 350 degrees F and let it preheat.
2. Meanwhile, take a large bowl, pour in milk, add applesauce, vinegar, sugar, oil, vanilla, and almond extract and then whisk until blended.
3. Take a medium bowl, place flour in it, add salt, baking powder, and soda and then stir until mixed.
4. Stir the flour mixture into the milk mixture until smooth batter comes together, and then spoon the mixture into a loaf pan lined with parchment paper.
5. Prepare streusel and for this, take a medium bowl, place flour in it, and then add sugar, salt, and cinnamon.
6. Stir until mixed, and then mix butter and oil with fingers until the crumble mixture comes together.
7. Spread the prepared streusel on top of the batter of the cake and then bake for 45 minutes until the top turn golden brown and cake have thoroughly cooked.
8. When done, let the cake rest in its pan for 10 minutes, remove it to cool completely and then cut it into slices.
9. Serve straight away.

Nutrition:

Calories: 259 Cal;

Fat: 10 g;

Protein: 3 g;

Carbs: 37 g;

Fiber: 1 g

Chocolate Marble Cake

Preparation Time: 15 Minutes

Cooking Time: 50 Minutes

Servings: 8

Ingredients:

- 1 ½ cup white whole-wheat flour
- 1 tablespoon flaxseed meal
- 2 ½ tablespoons cocoa powder
- ¼ teaspoon salt
- 4 tablespoons chopped walnuts
- 1 teaspoon baking powder
- 2/3 cup coconut sugar
- ¼ teaspoon baking soda
- 1 teaspoon vanilla extract, unsweetened
- 3 tablespoons peanut butter
- ¼ cup olive oil
- 1 cup almond milk, unsweetened

Directions:

1. Switch on the oven, then set it to 350 degrees F and let it preheat.
2. Meanwhile, take a medium bowl, place flour in it, add salt, baking powder, and soda in it and then stir until mixed.
3. Take a large bowl, pour in milk, add sugar, flaxseed, oil, and vanilla, whisk until sugar has dissolved, and then whisk in flour mixture until smooth batter comes together.
4. Spoon half of the prepared batter in a medium bowl, add cocoa powder and then stir until combined.
5. Add peanut butter into the other bowl and then stir until combined.
6. Take a loaf pan, line it with a parchment sheet, spoon half of the chocolate batter in it, and then spread it evenly.
7. Layer the chocolate batter with half of the peanut butter batter, cover with the remaining chocolate batter and then layer with the remaining peanut butter batter.
8. Make swirls into the batter with a toothpick, smooth the top with a spatula, sprinkle walnuts on top, and then bake for 50 minutes until done.

9. When done, let the cake rest in its pan for 10 minutes, then remove it to cool completely and cut it into slices.
10. Serve straight away.

Nutrition:

Calories: 299 Cal;

Fat: 14 g;

Protein: 6 g;

Carbs: 39 g;

Fiber: 3 g

Chocolate Chip Cookies

Preparation Time: 10 Minutes

Cooking Time: 10 Minutes

Servings: 11

Ingredients:

- 1 ¼ cups white whole-wheat flour
- 1 ½ tablespoon flax seeds
- ½ teaspoon baking soda
- ½ cup of coconut sugar
- ¼ teaspoon of sea salt
- ¼ cup powdered coconut sugar
- 1 teaspoon baking powder
- 2 teaspoons vanilla extract, unsweetened
- 4 ½ tablespoons water
- ½ cup of coconut oil
- 1 cup chocolate chips, vegan

Directions:

1. Take a large bowl, place flax seeds in it, stir in water and then let the mixture rest for 5 minutes until creamy.
2. Then add remaining ingredients into the flax seed's mixture except for flour and chocolate chips and then beat until light batter comes together.

3. Beat in flour, ¼ cup at a time, until smooth batter comes together, and then fold in chocolate chips.
4. Use an ice cream scoop to scoop the batter onto a baking sheet lined with parchment sheet with some distance between cookies and then bake for 10 minutes until cookies turn golden brown.
5. When done, let the cookies cool on the baking sheet for 3 minutes and then cool completely on the wire rack for 5 minutes.
6. Serve straight away.

Nutrition:

Calories: 141 Cal;

Fat: 7 g;

Protein: 1 g;

Carbs: 17 g;

Fiber: 2 g

Lemon Cake

Preparation Time: 10 Minutes

Cooking Time: 50 Minutes

Servings: 9

Ingredients:

- 1 ½ cup white whole-wheat flour
- 1 ½ teaspoon baking powder
- 2 tablespoons almond flour
- 1 lemon, zested
- ¼ teaspoon baking soda
- 1/8 teaspoon turmeric powder
- 1/3 teaspoon salt
- ¼ teaspoon vanilla extract, unsweetened
- 1/3 cup lemon juice
- ½ cup maple syrup
- ¼ cup olive oil

- ¼ cup of water
  For the Frosting:
- 1 tablespoon lemon juice
- 1/8 teaspoon salt
- ¼ cup maple syrup
- 2 tablespoons powdered sugar
- 6 ounces vegan cream cheese, softened

Directions:

1. Switch on the oven, then set it to 350 degrees F and let it preheat.
2. Take a large bowl, pour in water, lemon juice, and oil, add vanilla extract and maple syrup, and whisk until blended.
3. Whisk in flour, ¼ cup at a time, until smooth, and then whisk in almond flour, salt, turmeric, lemon zest, baking soda, and powder until well combined.
4. Take a loaf pan, grease it with oil, spoon prepared batter in it, and then bake for 50 minutes.
5. Meanwhile, prepare the frosting and for this, take a small bowl, place all of its ingredients in it, whisk until smooth, and then let it chill until required.
6. When the cake has cooked, let it cool for 10 minutes in its pan and then let it cool completely on the wire rack.
7. Spread the prepared frosting on top of the cake, slice the cake, and then serve.

Nutrition:

Calories: 275 Cal;

Fat: 12 g;

Protein: 3 g;

Carbs: 38 g;

Fiber: 1 g

Banana Muffins

Preparation Time: 10 Minutes

Cooking Time: 30 Minutes

Servings: 12

Ingredients:

- 1 ½ cups mashed banana
- 1 ½ cups and 2 tablespoons white whole-wheat flour, divided
- ¼ cup of coconut sugar
- ¾ cup rolled oats, divided
- 1 teaspoon ginger powder
- 1 tablespoon ground cinnamon, divided
- 2 teaspoons baking powder
- ½ teaspoon salt
- 1 teaspoon baking soda
- 1 tablespoon vanilla extract, unsweetened
- ½ cup maple syrup
- 1 tablespoon rum
- ½ cup of coconut oil

Directions:

1. Switch on the oven, then set it to 350 degrees F and let it preheat.
2. Meanwhile, take a medium bowl, place 1 ½ cup flour in it, add ½ cup oars, ginger, baking powder and soda, salt, and 2 teaspoons cinnamon and then stir until mixed.
3. Place ¼ cup of coconut oil in a heatproof bowl, melt it in the microwave oven and then whisk in maple syrup until combined.
4. Add mashed banana along with rum and vanilla, stir until combined, and then whisk this mixture into the flour mixture until smooth batter comes together.
5. Take a separate medium bowl, place remaining oats and flour in it, add cinnamon, coconut sugar, and coconut oil and then stir with a fork until crumbly mixture comes together.
6. Take a 12-cups muffin pan, fill evenly with prepared batter, top with oats mixture, and then bake for 30 minutes

until firm and the top turn golden brown.
7. When done, let the muffins cool for 5 minutes in its pan and then cool the muffins completely before serving.

Nutrition:

Calories: 240 Cal;

Fat: 9.3 g;

Protein: 2.6 g;

Carbs: 35.4 g;

Fiber: 2 g

No-Bake Cookies

Preparation Time: 30 Minutes

Cooking Time: 0 Minutes

Servings: 9

Ingredients:

- 1 cup rolled oats
- ¼ cup of cocoa powder
- 1/8 teaspoon salt
- 1 teaspoon vanilla extract, unsweetened
- ¼ cup and 2 tablespoons peanut butter, divided
- 6 tablespoons coconut oil, divided
- ¼ cup and 1 tablespoon maple syrup, divided

Directions:

1. Take a small saucepan, place it over low heat, add 5 tablespoons of coconut oil and then let it melt.
2. Whisk in 2 tablespoons peanut butter, salt, 1 teaspoon vanilla extract, and ¼ cup each of cocoa powder and maple syrup, and then whisk until well combined.

3. Remove pan from heat, stir in oats and then spoon the mixture evenly into 9 cups of a muffin pan.
4. Wipe clean the pan, return it over low heat, add remaining coconut oil, maple syrup, and peanut butter, stir until combined, and then cook for 2 minutes until thoroughly warmed.
5. Drizzle the peanut butter sauce over the oat mixture in the muffin pan and then let it freeze for 20 minutes or more until set.
6. Serve straight away.

Nutrition:

Calories: 213 Cal;

Fat: 14.8 g;

Protein: 4 g;

Carbs: 17.3 g;

Fiber: 2.1 g

Peanut Butter and Oat Bars

Preparation Time: 40 Minutes

Cooking Time: 8 Minutes

Servings: 8

Ingredients:

- 1 cup rolled oats
- 1/8 teaspoon salt
- ¼ cup chocolate chips, vegan
- ¼ cup maple syrup
- 1 cup peanut butter

Directions:

1. Take a medium saucepan, place it over medium heat, add peanut butter, salt, and maple syrup and then whisk until combined and thickened; this will take 5 minutes.

2. Remove pan from heat, place oats in a bowl, pour peanut butter mixture on it and then stir until well combined.
3. Take an 8-by-6 inches baking dish, line it with a parchment sheet, spoon the oats mixture in it, and then spread evenly, pressing the mixture into the dish.
4. Sprinkle the chocolate chips on top, press them into the bar mixture and then let the mixture rest in the refrigerator for 30 minutes or more until set.
5. When ready to eat, cut the bar mixture into even size pieces and then serve.

Nutrition:

Calories: 274 Cal;

Fat: 17 g;

Protein: 10 g;

Carbs: 19 g;

Fiber: 3 g

Baked Apples

Preparation Time: 5 Minutes

Cooking Time: 20 Minutes

Servings: 4

Ingredients:

- 6 medium apples, peeled, cut into chunks
- 1 teaspoon ground cinnamon
- 2 tablespoons melted coconut oil

Directions:

1. Switch on the oven, then set it to 350 degrees F and let it preheat.
2. Take a medium baking dish, and then spread apple pieces in it.

3. Take a small bowl, place coconut oil in it, stir in cinnamon, drizzle this mixture over apples and then toss until coated.
4. Place the baking dish into the oven and then bake for 20 minutes or more until apples turn soft, stirring halfway.
5. Serve straight away.

Nutrition:

Calories: 170 Cal;

Fat: 3.8 g;

Protein: 0.5 g;

Carbs: 31 g;

Fiber: 5.5 g

Chocolate Strawberry Shake

Preparation Time: 5 Minutes

Cooking Time: 0 Minutes

Servings: 2

Ingredients:

- 2 cups almond milk, unsweetened
- 4 bananas, peeled, frozen
- 4 tablespoons cocoa powder
- 2 cups strawberries, frozen

Directions:

1. Place all the ingredients into the jar of a high-speed food processor or blender in the order stated in the ingredients list and then cover it with the lid.
2. Pulse for 1 minute until smooth, and then serve.

Nutrition:

Calories: 208 Cal;

Fat: 0.2 g;

Protein: 12.4 g;

Carbs: 26.2 g;

Fiber: 1.4 g

Chocolate Clusters

Preparation Time: 15 Minutes

Cooking Time: 0 Minutes

Servings: 12

Ingredients:

- 1 cup chopped dark chocolate, vegan
- 1 cup cashews, roasted, salt
- 1 teaspoon sea salt flakes

Directions:

1. Take a large baking sheet, line it with wax paper, and then set aside until required.
2. Take a medium bowl, place chocolate in it, and then microwave for 1 minute.
3. Stir the chocolate and then continue microwaving it at 1-minute intervals until chocolate melts completely, stirring at every interval.
4. When melted, stir the chocolate to bring it to 90 degrees F and then stir in cashews.
5. Scoop the walnut-chocolate mixture on the prepared baking sheet, ½ tablespoons per cluster, and then sprinkle with salt.
6. Let the clusters stand at room temperature until harden and then serve.

Nutrition:

Calories: 79.4 Cal;

Fat: 6.6 g;

Protein: 1 g;

Carbs: 5.8 g;

Fiber: 1.1 g

Banana Coconut Cookies

Preparation Time: 40 Minutes

Cooking Time: 0 Minutes

Servings: 8

Ingredients:

- 1 ½ cup shredded coconut, unsweetened
- 1 cup mashed banana

Directions:

1. Switch on the oven, then set it to 350 degrees F and let it preheat.
2. Take a medium bowl, place the mashed banana in it and then stir in coconut until well combined.
3. Take a large baking sheet, line it with a parchment sheet, and then scoop the prepared mixture on it, 2 tablespoons of mixture per cookie.
4. Place the baking sheet into the refrigerator and then let it cool for 30 minutes or more until harden.
5. Serve straight away.

Nutrition:

Calories: 51 Cal;

Fat: 3 g;

Protein: 0.2 g;

Carbs: 4 g;

Fiber: 1 g

Chocolate Pots

Preparation Time: 4 Hours 10 Minutes

Cooking Time: 3 Minutes

Servings: 4

Ingredients:

- 6 ounces chocolate, unsweetened
- 1 cup Medjool dates, pitted
- 1 ¾ cups almond milk, unsweetened

Directions:

1. Cut the chocolate into small pieces, place them in a heatproof bowl and then microwave for 2 to 3 minutes until melt completely, stirring every minute.
2. Place dates in a blender, pour in the milk, and then pulse until smooth.
3. Add chocolate into the blender and then pulse until combined.
4. Divide the mixture into the small mason jars and then let them rest for 4 hours until set.
5. Serve straight away.

Nutrition:

Calories: 321 Cal;

Fat: 19 g;

Protein: 6 g;

Carbs: 34 g;

Fiber: 4 g

Maple and Tahini Fudge

Preparation Time: 2 Hours

Cooking Time: 3 Minutes

Servings: 15

Ingredients:

- 1 cup dark chocolate chips, vegan
- ¼ cup maple syrup
- ½ cup tahini

Directions:

1. Take a heatproof bowl, place chocolate chips in it and then microwave for 2 to 3

minutes until melt completely, stirring every minute.

2. When melted, remove the chocolate bowl from the oven and then whisk in maple syrup and tahini until smooth.

3. Take a 4-by-8 inches baking dish, line it with wax paper, spoon the chocolate mixture in it and then press it into the baking dish.

4. Cover with another sheet with wax paper, press it down until smooth, and then let the fudge rest for 1 hour in the freezer until set.

5. Then cut the fudge into 15 squares and serve.

Nutrition:

Calories: 110.7 Cal;

Fat: 5.3 g;

Protein: 2.2 g;

Carbs: 15.1 g;

Fiber: 1.6 g

Creaseless

Preparation Time: 5 Minutes

Cooking Time: 0 Minutes

Servings: 5

Ingredients:

- 3 tablespoons agave syrup
- 1 cup coconut milk, unsweetened
- ½ teaspoon vanilla extract, unsweetened
- 1 cup of orange juice

Directions:

1. Place all the ingredients in a food processor or blender and then pulse until combined.

2. Pour the mixture into five molds of Popsicle pan, insert a stick into each mold and then let it freeze for a minimum of 4 hours until hard.

3. Serve when ready.

Nutrition:

Calories: 152 Cal;

Fat: 10 g;

Protein: 1 g;

Carbs: 16 g;

Fiber: 1 g

Peanut Butter, Nut, and Fruit Cookies

Preparation Time: 30 Minutes

Cooking Time: 0 Minutes

Servings: 25

Ingredients:

- ¾ cup rolled oats
- ¼ cup chopped peanuts
- ½ cup coconut flakes, unsweetened
- ¼ cup and 2 tablespoons chopped cranberries, dried
- ¼ cup sliced almonds
- ¼ cup and 2 tablespoons raisins
- ¼ cup maple syrup
- ¾ cup peanut butter

Directions:

1. Take a baking sheet, line it with wax paper, and then set it aside until required.

2. Take a large bowl, place oats, almonds, and coconut flakes in it, add ¼ cup each of cranberries and raisins, and then stir until combined.

3. Add maple syrup and peanut butter, stir until well combined, and then scoop the

mixture on the prepared baking sheet with some distance between them.

4. Flatten each scoop of cookie mixture slightly, press remaining cranberries and raisins into each cookie, and then let it chill for 20 minutes until firm.
5. Serve straight away.

Nutrition:

Calories: 140 Cal;

Fat: 7 g;

Protein: 3 g;

Carbs: 18 g;

Fiber: 5 g

Chocolate Covered Dates

Preparation Time: 10 Minutes

Cooking Time: 3 Minutes

Servings: 8

Ingredients:

- 16 Medjool dates, pitted
- ½ teaspoon of sea salt
- ¾ cup almonds
- 1 teaspoon coconut oil
- 8 ounces chocolate chips, vegan

Directions:

1. Take a medium baking sheet, line it with parchment paper, and then set aside until required.
2. Place an almond into the pit of each date and then wrap the date tightly around it.
3. Place chocolate chips in a heatproof bowl, add oil, and then microwave for 2 to 3 minutes until chocolate melts, stirring every minute.
4. Working on one date at a time, dip each date into the chocolate mixture and

then place it onto the prepared baking sheet.

5. Sprinkle salt over the prepared dates and then let them rest in the refrigerator for 1 hour until chocolate is firm.
6. Serve straight away.

Nutrition:

Calories: 179 Cal;

Fat: 7.7 g;

Protein: 3 g;

Carbs: 28.5 g;

Fiber: 3 g

Hot Chocolate

Preparation Time: 5 Minutes

Cooking Time: 10 Minutes

Servings: 4

Ingredients:

- ¼ cup of cocoa powder
- 1/8 teaspoon salt
- ½ teaspoon vanilla extract, unsweetened
- ¼ cup of coconut sugar
- 3 cups almond milk, unsweetened

Directions:

1. Take a medium saucepan, add salt, sugar, and cocoa powder in it, whisk until combined, and then whisk in milk.
2. Place the pan over medium-high heat and then bring the milk mixture to a simmer and turn hot, continue whisking.
3. Divide the hot chocolate evenly into four mugs and then serve.

Nutrition:

Calories: 137 Cal;

Fat: 3 g;

Protein: 6 g;

Carbs: 21 g;

Fiber: 2 g

Vanilla Cupcakes

Preparation Time: 10 Minutes

Cooking Time: 20 Minutes

Servings: 18

Ingredients:

- 2 cups white whole-wheat flour
- 1 cup of coconut sugar
- ½ teaspoon salt
- 2 teaspoons baking powder
- 1 ¼ teaspoons vanilla extract, unsweetened
- ½ teaspoon baking soda
- 1 tablespoon apple cider vinegar
- ½ cup coconut oil, melted
- 1 ½ cups almond milk, unsweetened

Directions:

1. Switch on the oven, then set it to 350 degrees F, and then let it preheat.
2. Meanwhile, take a medium bowl, place vinegar in it, stir in milk, and then let it stand for 5 minutes until curdled.
3. Take a large bowl, place flour in it, add salt, baking soda and powder, and sugar and then stir until mixed.
4. Take a separate large bowl, pour in curdled milk mixture, add vanilla and coconut oil and then whisk until combined.
5. Whisk almond milk mixture into the flour mixture until smooth batter comes together, and then spoon the mixture

into two 12-cups muffin pans lined with muffin cups.
6. Bake the muffins for 15 to 20 minutes until firm and the top turn golden brown, and then let them cool on the wire rack completely.
7. Serve straight away.

Nutrition:

Calories: 152.4 Cal;

Fat: 6.4 g;

Protein: 1.5 g;

Carbs: 22.6 g;

Fiber: 0.5 g

Stuffed Dried Figs

Preparation Time: 20 Minutes

Cooking Time: 0 Minutes

Servings: 4

Ingredients:

- 12 dried figs
- 2 Tbsps. thyme honey
- 2 Tbsps. sesame seeds
- 24 walnut halves

Directions:

1. Cut off the tough stalk ends of the figs.
2. Slice open each fig.
3. Stuff the fig openings with two walnut halves and close
4. Arrange the figs on a plate, drizzle with honey, and sprinkle the sesame seeds on it.
5. Serve.

Nutrition:

Calories: 110kcal

Carbs: 26

Fat: 3g,

Protein: 1g

Feta Cheesecake

Preparation Time: 30 Minutes

Cooking Time: 90 Minutes

Servings: 12

Ingredients:

- 2 cups graham cracker crumbs (about 30 crackers)
- ½ tsp ground cinnamon
- 6 tbsps. unsalted butter, melted
- ½ cup sesame seeds, toasted
- 12 ounces cream cheese, softened
- 1 cup crumbled feta cheese
- 3 large eggs
- 1 cup of sugar
- 2 cups plain yogurt
- 2 tbsps. grated lemon zest
- 1 tsp vanilla

Directions:

1. Set the oven to 350°F.
2. Mix the cracker crumbs, butter, cinnamon, and sesame seeds with a fork. Move the combination to a springform pan and spread until it is even. Refrigerate.
3. In a separate bowl, mix the cream cheese and feta. With an electric mixer, beat both kinds of cheese together. Add the eggs one after the other, beating the mixture with each new addition. Add sugar, then keep beating until creamy. Mix in yogurt, vanilla, and lemon zest.
4. Bring out the refrigerated springform and spread the batter on it. Then place it in a baking pan. Pour water in the pan till it is halfway full.
5. Bake for about 50 minutes. Remove cheesecake and allow it to cool. Refrigerate for at least 4 hours.
6. It is done. Serve when ready.

Nutrition:

Calories: 98kcal

Carbs: 7g

Fat: 7g

Protein: 3g

Pear Croustade

Preparation Time: 30 Minutes

Cooking Time: 60 Minutes

Servings: 10

Ingredients:

- 1 cup plus 1 tbsp. all-purpose flour, divided
- 4 ½ tbsps. sugar, divided
- 1/8 tsp salt
- 6 tbsps. unsalted butter, chilled, cut into ½ inch cubes
- 1 large-sized egg, separated
- 1 1/2 tbsps. ice-cold water
- 3 firm, ripe pears (Bosc), peeled, cored, sliced into ¼ inch slices 1 tbsp. fresh lemon juice
- 1/3 tsp ground allspice
- 1 tsp anise seeds

Directions:

1. Pour 1 cup of flour, 1 ½ Tbsps. of sugar, butter, and salt into a food processor and combine the ingredients by pulsing.
2. Whisk the yolk of the egg and ice water in a separate bowl. Mix the egg mixture with the flour mixture. It will form a dough, wrap it, and set aside for an hour.

3. Set the oven to 400°F.
4. Mix the pear, sugar, leftover flour, allspice, anise seed, and lemon juice in a large bowl to make a filling.
5. Arrange the filling on the center of the dough.
6. Bake for about 40 minutes. Cool for about 15 minutes before serving.

Nutrition:

Calories: 498kcal

Carbs: 32g

Fat: 32g

Protein: 18g

Melomakarona

Preparation Time: 20 Minutes

Cooking Time: 45 Minutes

Servings: 20

Ingredients:

- 4 cups of sugar, divided
- 4 cups of water
- 1 cup plus 1 tbsp. honey, divided
- 1 (2-inch) strip orange peel, pith removed
- 1 cinnamon stick
- ½ cup extra-virgin olive oil
- ¼ cup unsalted butter,
- ¼ cup Metaxa brandy or any other brandy
- 1 tbsp. grated
- Orange zest
- ¾ cup of orange juice
- ¼ tsp baking soda
- 3 cups pastry flour
- ¾ cup fine semolina flour
- 1 ½ tsp baking powder
- 4 tsp ground cinnamon, divided
- 1 tsp ground cloves, divided
- 1 cup finely chopped walnut
- 1/3 cup brown sugar

Directions:

1. Mix 3 ½ cups of sugar, 1 cup honey, orange peel, cinnamon stick, and water in a pot and heat it for about 10 minutes.
2. Mix the sugar, oil, and butter for about minutes, then add the brandy, leftover honey, and zest. Then add a mixture of baking soda and orange juice. Mix thoroughly.
3. In a distinct bowl, blend the pastry flour, baking powder, semolina, 2 tsp of cinnamon, and ½ tsp. of cloves. Add the mixture to the mixer slowly. Run the mixer until the ingredients form a dough. Cover and set aside for 30 minutes.
4. Set the oven to 350°F
5. With your palms, form small oval balls from the dough. Make a total of forty balls.
6. Bake the cookie balls for 30 minutes, then drop them in the prepared syrup.
7. Create a mixture with the walnuts, leftover cinnamon, and cloves. Spread the mixture on the top of the baked cookies.
8. Serve the cookies or store them in a closed-lid container.

Nutrition:

Calories: 294kcal

Carbs: 44g

Fat: 12g

Protein: 3g

Loukoumades (Fried Honey Balls)

Preparation Time: 20 Minutes

Cooking Time: 45 Minutes

Servings: 10

Ingredients:

- 2 cups of sugar
- 1 cup of water
- 1 cup honey
- 1 ½ cups tepid water
- 1 tbsp. brown sugar
- ¼ cup of vegetable oil
- 1 tbsp. active dry yeast
- 1 ½ cups all-purpose flour, 1 cup cornstarch, ½ tsp salt
- Vegetable oil for frying
- 1 ½ cups chopped walnuts
- ¼ cup ground cinnamon

Directions:

1. Boil the sugar and water on medium heat. Add honey after 10 minutes. cool and set aside.
2. Mix the tepid water, oil, brown sugar,' and yeast in a large bowl. Allow it to sit for 10 minutes. In a distinct bowl, blend the flour, salt, and cornstarch. With your hands mix the yeast and the flour to make a wet dough. Cover and set aside for 2 hours.
3. Fry in oil at 350°F. Use your palm to measure the sizes of the dough as they are dropped in the frying pan. Fry each batch for about 3-4 minutes.
4. Immediately the loukoumades are done frying, drop them in the prepared syrup.
5. Serve with cinnamon and walnuts.

Nutrition:

Calories: 355kcal

Carbs: 64g

Fat: 7g

Protein: 6g

Crème Caramel

Preparation Time: 60 Minutes

Cooking Time: 60 Minutes

Servings: 12

Ingredients:

- 5 cups of whole milk
- 2 tsp vanilla extract
- 8 large egg yolks
- 4 large-sized eggs
- 2 cups sugar, divided
- ¼ cup 0f water

Directions:

1. Preheat the oven to 350°F
2. Heat the milk with medium heat wait for it to be scalded.
3. Mix 1 cup of sugar and eggs in a bowl and add it to the eggs.
4. With a nonstick pan on high heat, boil the water and remaining sugar. Do not stir, instead whirl the pan. When the sugar forms caramel, divide it into ramekins.
5. Divide the egg mixture into the ramekins and place in a baking pan. Increase water to the pan until it is half full. Bake for 30 minutes.
6. Remove the ramekins from the baking pan, cool, then refrigerate for at least 8 hours.
7. Serve.

Nutrition:

Calories: 110kcal

Carbs: 21g

Fat: 1g

Protein: 2g

Galaktoboureko

Preparation Time: 30 Minutes

Cooking Time: 90 Minutes

Servings: 12

Ingredients:

- 4 cups sugar, divided
- 1 tbsp. fresh lemon juice
- 1 cup of water
- 1 Tbsp. plus 1 ½ tsp grated lemon zest, divided into 10 cups
- Room temperature whole milk
- 1 cup plus 2 tbsps. unsalted butter, melted and divided into 2
- Tbsps. vanilla extract
- 7 large-sized eggs
- 1 cup of fine semolina
- 1 package phyllo, thawed and at room temperature

Directions:

1. Preheat oven to 350°F
2. Mix 2 cups of sugar, lemon juice, 1 ½ tsp of lemon zest, and water. Boil over medium heat. Set aside.
3. Mix the milk, 2 Tbsps. of butter, and vanilla in a pot and put-on medium heat. Remove from heat when milk is scalded
4. Mix the eggs and semolina in a bowl, then add the mixture to the scalded milk. Put the egg-milk mixture on medium heat. Stir until it forms a custard-like material.
5. Brush butter on each sheet then arrange all over the baking pan until everywhere is covered. Spread the custard on the bottom pile phyllo
6. Arrange the buttered phyllo all over the top of the custard until every inch is covered.
7. Bake for about 40 minutes. cover the top of the pie with all the prepared syrup. Serve.

Nutrition:

Calories: 393kcal

Carbs: 55g

Fat: 15g

Protein: 8g

Kourabiedes Almond Cookies

Preparation Time: 20 Minutes

Cooking Time: 50 Minutes

Servings: 20

Ingredients:

- 1 ½ cups unsalted butter, clarified, at room temperature 2 cups
- Confectioners' sugar, divided
- 1 large egg yolk
- 2 tbsps. brandy
- 1 1/2 tsp baking powder
- 1 tsp vanilla extract
- 5 cups all-purpose flour, sifted
- 1 cup roasted almonds, chopped

Directions:

1. Preheat the oven to 350°F
2. Thoroughly mix butter and ½ cup of sugar in a bowl. Add in the egg after a while. Create a brandy mixture by mixing the brandy and baking powder. Add the mixture to the egg, add vanilla, then keep beating until the ingredients are properly blended
3. Add flour and almonds to make a dough.
4. Roll the dough to form crescent shapes. You should be able to get about 40 pieces. Place the pieces on a baking sheet, then bake in the oven for 25 minutes.
5. Allow the cookies to cool, then coat them with the remaining confectioner's sugar.

6. Serve.

Nutrition:

Calories: 102kcal

Carbs: 10g

Fat: 7g

Protein: 2g

Ekmek Kataifi

Preparation Time: 30 Minutes

Cooking Time: 45 Minutes

Servings: 10

Ingredients:

- 1 cup of sugar
- 1 cup of water
- 2 (2-inch) strips lemon peel, pith removed
- 1 tbsp. fresh lemon juice
- ½ cup plus 1 tbsp. unsalted butter, melted
- ½lbs. frozen kataifi pastry, thawed, at room temperature
- 2 ½ cups whole milk
- ½ tsp. ground mastiha
- 2 large eggs
- ¼ cup fine semolina
- 1 tsp. of cornstarch
- ¼ cup of sugar
- ½ cup sweetened coconut flakes
- 1 cup whipping cream
- 1 tsp. vanilla extract
- 1 tsp. powdered milk
- 3 tbsps. of confectioners' sugar
- ½ cup chopped unsalted pistachios

Directions:

1. Set the oven to 350°F. Grease the baking pan with 1. Tbsp of butter.

2. Put a pot on medium heat, then add water, sugar, lemon juice, lemon peel. Leave to boil for about 10 minutes. Reserve.
3. Untangle the kataifi, coat with the leftover butter, then place in the baking pan.
4. Mix the milk and mastiha, then place it on medium heat. Remove from heat when the milk is scalded, then cool the mixture.
5. Mix the eggs, cornstarch, semolina, and sugar in a bowl, stir thoroughly, then whisk the cooled milk mixture into the bowl.
6. Transfer the egg and milk mixture to a pot and place on heat. Wait for it to thicken like custard, then add the coconut flakes and cover it with a plastic wrap. Cool.
7. Spread the cooled custard-like material over the kataifi. Place in the refrigerator for at least 8 hours.
8. Strategically remove the kataifi from the pan with a knife. Take it away in such a way that the mold faces up.
9. Whip a cup of cream, add 1 tsp. vanilla, 1tsp. powdered milk, and 3 tbsps. Of sugar. Spread the mixture all over the custard, wait for it to harden, then flip and add the leftover cream mixture to the kataifi side.
10. Serve.

Nutrition:

Calories: 649kcal

Carbs: 37g

Fat: 52g

Protein: 11g

Revani Syrup Cake

Preparation Time: 30 Minutes

Cooking Time: 3 Hours

Servings: 24

Ingredients:

- 1 tbsp. unsalted butter
- 2 tbsps. all-purpose flour
- 1 cup ground rusk or bread crumbs
- 1 cup fine semolina flour
- ¾ cup ground toasted almonds
- 3 tsp baking powder
- 16 large eggs
- 2 tbsps. vanilla extract
- 3 cups of sugar, divided
- 3 cups of water
- 5 (2-inch) strips lemon peel, pith removed
- 3 tbsps. fresh lemon juice
- 1 oz of brandy

Directions:

1. Preheat the oven to 350°F. Grease the baking pan with 1 Tbsp. of butter and flour.
2. Mix the rusk, almonds, semolina, baking powder in a bowl.
3. In another bowl, mix the eggs, 1 cup of sugar, vanilla, and whisk with an electric mixer for about 5 minutes. Add the semolina mixture to the eggs and stir.
4. Pour the stirred batter into the greased baking pan and place in the preheated oven.
5. With the remaining sugar, lemon peels, and water make the syrup by boiling the mixture on medium heat. Add the lemon juice after 6 minutes, then cook for 3 minutes. Remove the lemon peels and set the syrup aside.
6. After the cake is done in the oven, spread the syrup over the cake.
7. Cut the cake as you please and serve.

Nutrition:

Calories: 348kcal

Carbs: 55g

Fat: 9g

Protein: 5g

Almonds and Oats Pudding

Preparation Time: 10 Minutes

Cooking Time: 15 Minutes

Servings: 4

Ingredients:

- 1 tablespoon lemon juice
- Zest of 1 lime
- 1 and ½ cups of almond milk
- 1 teaspoon almond extract
- ½ cup oats
- 2 tablespoons stevia
- ½ cup silver almonds, chopped

Directions:

1. In a pan, blend the almond milk plus the lime zest and the other ingredients, whisk, bring to a simmer and cook over medium heat for 15 minutes.
2. Split the mix into bowls then serve cold.

Nutrition:

Calories 174

Fat 12.1

Fiber 3.2

Carbs 3.9

Protein 4.8

Chocolate Cups

Preparation Time: 2 Hours

Cooking Time: 0 Minutes

Servings: 6

Ingredients:

- ½ cup avocado oil
- 1 cup, chocolate, melted
- 1 teaspoon matcha powder
- 3 tablespoons stevia

Directions:

1. In a bowl, mix the chocolate with the oil and the rest of the ingredients.
2. Whisk well and divide into cups.
3. Keep in the freezer for 2 hours before serving.

Nutrition:

Calories 174

Fat 9.1

Fiber 2.2

Carbs 3.9

Protein 2.8

Mango Bowls

Preparation Time: 30 Minutes

Cooking Time: 0 Minutes

Servings: 4

Ingredients:

- 3 cups mango, cut into medium chunks
- ½ cup of coconut water
- ¼ cup stevia
- 1 teaspoon vanilla extract

Directions:

1. In a blender, blend the mango plus the rest of the ingredients, pulse well.
2. Divide into bowls and serve cold.

Nutrition:

Calories 122

Fat 4

Fiber 5.3

Carbs 6.6

Protein 4.5

Cocoa and Pears Cream

Preparation Time: 10 Minutes

Cooking Time: 0 Minutes

Servings: 4

Ingredients:

- 2 cups heavy creamy
- 1/3 cup stevia
- ¾ cup cocoa powder
- 6 ounces dark chocolate, chopped
- Zest of 1 lemon
- 2 pears, chopped

Directions:

1. In a blender, blend the cream plus the stevia and the rest of the ingredients.
2. Blend well.
3. Divide into cups and serve cold.

Nutrition:

Calories 172

Fat 5.6

Fiber 3.5

Carbs 7.6

Protein 4

Pineapple Pudding

Preparation Time: 10 Minutes

Cooking Time: 40 Minutes

Servings: 4

Ingredients:

- 3 cups almond flour
- ¼ cup olive oil
- 1 teaspoon vanilla extract
- 2 and ¼ cups stevia
- 3 eggs, whisked
- 1 and ¼ cup natural apple sauce
- 2 teaspoons baking powder
- 1 and ¼ cups of almond milk
- 2 cups pineapple, chopped
- Cooking spray

Directions:

1. In a bowl, blend the almond flour plus the oil and the rest of the ingredients except the cooking spray and stir well.
2. Grease a cake pan with the cooking spray, pour the pudding mix inside, introduce in the oven and bake at 370 degrees F for 40 minutes.
3. Serve the pudding cold.

Nutrition:

Calories 223

Fat 8.1

Fiber 3.4

Carbs 7.6

Protein 3.4

Lime Vanilla Fudge

Preparation Time: 3 Hours

Cooking Time: 0 Minutes

Servings: 6

Ingredients:

- 1/3 cup cashew butter
- 5 tablespoons lime juice

- ½ teaspoon lime zest, grated
- 1 tablespoons stevia

Directions:

1. In a bowl, mix the cashew butter with the other ingredients and whisk well.
2. Line a muffin tray with parchment paper, scoop 1 tablespoon of lime fudge mix in each of the muffin tins and keep in the freezer for 3 hours before serving.

Nutrition:

Calories 200

Fat 4.5

Fiber 3.4

Carbs 13.5

Protein 5

Mixed Berries Stew

Preparation Time: 10 Minutes

Cooking Time: 15 Minutes

Servings: 6

Ingredients:

- Zest of 1 lemon, grated
- Juice of 1 lemon
- ½ pint blueberries
- 1-pint strawberries halved
- 2 cups of water
- 2 tablespoons stevia

Directions:

1. In a pan, blend the berries plus the water, stevia and the other ingredients.
2. Bring to a simmer, cook over medium heat for 15 minutes.
3. Divide into bowls and serve cold.

Nutrition:

Calories 172

Fat 7

Fiber 3.4

Carbs 8

Protein 2.3

Orange and Apricots Cake

Preparation Time: 10 Minutes

Cooking Time: 20 Minutes

Servings: 8

Ingredients:

- ¾ cup stevia
- 2 cups almond flour
- ¼ cup olive oil
- ½ cup almond milk
- 1 teaspoon baking powder
- 2 eggs
- ½ teaspoon vanilla extract
- Juice and zest of 2 oranges
- 2 cups apricots, chopped

Directions:

1. In a bowl, blend the stevia plus the flour and the rest of the ingredients, whisk and pour into a cake pan lined with parchment paper.
2. Introduce in the oven at 375 degrees F, bake for 20 minutes.
3. Cool down, slice and serve.

Nutrition:

Calories 221

Fat 8.3

Fiber 3.4

Carbs 14.5

Protein 5

Blueberry Cake

Preparation Time: 10 Minutes

Cooking Time: 30 Minutes

Servings: 6

Ingredients:

- 2 cups almond flour
- 3 cups blueberries
- 1 cup walnuts, chopped
- 3 tablespoons stevia
- 1 teaspoon vanilla extract
- 2 eggs, whisked
- 2 tablespoons avocado oil
- 1 teaspoon baking powder
- Cooking spray

Directions:

1. In a bowl, blend the flour plus the blueberries, walnuts and the other ingredients except for the cooking spray, and stir well.
2. Grease a cake pan with the cooking spray, pour the cake mix inside, introduce everything in the oven at 350 degrees F and bake for 30 minutes.
3. Cool the cake down, slice and serve.

Nutrition:

Calories 225

Fat 9

Fiber 4.5

Carbs 10.2

Protein 4.5

Almond Peaches Mix

Preparation Time: 10 Minutes

Cooking Time: 10 Minutes

Servings: 4

Ingredients:

- 1/3 cup almonds, toasted
- 1/3 cup pistachios, toasted
- 1 teaspoon mint, chopped
- ½ cup of coconut water
- 1 teaspoon lemon zest, grated
- 4 peaches, halved
- 2 tablespoons stevia

Directions:

1. In a pan, combine the peaches with the stevia and the rest of the ingredients.
2. Simmer over medium heat for 10 minutes.
3. Divide into bowls and serve cold.

Nutrition:

Calories 135

Fat 4.1

Fiber 3.8

Carbs 4.1

Protein 2.3

Spiced Peaches

Preparation Time: 5 minutes

Cooking Time: 10 minutes

Servings: 2

Ingredients:

- Canned peaches with juices – 1 cup
- Cornstarch – ½ tsp.
- Ground cloves – 1 tsp.
- Ground cinnamon – 1 tsp.
- Ground nutmeg – 1 tsp.
- Zest of ½ lemon
- Water – ½ cup

Directions:

1. Drain peaches.
2. Combine cinnamon, cornstarch, nutmeg, ground cloves, and lemon zest in a pan on the stove.
3. Heat on medium heat and add peaches.
4. Bring to a boil, decrease the heat then simmer for 10 minutes.
5. Serve.

Nutrition:

Calories: 70;

Fat: 0g;

Carb: 14g;

Phosphorus: 23mg;

Potassium: 176mg;

Sodium: 3mg;

Protein: 1g

Pumpkin Cheesecake Bar

Preparation Time: 10 minutes

Cooking Time: 50 minutes

Servings: 4

Ingredients:

- Unsalted butter – 2 ½ Tbsps.
- Cream cheese – 4 oz.
- All-purpose white flour – ½ cup
- Golden brown sugar – 3 Tbsps.
- Granulated sugar – ¼ cup
- Pureed pumpkin – ½ cup
- Egg whites - 2
- Ground cinnamon – 1 tsp.
- Ground nutmeg – 1 tsp.
- Vanilla extract – 1 tsp.

Directions:

1. Preheat the oven to 350F.

2. Mix brown sugar and flour in a container.
3. Mix in the butter to form 'breadcrumbs.'
4. Place ¾ of this mixture in a dish.
5. Bake in the oven for 15 minutes. Remove and cool.
6. Lightly whisk the egg and fold in the cream cheese, sugar, pumpkin, cinnamon, nutmeg, and vanilla until smooth.
7. Pour this mixture over the oven-baked base and sprinkle with the rest of the breadcrumbs from earlier.
8. Bake for 30 to 35 minutes more.
9. Cool, slice, and serve.

Nutrition:

Calories: 248;

Fat: 13g;

Carb: 33g;

Phosphorus: 67mg;

Potassium: 96mg;

Sodium: 146mg;

Protein: 4g

Blueberry Mini Muffins

Preparation Time: 10 minutes

Cooking Time: 35 minutes

Servings: 4

Ingredients:

- Egg whites – 3
- All-purpose white flour – ¼ cup
- Coconut flour – 1 Tbsp.
- Baking soda – 1 tsp.
- Nutmeg – 1 Tbsp. grated
- Vanilla extract – 1 tsp.
- Stevia – 1 tsp.
- Fresh blueberries – ¼ cup

Directions:

1. Preheat the oven to 325F.
2. Mix all the ingredients in a bowl.
3. Divide the batter into four and spoon into a lightly oiled muffin tin.
4. Bake in the oven for 15 to 20 minutes or until cooked through.
5. Cool and serve.

Nutrition:

Calories: 62;

Fat: 0g;

Carb: 9g;

Phosphorus: 103mg;

Potassium: 65mg;

Sodium: 62mg;

Protein: 4g;

Vanilla Custard

Preparation Time: 7 minutes

Cooking Time: 10 minutes

Servings: 10

Ingredients:

- Egg – 1
- Vanilla – 1/8 tsp.
- Nutmeg – 1/8 tsp.
- Almond milk – ½ cup
- Stevia - 2 Tbsp.

Directions:

1. Scald the milk, then let it cool a little.
2. Break the egg into a bowl and beat it with the nutmeg.
3. Add the scalded milk, the vanilla, and the sweetener to taste. Mix well.

4. Place the bowl in a baking pan filled with ½ deep of water.
5. Bake for 30 minutes at 325F.
6. Serve.

Nutrition:

Calories: 167.3;

Fat: 9g;

Carb: 11g;

Phosphorus: 205mg;

Potassium: 249mg;

Sodium: 124mg;

Protein: 10g;

Chocolate Chip Cookies

Preparation Time: 7 minutes

Cooking Time: 10 minutes

Servings: 10

Ingredients:

- Semi-sweet chocolate chips – ½ cup
- Baking soda – ½ tsp.
- Vanilla – ½ tsp.
- Egg – 1
- Flour – 1 cup
- Margarine – ½ cup
- Stevia – 4 tsp.

Directions:

1. Sift the dry ingredients.
2. Cream the margarine, stevia, vanilla, and egg with a whisk.
3. Add flour mixture and beat well.

4. Stir in the chocolate chips, then drop a teaspoonful of the mixture over a greased baking sheet.
5. Bake the cookies for about 10 minutes at 375F.
6. Cool and serve.

Nutrition:

Calories: 106.2;

Fat: 7g;

Carb: 8.9g;

Phosphorus: 19mg;

Potassium: 28mg;

Sodium: 98mg;

Protein: 1.5g;

Baked Peaches with Cream Cheese

Preparation Time: 10 minutes

Cooking Time: 15 minutes

Servings: 4

Ingredients:

- Plain cream cheese – 1 cup
- Crushed meringue cookies – ½ cup
- Ground cinnamon – ¼ tsp.
- Pinch ground nutmeg
- Canned peach halves – 8, in juice
- Honey – 2 Tbsp.

Directions:

1. Preheat the oven to 350F.
2. Line a baking sheet with parchment paper. Set aside.
3. In a small bowl, stir together the meringue cookies, cream cheese, cinnamon, and nutmeg.

4. Spoon the cream cheese mixture evenly into the cavities in the peach halves.
5. Place the peaches on the baking sheet and bake for 15 minutes or until the fruit is soft and the cheese is melted.
6. Remove the peaches from the baking sheet onto plates.
7. Drizzle with honey and serve.

Nutrition:

Calories: 260;

Fat: 20;

Carb: 19g;

Phosphorus: 74mg;

Potassium: 198mg;

Sodium: 216mg;

Protein: 4g;

Bread Pudding

Preparation Time: 15 minutes

Cooking Time: 40 minutes

Servings: 6

Ingredients:

- Unsalted butter, for greasing the baking dish
- Plain rice milk – 1 ½ cups
- Eggs – 2
- Egg whites – 2
- Honey – ¼ cup
- Pure vanilla extract – 1 tsp.
- Cubed white bread – 6 cups

Directions:

1. Grease an 8-by-8-inch baking dish with butter. Set it aside.
2. In a bowl, whisk together the eggs, egg whites, rice milk, honey, and vanilla.

3. Add the bread cubes and stir until the bread is coated.
4. Transfer the mixture to the baking dish and cover with plastic wrap.
5. Store the dish in the refrigerator for at least 3 hours.
6. Preheat the oven to 325F.
7. Take away the plastic wrap from the baking dish, bake the pudding for 35 to 40 minutes, or golden brown.
8. Serve.

Nutrition:

Calories: 167;

Fat: 3g;

Carb: 30g;

Phosphorus: 95mg;

Potassium: 93mg;

Sodium: 189mg;

Protein: 6g;

Strawberry Ice Cream

Preparation Time: 5 minutes

Cooking Time: 5 minutes

Servings: 3

Ingredients:

- Stevia – ½ cup
- Lemon juice – 1 Tbsp.
- Non-dairy coffee creamer – ¾ cup
- Strawberries – 10 oz.
- Crushed ice – 1 cup

Directions:

1. Blend everything in a blender until smooth.
2. Freeze until frozen.
3. Serve.

Nutrition:

Calories: 94.4;

Fat: 6g;

Carb: 8.3g;

Phosphorus: 25mg;

Potassium: 108mg;

Sodium: 25mg;

Protein: 1.3g;

Cinnamon Custard

Preparation Time: 20 minutes

Cooking Time: 1 hour

Servings: 6

Ingredients:

- Unsalted butter, for greasing the ramekins
- Plain rice milk – 1 ½ cups
- Eggs – 4
- Granulated sugar – ¼ cup
- Pure vanilla extract – 1 tsp.
- Ground cinnamon – ½ tsp.
- Cinnamon sticks for garnish

Directions:

1. Preheat the oven to 325F.
2. Lightly grease six ramekins and place them in a baking dish. Set aside.
3. In a large bowl, whisk together the eggs, rice milk, sugar, vanilla, and cinnamon until the mixture is smooth.
4. Pour the mixture through a fine sieve into a pitcher.
5. Evenly divide the custard mixture among the ramekins.
6. Fill the baking dish with hot water until the water reaches halfway up the sides of the ramekins.

7. Bake for 1 hour or until the custards are set, and a knife inserted in the center comes out clean.
8. Remove the custards from the oven and take the ramekins out of the water.
9. Cool on the wire racks for 1 hour, then chill for 1 hour.
10. Garnish with cinnamon sticks and serve.

Nutrition:

Calories: 110;

Fat: 4g;

Carb: 14g;

Phosphorus: 100mg;

Potassium: 64mg;

Sodium: 71mg;

Protein: 4g;

Raspberry Brule

Preparation Time: 15 minutes

Cooking Time: 1 minute

Servings: 4

Ingredients:

- Light sour cream – ½ cup
- Plain cream cheese – ½ cup
- Brown sugar – ¼ cup, divided
- Ground cinnamon – ¼ tsp.
- Fresh raspberries – 1 cup

Directions:

1. Preheat the oven to broil.
2. In a bowl, beat together the cream cheese, sour cream, 2 tbsp. brown sugar and cinnamon for 4 minutes or until the mixture are very smooth and fluffy.

3. Evenly divide the raspberries among 4 (4-ounce) ramekins.
4. Spoon the cream cheese mixture over the berries and smooth the tops.
5. Sprinkle ½ tbsp. brown sugar evenly over each ramekin.
6. Place the ramekins on a baking sheet and broil 4 inches from the heating element until the sugar is caramelized and golden brown.
7. Cool and serve.

Nutrition:

Calories: 188;

Fat: 13g;

Carb: 16g;

Phosphorus: 60mg;

Potassium: 158mg;

Sodium: 132mg;

Tart Apple Granita

Preparation time: 15 minutes, plus 4 hours freezing time
Cooking time: 0
Servings: 4
Ingredients:

- ½ cup granulated sugar
- ½ cup of water
- 2 cups unsweetened apple juice
- ¼ cup freshly squeezed lemon juice

Directions:

1. In a small saucepan over medium-high heat, heat the sugar and water.

2. Bring the mixture to a boil and then reduce the heat to low. Let it simmer for about 15 minutes or until the liquid has reduced by half.

3. Remove the pan from the heat and pour the liquid into a large shallow metal pan.

4. Let the liquid cool for about 30 minutes, and then stir in the apple juice and lemon juice.

5. Place the pan in the freezer.

6. After 1 hour, run a fork through the liquid to break up any ice crystals that have formed. Scrape down the sides as well.

7. Place the pan back in the freezer and repeat the stirring and scraping every 20 minutes, creating slush.

8. Serve when the mixture is completely frozen and looks like crushed ice, after about 3 hours.

Nutrition:

Calories: 157;

Fat: 0g;

Carbohydrates: 0g;

Phosphorus: 10mg;

Potassium: 141mg;

Sodium: 5mg;

Protein: 0g

Lemon-Lime Sherbet

Preparation time: 5 minutes, plus 3 hours chilling time
Cooking time: 15 minutes
Servings: 2
Ingredients:

- 2 cups of water
- 1 cup granulated sugar
- 3 tablespoons lemon zest, divided
- ½ cup freshly squeezed lemon juice
- Zest of 1 lime

- Juice of 1 lime
- ½ cup heavy (whipping) cream

Directions:

1. Place a large saucepan over medium-high heat and add the water, sugar, and two tablespoons of the lemon zest.

2. Bring the mixture to a boil and then reduce the heat and simmer for 15 minutes.

3. Transfer the mixture to a large bowl and add the remaining 1 tablespoon lemon zest, the lemon juice, lime zest, and lime juice.

4. Chill the mixture in the fridge until completely cold, about 3 hours.

5. Whisk in the heavy cream and transfer the mixture to an ice cream maker.

6. Freeze according to the manufacturer's instructions.

Nutrition:

Calories: 151;

Fat: 6g;

Carbohydrates: 26g;

Phosphorus: 10mg;

Potassium: 27mg;

Sodium: 6mg;

Protein: 0g

Pavlova with Peaches

Preparation time: 30 minutes
Cooking time: 1 hour, plus cooling time
Servings: 3
Ingredients:

- 4 large egg whites, at room temperature
- ½ teaspoon cream of tartar
- 1 cup superfine sugar
- ½ teaspoon pure vanilla extract
- 2 cups drained canned peaches in juice

Directions:

1. Preheat the oven to 225°F.

2. Line a baking sheet with parchment paper; set aside.

3. In a large bowl, beat the egg whites for about 1 minute or until soft peaks form.

4. Beat in the cream of tartar.

5. Add the sugar, one tablespoon at a time, until the egg whites are very stiff and glossy. Do not overbeat.

6. Beat in the vanilla.

7. Evenly spoon the meringue onto the baking sheet so that you have eight rounds.

8. Use the back of the spoon to create an indentation in the middle of each round.

9. Bake the meringues for about 1 hour or until a light brown crust form.

10. Turn off the oven and let the meringues stand, still in the oven, overnight.

11. Remove the meringues from the sheet and place them on serving plates.

12. Spoon the peaches, dividing evenly into the centers of the meringues and serve.

13. Store any unused meringues in a sealed container at room temperature for up to 1 week.

Nutrition:

Calories: 132;

Fat: 0g;

Carbohydrates: 32g;

Phosphorus: 7mg;

Potassium: 95mg;

Sodium: 30mg;

Protein: 2g

Tropical Vanilla Snow Cone

Preparation time: 15 minutes, plus freezing time

Cooking time: 0 minutes

Servings: 2

Ingredients:

- 1 cup pineapple
- 1 cup of frozen strawberries
- 6 tablespoons water
- 2 tablespoons granulated sugar
- 1 tablespoon vanilla extract

Directions:

1. In a large saucepan, mix together the peaches, pineapple, strawberries, water, and sugar over medium-high heat and bring to a boil.

2. Reduce the heat to low and simmer the mixture, occasionally stirring, for 15 minutes.

3. Remove from the heat and let the mixture cool completely, for about 1 hour.

4. Stir in the vanilla and transfer the fruit mixture to a food processor or blender.

5. Purée until smooth, and pour the purée into a 9-by-13-inch glass baking dish.

6. Cover and place the dish in the freezer overnight.

7. When the fruit mixture is completely frozen, use a fork to scrape the sorbet until you have flaked flavored ice.

8. Scoop the ice flakes into four serving dishes.

Nutrition:

Calories: 92;

Fat: 0g;

Carbohydrates: 22g;

Phosphorus: 17mg;

Potassium: 145mg;

Sodium: 4mg;

Protein: 1g

Rhubarb Crumble

Preparation time: 15 minutes
Cooking time: 30 minutes
Servings: 6
Ingredients:

- Unsalted butter, for greasing the baking dish
- 1 cup all-purpose flour
- ½ cup brown sugar
- ½ teaspoon ground cinnamon
- ½ cup unsalted butter, at room temperature
- 1 cup chopped rhubarb
- 2 apples, peeled, cored, and sliced thin
- 2 tablespoons granulated sugar
- 2 tablespoons water

Directions:

1. Preheat the oven to 325°F.

2. Lightly grease an 8-by-8-inch baking dish with butter; set aside.

3. In a small bowl, stir together the flour, sugar, and cinnamon until well combined.

4. Add the butter and rub the mixture between your fingers until it resembles coarse crumbs.

5. In a medium saucepan, mix together the rhubarb, apple, sugar, and water over medium heat and cook for about 20 minutes or until the rhubarb is soft.

6. Spoon the fruit mixture into the baking dish and evenly top with the crumble.

7. Bake the crumble for 20 to 30 minutes or until golden brown.

8. Serve hot.

Nutrition:

Calories: 450;

Fat: 23g;

Carbohydrates: 60g;

Phosphorus: 51mg;

Potassium: 181mg;

Sodium: 10mg;

Protein: 4g

Gingerbread Loaf

Preparation time: 20 minutes

Cooking time: 1 hour

Servings: 16

Ingredients:

- Unsalted butter, for greasing the baking dish
- 3 cups all-purpose flour
- ½ teaspoon Ener-G baking soda substitute
- 2 teaspoons ground cinnamon
- 1 teaspoon ground allspice
- ¾ cup granulated sugar
- 1¼ cups plain rice milk
- 1 large egg
- ¼ cup olive oil
- 2 tablespoons molasses
- 2 teaspoons grated fresh ginger
- Powdered sugar, for dusting

Directions:

1. Preheat the oven to 350°F.

2. Lightly grease a 9-by-13-inch baking dish with butter; set aside.

3. In a large bowl, sift together the flour, baking soda substitute, cinnamon, and allspice.

4. Stir the sugar into the flour mixture.

5. In medium bowl, whisk together the milk, egg, olive oil, molasses, and ginger until well blended.

6. Make a well in the center of the flour mixture and pour in the wet ingredients.

7. Mix until just combined, taking care not to overmix.

8. Pour the batter into the baking dish and bake for about 1 hour or until a wooden pick inserted in the middle comes out clean.

9. Serve warm with a dusting of powdered sugar.

Nutrition:

Calories: 232;

Fat: 5g;

Carbohydrates: 42g;

Phosphorus: 54mg;

Potassium: 104mg;

Sodium: 18mg;

Protein: 4g

Elegant Lavender Cookies

Preparation time: 10 minutes
Cooking time: 15 minutes
Servings: Makes 24 cookies

Ingredients:

- 5 dried organic lavender flowers, the entire top of the flower
- ½ cup granulated sugar
- 1 cup unsalted butter, at room temperature
- 2 cups all-purpose flour
- 1 cup of rice flour

Directions:

1. Strip the tiny lavender flowers off the main stem carefully and place the flowers and granulated sugar into a food processor or blender. Pulse until the mixture is finely chopped.

2. In a medium bowl, cream together the butter and lavender sugar until it is very fluffy.

3. Mix the flours into the creamed mixture until the mixture resembles fine crumbs.

4. Gather the dough together into a ball and then roll it into a long log.

5. Wrap the cookie dough in plastic and refrigerate it for about 1 hour or until firm.

6. Preheat the oven to 375°F.

7. Slice the chilled dough into ¼-inch rounds and refrigerate it for 1 hour or until firm.

8. Bake the cookies for 15 to 18 minutes or until they are a very pale, golden brown.

9. Let the cookies cool.

10. Store the cookies at room temperature in a sealed container for up to 1 week.

Nutrition:

Calories: 153;

Fat: 9g;

Carbohydrates: 17g;

Phosphorus: 18mg;

Potassium: 17mg;

Sodium: 0mg;

Protein: 1g

Carob Angel Food Cake

Preparation time: 30 minutes
Cooking time: 30 minutes
Servings: 16
Ingredients:

- ¾ cup all-purpose flour
- ¼ cup carob flour
- 1½ cups sugar, divided
- 12 large egg whites, at room temperature
- 1½ teaspoons cream of tartar
- 2 teaspoons vanilla

Directions:

1. Preheat the oven to 375°F.

2. In a medium bowl, sift together the all-purpose flour, carob flour, and ¾ cup of the sugar; set aside.

3. Beat the egg whites and cream of tartar with a hand mixer for about 5 minutes or until soft peaks form.

4. Add the remaining ¾ cup sugar by the tablespoon to the egg whites until all the sugar is used up and stiff peaks form.

5. Fold in the flour mixture and vanilla.

6. Spoon the batter into an angel food cake pan.

7. Run a knife through the batter to remove any air pockets.

8. Bake the cake for about 30 minutes or until the top springs back when pressed lightly.

9. Invert the pan onto a wire rack to cool.

10. Run a knife around the rim of the cake pan and remove the cake from the pan.

Nutrition:

Calories: 113;

Fat: 0g;

Carbohydrates: 25g;

Phosphorus: 11mg;

Potassium: 108mg;

Sodium: 42mg;

Protein: 3g

Old-Fashioned Apple Kuchen

Preparation time: 25 minutes
Cook time: 1 hour
Servings: 16
Ingredients:
- Unsalted butter, for greasing the baking dish
- 1 cup unsalted butter, at room temperature

- 2 cups granulated sugar
- 2 eggs, beaten
- 2 teaspoons pure vanilla extract
- 2 cups all-purpose flour
- 1 teaspoon Ener-G baking soda substitute
- 2 teaspoons ground cinnamon
- ½ teaspoon ground nutmeg
- Pinch ground allspice
- 2 large apples, peeled, cored, and diced (about 3 cups)

Directions:

1. Preheat the oven to 350°F.

2. Grease a 9-by-13-inch glass baking dish; set aside.

3. Cream together the butter and sugar with a hand mixer until light and fluffy, for about 3 minutes.

4. Add the eggs and vanilla and beat until combined, scraping down the sides of the bowl, about 1 minute.

5. In a small bowl, stir together the flour, baking soda substitute, cinnamon, nutmeg, and allspice.

6. Add the dry ingredients to the wet ingredients and stir to combine.

7. Stir in the apple and spoon the batter into the baking dish.

8. Bake for about 1 hour or until the cake is golden.

9. Cool the cake on a wire rack.

10. Serve warm or chilled.

Nutrition:

Calories: 368;

Fat: 16g;

Carbohydrates: 53g;

Phosphorus: 46mg;

Potassium: 68mg;

Sodium: 15mg;

Protein: 3g

Dark Chocolate and Cherry Trail Mix

Preparation time: 5 minutes

Cooking time: 5 minutes

Servings: Makes 3 cups (¼ cup per serving)

Ingredients:

- 1 cup unsalted almonds
- 2/3 cup dried cherries
- ½ cup walnuts
- ½ cup sweet cinnamon-roasted chickpeas
- ¼ cup dark chocolate chips

Directions:

1. Combine the almonds, cherries, walnuts, chickpeas, and chocolate chips in an airtight container.
2. Store at room temperature for up to 1 week or in the freezer for up to 3 months.

Nutrition:

Calories: 174;

Total Fat: 12g;

Saturated Fat: 2g;

Cholesterol: 0mg;

Sodium: 18mg;

Carbohydrates: 16g;

Fiber: 4g;

"Rugged" Coconut Balls

Preparation Time: 10minutes

Cooking time: 0minutes

Servings: 3

Ingredients:

- 1/3 cup coconut oil melted
- 1/3 cup coconut butter softened
- 2 oz. coconut, finely shredded, unsweetened
- 4 Tbsp. coconut palm sugar
- 1/2 cup shredded coconut

Directions:

1. Combine all ingredients in a blender.
2. Blend until soft and well combined.
3. Do a small ball roll in shredded coconut.
4. Place on a sheet lined with parchment paper and refrigerate overnight.
5. Keep coconut balls into sealed container in fridge up to one week.

Nutrition:

Calories 226.89

Calories from Fat 190.39 |

Total Fat 21.6g

Saturated Fat 19.84g

Cholesterol 0mg

Sodium 17.19mg

Potassium 45mg

Total Carbohydrates 9g

Fiber 1.16g

Sugar 5.7g

Protein 1g

Almond - Choco Cake

Preparation Time: 10minutes

Cooking time: 45minutes

Servings: 5

Ingredients:

- 1 1/2 cups of almond flour
- 1/3 cup almonds finely chopped
- 1/4 cup of cocoa powder unsweetened
- Pinch of salt
- 1/2 tsp. baking soda
- 2 Tbsp. almond milk
- 1/2 cup Coconut oil melted
- 2 tsp. pure vanilla extract
- 1/3 cup brown sugar (packed)

Directions:

1. Preheat oven to 350 F.
2. Set the pan, and grease with a little melted coconut oil; set aside.
3. Stir the almond flour, chopped almonds, cocoa powder, salt, and baking soda in a bowl.
4. In a separate bowl, stir the remaining ingredients.
5. Merge the almond flour mixture with the almond milk mixture and stir well.
6. Place batter in a prepared cake pan.
7. Bake for 30 to 32 minutes...
8. Store the cake-slices a freezer, tightly wrapped in a double layer of plastic wrap and a layer of foil. It will keep on this way for up to a month.

Nutrition:

Calories 326.89

Calories from Fat 165.39 |

Total Fat 34.6g

Saturated Fat 29.84g

Cholesterol 0mg

Sodium 18.19mg

Potassium 45mg

Total Carbohydrates 9g

Fiber 1.16g

Sugar 5.7g

Protein 1g

Banana-Almond Cake

Preparation Time: 10minutes

Cooking time: 45minutes

Servings: 5

Ingredients

- 4 ripe bananas in chunks
- 3 Tbsps. honey or maple syrup
- 1 tsp. pure vanilla extract
- 1/2 cup almond milk
- 3/4 cup of self-rising flour
- 1 tsp. cinnamon
- 1 tsp. baking powder
- 1 pinch of salt
- 1/3 cup of almonds finely chopped

- Almond slices for decoration

Directions:

1. Preheat the oven to 400 F (air mode).
2. Oil a cake mold; set aside.
3. Add bananas into a bowl and mash with the fork.
4. Add honey, vanilla, almond, and stir well.
5. In a separate bowl, stir flour, cinnamon, baking powder, salt, the almonds broken, and mix with a spoon.
6. Transfer the mixture to prepared cake mold and sprinkle with sliced almonds.
7. Bake for 40-45 minutes.
8. Remove from the oven, and allow the cake to cool completely.
9. Cut cake into slices, place in tin foil, or an airtight container, and keep refrigerated up to one week.

Nutrition:

Calories 326.89

Calories from Fat 145.39 |

Total Fat 24.6g

Saturated Fat 12.84g

Cholesterol 0mg

Sodium 20.19mg

Potassium 32

Total Carbohydrates 9g

Fiber 1.16g

Sugar 5.7g

Protein 1g

Banana-Coconut Ice Cream

Preparation Time: 15minutes

Cooking time: 0minutes

Servings: 5

Ingredients

- 1 cup coconut cream
- 1/2 cup Inverted sugar
- 2 large frozen bananas (chunks)
- 3 Tbsp. honey extracted
- 1/4 tsp. cinnamon powder

Directions:

1. Do the coconut cream with the inverted sugar in a bowl.
2. In a separate bowl, beat the banana with honey and cinnamon.
3. Incorporate the coconut whipped cream and banana mixture; stir well.
4. Cover the bowl and let cool in the refrigerator over the night.
5. Stir the mixture 3 to 4 times to avoid crystallization.
6. Keep frozen 1 to 2 months.

Nutrition:

Calories 126.89

Calories from Fat 245.39 |

Total Fat 34.6g

Saturated Fat 12.84g

Cholesterol 0mg

Sodium 20.19mg

Potassium 32

Total Carbohydrates 9g

Fiber 1.16g

Sugar 5.7g

Protein 1g

Coconut Butter Clouds Cookies

Preparation Time: 15minutes

Cooking time: 25minutes

Servings: 5

Ingredients

- 1/2 cup coconut butter softened
- 1/2 cup peanut butter softened
- 1/2 cup of granulated sugar
- 1/2 cup of brown sugar
- 2 Tbsp. chia seeds soaked in 4 tablespoons water
- 1/2 tsp. pure vanilla extract
- 1/2 tsp. baking soda
- 1/4 tsp. salt
- 1 cup of all-purpose flour

Directions:

1. Preheat oven to 360 F.
2. Add coconut butter, peanut butter, and both sugars in a mixing bowl.
3. Beat with a mixer until soft and sugar combined well.
4. Add soaked chia seeds and vanilla extract; beat.
5. Add baking soda, salt, and flour; beat until all ingredients are combined well.

6. With your hands, shape dough into cookies.
7. Arrange your cookies onto a baking sheet, and bake for about 10 minutes.
8. Remove cookies from the oven and allow cooling completely.
9. Sprinkle with icing sugar and enjoy your cookies.
10. Place cookies in an airtight container and keep refrigerated up to 10 days.
11. Nutrition:

Calories 226.89

Calories from Fat 255.39 |

Total Fat 34.6g

Saturated Fat 12.84g

Cholesterol 0mg

Sodium 10.19mg

Potassium 22

Total Carbohydrates 10g

Fiber 1.16g

Sugar 7.7g

Protein 5g

Choco Mint Hazelnut Bars

Preparation Time: 15minutes

Cooking time: 35minutes

Servings: 4

Ingredients

- 1/2 cup coconut oil, melted
- 4 Tbsp. cocoa powder
- 1/4 cup almond butter

- 3/4 cup brown sugar - (packed)
- 1 tsp. vanilla extract
- 1 tsp. pure peppermint extract
- Pinch of salt
- 1 cup shredded coconut
- 1 cup hazelnuts sliced

Directions:

1. Slice the hazelnuts in a food processor
2. Boil the and place it on low heat.
3. Put the coconut oil, cacao powder, almond butter, brown sugar, vanilla, peppermint extract, and salt in the top of a double boiler over hot (not boiling) water and constantly stir for 10 minutes.
4. Add hazelnuts and shredded coconut to the melted mixture and stir together.
5. Pour the mixture in a dish lined with parchment and freeze for several hours.
6. Remove from the freezer and cut into bars.
7. Store in airtight container or freezer bag in a freezer.
8. Let the bars at room temperature for 10 to 15 minutes before eating.

Nutrition:

Calories 126.89

Calories from Fat 155.39 |

Total Fat 34.6g

Saturated Fat 18.84g

Cholesterol 0mg

Sodium 15.19mg

Potassium 32

Total Carbohydrates 10g

Fiber 1.16g

Sugar 7.7g

Protein 5g

Coco-Cinnamon Balls

Preparation Time: 15minutes

Cooking time: 35minutes

Servings: 4

Ingredients

- 1 cup coconut butter softened
- 1 cup coconut milk canned
- 1 tsp. pure vanilla extract
- 3/4 tsp. cinnamon
- 1/2 tsp. nutmeg
- 2 Tbsp. coconut palm sugar (or granulated sugar)
- 1 cup coconut shreds

Directions:

1. Combine all ingredients (except the coconut shreds) in a heated bath - bain-marie.
2. Cook and stir until all ingredients are soft and well combined.
3. Remove bowl from heat, place into a bowl, and refrigerate until the mixture firmed up.
4. Form cold coconut mixture into balls, and roll each ball in the shredded coconut.

5. Store into a sealed container, and keep refrigerated up to one week.

Nutrition:

Calories 136.89

Fat 235.39 |

Total Fat 24.6g

Saturated Fat 19.84g

Cholesterol 0mg

Sodium 15.19mg

Potassium 32

Total Carbohydrates 10g

Fiber 2.16g

Sugar 7.7g

Protein 5g

Express Coconut Flax Pudding

Preparation Time: 15minutes

Cooking time: 25minutes

Servings: 4

Ingredients

- 1 Tbsp. coconut oil softened
- 1 Tbsp. coconut cream
- 2 cups coconut milk canned
- 3/4 cup ground flax seed
- 4 Tbsp. coconut palm sugar (or to taste)

Directions:

1. Press SAUTÉ button on your Instant Pot
2. Add coconut oil, coconut cream, coconut milk, and ground flaxseed.

3. Stir about 5 - 10 minutes.
4. Close lid into place and Start.
5. When the timer beeps, press "Cancel" and carefully flip the Quick Release valve to let the pressure out.
6. Add the palm sugar and stir well.
7. Taste and adjust sugar to taste.
8. Allow pudding to cool down completely.
9. Set the pudding in an airtight container and refrigerate for up to 2 weeks.

Nutrition:

Calories 126.89

Calories from Fat 124.39 |

Total Fat 14.6g

Saturated Fat 17.84g

Cholesterol 0mg

Sodium 18.19mg

Potassium 22

Total Carbohydrates 10g

Fiber 2.16g

Sugar 7.7g

Protein 5g

Full-Flavored Vanilla Ice Cream

Preparation Time: 15minutes

Cooking time: 0minutes

Servings: 4

Ingredients

- 1 1/2 cups canned coconut milk
- 1 cup coconut whipping cream

- 1 frozen banana cut into chunks
- 1 cup vanilla sugar
- 3 Tbsp. apple sauce
- 2 tsp. pure vanilla extract
- 1 tsp. Xanthan gum or agar-agar thickening agent

Directions:

1. Merge all ingredients; process until all ingredients combined well.
2. Place the ice cream mixture in a freezer-safe container with a lid over.
3. Freeze for at least 4 hours.
4. Remove frozen mixture to a bowl and beat with a mixer to break up the ice crystals.
5. Repeat this process 3 to 4 times.
6. Let the ice cream at room temperature for 15 minutes before serving.

Nutrition:

Calories 126.89

Calories from Fat 134.39 |

Total Fat 15.6g

Saturated Fat 19.84g

Cholesterol 0mg

Sodium 28.19mg

Potassium 22

Total Carbohydrates 10g

Fiber 2.16g

Sugar 7.7g

Protein 5g

Irresistible Peanut Cookies

Preparation Time: 20minutes

Cooking time: 0minutes

Servings: 6

Ingredients

- 4 Tbsp. all-purpose flour
- 1 tsp. baking soda
- Pinch of salt
- 1/3 cup granulated sugar
- 1/3 cup peanut butter softened
- 3 Tbsp. applesauce
- 1/2 tsp. pure vanilla extract

Directions:

1. Preheat oven to 350 F.
2. Combine the flour, baking soda, salt, and sugar in a mixing bowl; stir.
3. Merge all remaining ingredients
4. Roll dough into cookie balls/patties.
5. Arrange your cookies onto greased (with oil or cooking spray) baking sheet.
6. Let cool before removing from tray.
7. Take out cookies from the tray and let cool completely.
8. Place your peanut butter cookies in an airtight container, and keep refrigerated up to 10 days.

Nutrition:

Calories 116.89

Calories from Fat 114.39 |

Total Fat 18.6g

Saturated Fat 20.84g

Cholesterol 0mg

Sodium 12.19mg

Potassium 22

Total Carbohydrates 10g

Fiber 2.16g

Sugar 7.7g

Protein 5g

Murky Almond Cookies

Preparation Time: 10minutes

Cooking time: 15minutes

Servings: 6

Ingredients

- 4 Tbsp. cocoa powder
- 2 cups almond flour
- 1/4 tsp. salt
- 1/2 tsp. baking soda
- 5 Tbsp. coconut oil melted
- 2 Tbsp. almond milk
- 1 1/2 tsp. almond extract
- 1 tsp. vanilla extract
- 4 Tbsp. corn syrup or honey

Directions:

1. Preheat oven to 340 F degrees.
2. Grease a large baking sheet; set aside.
3. Merge the cocoa powder, almond flour, salt, and baking soda.
4. Merge the melted coconut oil, almond milk; almond and vanilla extract, and corn syrup or honey.
5. Merge the almond flour mixture with the almond milk mixture and stir well.
6. Roll tablespoons of the dough into balls, and arrange onto a prepared baking sheet.
7. Bake for 12 to 15 minutes.
8. Remove from the oven and transfer onto a plate lined with a paper towel.
9. Allow cookies to cool down completely and store in an airtight container at room temperature for about four days.

Nutrition:

Calories 16.89

Calories from Fat 19.39 |

Total Fat 18.6g

Saturated Fat 20.84g

Cholesterol 0mg

Sodium 12.19mg

Potassium 22

Total Carbohydrates 10g

Fiber 2.16g

Sugar 7.7g

Protein 5g

Orange Semolina Halva

Preparation Time: 10minutes

Cooking time: 25minutes

Servings: 6

Ingredients

- 6 cups fresh orange juice
- Zest from 3 oranges
- 3 cups brown sugar
- 1 1/4 cup semolina flour
- 1 Tbsp. almond butter (plain, unsalted)
- 4 Tbsp. ground almond
- 1/4 tsp. cinnamon

Directions:

1. Heat the orange juice, orange zest with brown sugar in a pot.
2. Let the sugar dissolved.
3. Add the semolina flour and cook over low heat for 15 minutes; stir occasionally.
4. Add almond butter, ground almonds, and cinnamon, and stir well.
5. Cook, frequently stirring, for further 5 minutes.
6. Transfer the halva mixture into a mold, let it cool and refrigerate for at least 4 hours.
7. Keep refrigerated in a sealed container for one week.

Nutrition:

Calories 16.89

Calories from Fat 19.39 |

Total Fat 18.6g

Saturated Fat 20.84g

Cholesterol 0mg

Sodium 12.19mg

Potassium 22

Total Carbohydrates 10g

Fiber 2.16g

Sugar 7.7g

Protein 5g

Seasoned Cinnamon Mango Popsicles

Preparation Time: 15minutes

Cooking time: 0minutes

Servings: 6

Ingredients

- 1 1/2 cups of mango pulp
- 1 mango cut in cubes
- 1 cup brown sugar (packed)
- 2 Tbsp. lemon juice freshly squeezed
- 1 tsp. cinnamon
- 1 pinch of salt

Directions:

1. Add all ingredients into your blender.
2. Blend until brown sugar dissolved.
3. Pour the mango mixture evenly in Popsicle molds or cups.
4. Insert sticks into each mold.
5. Place molds in a freezer, and freeze for at least 5 to6 hours.
6. Before serving, un-mold easy your popsicles placing molds under lukewarm water.

Nutrition:

Calories 16.89

Calories from Fat 19.39 |

Total Fat 18.6g

Saturated Fat 20.84g

Cholesterol 0mg

Sodium 12.19mg

Potassium 22

Total Carbohydrates 10g

Fiber 2.16g

Sugar 7.7g

Protein 5g

Strawberry Molasses Ice Cream

Preparation Time: 20minutes

Cooking time: 0minutes

Servings: 9

Ingredients

- 1 lb. strawberries
- 3/4 cup coconut palm sugar
- 1 cup coconut cream
- 1 Tbsp. molasses
- 1 tsp. balsamic vinegar
- 1/2 tsp. agar-agar
- 1/2 tsp. pure strawberry extract

Directions:

1. Add strawberries, date sugar, and the balsamic vinegar in a blender; blend until completely combined.

2. Place the mixture in the refrigerator for one hour.

3. In a mixing bowl, beat the coconut cream with an electric mixer to make a thick mixture.

4. Add molasses, balsamic vinegar, agar-agar, and beat for further one minute or until combined well.

5. Add the strawberry mixture and beat again for 2 minutes.

6. Pour ice cream mix into an ice cream maker, turn on the machine, and churn according to manufacturer's directions.

7. Keep frozen in a freezer-safe container (with plastic film and lid over).

Nutrition:

Calories 16.89

Calories from Fat 19.39 |

Total Fat 18.6g

Saturated Fat 20.84g

Cholesterol 0mg

Sodium 12.19mg

Potassium 22

Total Carbohydrates 10g

Fiber 2.16g

Sugar 7.7g

Protein 5g

Strawberry-Mint Sorbet

Preparation Time: 15minutes

Cooking time: 0minutes

Servings: 6

Ingredients

- 1 cup of granulated sugar
- 1 cup of orange juice
- 1 lb. frozen strawberries

- 1 tsp. pure peppermint extract

Directions:

1. Add sugar and orange juice in a saucepan.
2. Stir over high heat and boil for 5 minutes or until sugar dissolves.
3. Remove from the heat and let it cool down.
4. Add strawberries into a blender, and blend until smooth.
5. Pour syrup into strawberries, add peppermint extract and stir until all ingredients combined well.
6. Transfer mixture to a storage container, cover tightly, and freeze until ready to serve.

Nutrition:

Calories 16.89

Calories from Fat 1.39 |

Total Fat 12.6g

Saturated Fat 2.84g

Cholesterol 0mg

Sodium 1.19mg

Potassium 22

Total Carbohydrates 10g

Fiber 2.16g

Sugar 33g

Protein 5g

Vegan Choco - Hazelnut Spread

Preparation Time: 15minutes

Cooking time: 0minutes

Servings: 5

Ingredients

- 1 cup hazelnuts soaked
- 4 Tbsp. dry cacao powder
- 4 Tbsp. Maple syrup
- 1 tsp. pure vanilla extract
- 1/4 tsp. kosher salt
- 4 Tbsp. almond milk

Directions:

1. Soak hazelnuts with water overnight.
2. Add soaked hazelnuts along with all remaining ingredients in a food processor.
3. Process for about 10 minutes or until a cream gets the desired consistency.
4. Keep the spread in a sealed container refrigerated up to 2 weeks.

Nutrition:

Calories 16.89

Calories from Fat 4.39 |

Total Fat 6.6g

Saturated Fat 3.84g

Cholesterol 0mg

Sodium 5.19mg

Potassium 22

Total Carbohydrates 10g

Fiber 2.16g

Sugar 43g

Protein 5g

Vegan Exotic Chocolate Mousse

Preparation Time: 10minutes

Cooking time: 0minutes

Servings: 4

Ingredients:

- 2 frozen bananas chunks
- 2 avocados
- 1/3 cup of dates
- 4 Tbsp. cocoa powder
- 1/2 cup of fresh orange juice
- Zest, from 1 orange

Directions:

1. Add bananas, avocado, and dates in a food processor.
2. Process for about 2 to 3 minutes until combined well.
3. Add cocoa powder, orange juice, and orange zest; process for further one minute.
4. Place cream in a glass jar or container and keep refrigerated up to one week.
5. Nutrition: Facts

Nutrition:

Calories 16.89

Calories from Fat 4.39 |

Total Fat 5.6g

Saturated Fat 2.84g

Cholesterol 0mg

Sodium 7.19mg

Potassium 32

Total Carbohydrates 10g

Fiber 2.16g

Sugar 43g

Protein 5g

Vegan Lemon Pudding

Preparation Time: 20minutes

Cooking time: 0minutes

Servings: 6

Ingredients

- 2 cups almond milk
- 3 Tbsp. of corn flour
- 2 Tbsp. of all-purpose flour
- 1 cup of sugar granulated
- 1/4 cup almond butter (plain, unsalted)
- 1 tsp. lemon zest
- 1/3 cup fresh lemon juice

Directions:

1. Add the almond milk with corn flour, flour, and sugar in a saucepan.
2. Cook, frequently stirring, until sugar dissolved, and all ingredients combine well (for about 5 to 7 minutes over medium heat).
3. Add the almond butter, lemon zest, and lemon juice.
4. Cook, frequently stirring, for further 5 to 6 minutes.
5. Remove the lemon pudding from the heat and allow it to cool completely.
6. Pour into the sealed container and keep refrigerated up to one week.

Nutrition:

Calories 16.89

Calories from Fat 7.39 |

Total Fat 3.6g

Saturated Fat 1.84g

Cholesterol 0mg

Sodium 7.19mg

Potassium432

Total Carbohydrates 20g

Fiber 1.16g

Sugar 24g

Protein 5g

Vitamin Blast Tropical Sherbet

Preparation Time: 15minutes

Cooking time: 0minutes

Servings: 8

Ingredients

- 4 cups mangos pitted and cut into 1/2-inch dice
- 1 papaya cut into 1/2-inch dice
- 1/4 cup granulated sugar or honey (optional)
- 1 cup pineapple juice canned
- 1/4 cup coconut milk
- 2 Tbsp. coconut cream
- 1 fresh lime juice

Directions:

1. Add all ingredients into your food processor; process until all ingredients smooth and combine well.
2. Put the mixture to a bowl, and cover
3. Remove the sherbet mixture from the fridge, stir well, and pour in a freezer-safe container (with plastic film and lid over).
4. Keep frozen.
5. Let the sherbet at room temperature for 15 minutes before serving.

Nutrition:

Calories 16.89

Calories from Fat 9.39 |

Total Fat 2.6g

Saturated Fat 3.84g

Cholesterol 0mg

Sodium 7.15mg

Potassium132

Total Carbohydrates 15g

Fiber 1.16g

Sugar 24g

Protein 5g

Walnut Vanilla Popsicles

Preparation Time: 15minutes

Cooking time: 0minutes

Servings: 7

Ingredients

- 1 1/2 cup finely sliced walnuts
- 4 cups of almond milk

- 4 Tbsp. brown sugar (packed)

- 1 scoop protein powder (pea or soy)

- 2 tsp. pure vanilla extract

Directions:

1. Add all ingredients in your high-speed blender and blend until smooth and combined well.

2. Pour the mixture in Popsicle molds and insert the wooden stick into the middle of each mold.

3. Freeze until your ice popsicles are completely frozen.

4. Serve and enjoy!

Nutrition:

Calories 16.89

Calories from Fat 9.39 |

Total Fat 2.6g

Saturated Fat 3.84g

Cholesterol 0mg

Sodium 7.15mg

Potassium122

Total Carbohydrates 15g

Fiber 1.16g

Sugar 34g

Protein 5g

Conclusion

Thank you for your support on this book. As we end here are some tips for success in Pegan Diet:

1. Reduce the intake of unhealthy foods

In Pegan Diet, the focus is not to cut out any foods in particular. The goal is to reduce the intake of unhealthy foods and increase the intake of healthy foods.

2. Eat a lot of vegetables and fruit

You should eat a lot of vegetables and fruit because they are good sources of vitamins, minerals and fiber.

3. Eat less sodium

Reducing the intake of sodium will improve your cardiovascular health.

4. Eat less saturated fats

Reducing the intake of saturated fats will help you lose weight. You should try to substitute saturated fats with "good" fats (unsaturated fats).

5. Eat healthy proteins

Although it is possible to eat animal protein in Pegan Diet, you should still limit the intake of animal foods and eat more plant-based protein sources instead (e.g., soy products, nuts, beans). Incorporate more protein, including beans, lentils and tofu into your diet.

6. Eat healthy fats

Instead of relying on oils (e.g., vegetable oils, corn oil, etc.), use healthy fats like avocado, nuts and seeds to get the same flavor and texture effect.

6. Don't drink too much alcohol

Drinking too much alcohol is not good for your health. It will make you gain weight and increase the risk of developing serious diseases.

7. Reduce the intake of refined carbs

Reduce your intake of refined carbs (e.g., white bread, white rice). Replace them with whole grains instead (e.g., whole wheat bread, brown rice).

8. Reduce sugars and grains

Reduce your intake of sugars and grains. If your body is sensitive to gluten, you should try to avoid gluten-containing foods (e.g., wheat, rye, barley).

9. Eat more herbs

Herbs are rich in nutrients and have many health benefits. Include more fresh herbs in your cooking or eat them as snacks with breads or crackers.

10. Drink a lot of water

Drinking a lot of water will help you stay hydrated and keep your body flushed out, which will help you feel less hungry and lose weight. Drinking more water will also help improve digestion.

11. Don't go on extreme diets

Don't go on extreme diets that cut out entire food groups altogether (e.g., cutting out all desserts, or all carbs). Rather, you should focus on reducing the intake of unhealthy foods.

12. Don't be afraid to eat

Research has shown that having a positive attitude towards food can help you lose more weight and keep it off for longer. So instead of being fearful towards certain types of food, try to enjoy your meals and appreciate the tastes of different foods. A positive approach will reduce your stress levels and make it easier for you to stick to your goals.

13. Avoid processed food or anything that contains high levels of salt, sugar or fat

You should avoid processed food or anything that contains high levels of salt, sugar or fat. Processing can lead to the addition of unhealthy additives into your food, which will make it much harder for you to lose weight.

14. Be realistic

It is important to be realistic in your goals (e.g., don't expect to lose 2 kg a week without changing your lifestyle) and have a plan that is reasonable and achievable.

15. Have more than one weight loss goal

When you have multiple weight loss goals, you will find it easier to focus on various aspects of your health and lose weight faster too. For example, if there are two aspects you care about (e.g., lose weight and improve cardiovascular health), you can have one goal for each of them.

16. Don't be afraid to ask for help

When you are trying to achieve a lifestyle change, it is important to know that you are not alone in your efforts. Whenever you feel like quitting, ask for help or seek out support from friends and family members to help keep yourself on track with your goals.

17. Prepare ahead of time

Prepare a healthy meal in advance at the start of each week when you have more time and fewer distractions (e.g., weekends). This way, it will be easier for you to stick to your diet during the week when things can get hectic at work or school.

Again, thank you and good luck.

CPSIA information can be obtained
at www.ICGtesting.com
Printed in the USA
LVHW060345230421
685283LV00015B/796